THE
PRIMAL
BLUEPRINT

MARK SISSON

Critical Acclaim for *The Primal Blueprint*

The Primal Blueprint is dense with options and can't-fail lifestyle transitioning tips. We're all constantly presented with many different avenues to wellbeing; Mark Sisson outlines steps on these paths, keeping it simple and actionable, and the improvements sustainable.

> — **Katy Bowman**
> Nutritious Movement guru, author of *Move Your DNA*

❖

Mark Sisson is a pioneer in the evolutionary health movement and a bona fide fat-burning beast. If you want to learn from the best, *The Primal Blueprint* is required reading. So drop that sandwich and pick up this book. You're going to love it!

> — **Abel James**, *New York Times* best-selling author of *The Wild Diet* and award-winning host of *Fat Burning Man*

❖

If I think back about books, people, and experiences that have influenced and shaped me, it's hard to think of a book (*The Primal Blueprint*) and person (Mark Sisson) that have had greater impact on my life. *The Primal Blueprint* was not only one of the first books on the scene with the emergence of paleo/primal/ancestral health, it has also stood the test of time. That's pretty remarkable given how rapidly we gain new information and insights these days. Millions of people have improved their lives via Mark's work, and I certainly count myself amongst those who live a better life because of *The Primal Blueprint* and Mark's passion for all things health.

> — **Robb Wolf**, former research biochemist and *New York Times* best-selling author of *The Paleo Solution: The Original Human Diet*

The Primal Blueprint impacted the way I practice medicine more than any medical textbook or journal I've ever read. I came out of medical training ill-equipped to manage the deluge of lifestyle-induced chronic health conditions I encountered in my patients. My greatest weapon at that time was my prescription pad. *The Primal Blueprint* changed that completely. It not only transformed my own health, but gave me a template to help manage and actually reverse diseases in my patients. Mark masterfully weaves together complex exercise and nutrition science, ancestral health, and his profound, yet practical wisdom gained from his years of being an elite athlete and a normal human being who suffered physical and mental burnout. The result is an elegant, yet simple solution to optimal health that is now not only the gold standard in the world of health and fitness, but is also having a growing impact on physicians and health practitioners around the world.

> — **Dr. Ronesh Sinha**, author of *The South Asian Health Solution* and Palo Alto Medical Foundation Director of Corporate Wellness for Sutter Health in Silicon Valley

❖

Far and away, the most important health concept in the *The Primal Blueprint* is that the metabolic state of burning fat is essential to normal health. We often think of exercise as a way to burn fat, but if your diet does not contain the right nutrients, you will not burn fat optimally. I regularly recommend this book to patients at my weight-loss clinic—it offers a safe, sensible, and comprehensive plan for a complete lifestyle transformation. By following such recommendations for diet, exercise, and lifestyle, I have seen patients double their fat-burning capacity in four weeks. Years of clinical experience has taught me that fat burning is the biggest factor in determining long-term weight-management success as well as moderation of disease risk factors.

> — **Dr. Cate Shanahan** (DrCate.com), author of *Deep Nutrition* and *Food Rules,* Science Director of the Los Angeles Lakers PRO Nutrition program

Reading *The Primal Blueprint* and adopting a primal lifestyle saved my life, as I was struggling with weight issues, food addictions, adrenal fatigue, and unresolved thyroid disease despite extensive medical intervention. I thought I was eating extremely healthy, and exercising optimally, but the results were exhaustion, weight gain, and blood work showing conditions of pre-diabetes and thyroid dysfunction. Going primal helped eliminate my health problems relatively quickly and easily. I became fat-adapted, energetic, healthy, happy, and free of suffering for the first time in years. If you are pre-diabetic, have extra weight to lose, or have an unhealthy relationship with food, going primal can help you break free from your struggles and promote the optimal gene expression that you deserve.

— **Elle Russ,** author of *The Paleo Thyroid Solution,*
host of *Primal Blueprint Podcast*

※

Mark Sisson is a natural born coach. His long career as a personal trainer and coach of elite endurance athletes has infused his Primal Blueprint message with inspiration, support, and sensitivity. As you read *The Primal Blueprint*, it feels like Mark is there with you every step of the way offering personal guidance and a gentle, supportive touch.

— **Christine Hassler, M.A.**, best-selling author
of *Expectation Hangover,* keynote speaker,
podcast host and Coaching Director of the
Primal Health Coach certification program

※

Mark Sisson's influence has extended across the globe and been a great inspiration for us in promoting the big picture of healthy eating, exercise, and lifestyle principles here in the United Kingdom. Unlike so many diet and fitness gurus with extreme, overly-stressful programs, *The Primal Blueprint* offers a sensible approach to lifestyle change, one that allows you to express your personal preferences and have fun along the way.

— **Keris Marsden and Matt Whitmore,** London,
England-based authors of *Paleo Primer* and
Paleo Primer: Second Helping

Mark Sisson and *The Primal Blueprint* played an instrumental role in launching the ancestral health movement many years ago. I notice in my functional medicine practice that many people respond to simple lifestyle changes that honor our evolutionary development—doing things like ditching grains, sugars, and refined vegetable oils, consuming more nutrient-dense plant and animal foods, getting sensible exercise instead of overdoing it, and placing more emphasis on sleep. *The Primal Blueprint* covers all the bases to leading a healthy lifestyle. It's at the top of my recommended reading list for anyone interested in reclaiming their health with diet and lifestyle change.

> — **Chris Kresser**, author of *The Paleo Cure* and *Your Personal Paleo Code*, and Co-director and President of California Center for Functional Medicine

❋

As a former professional athlete like Mark Sisson, I understand how pursuing competitive athletic goals can actually compromise your health instead of support it. *The Primal Blueprint* helped me reframe my perspective about what being healthy really means and helped me embrace a broader perspective of fitness. Mark is a guy who has been there and done that; his credibility is excellent, as is his research to support his ideas. If you are looking to get healthy and fit, then get *The Primal Blueprint*.

> — **Lewis Howes**, *New York Times* best-selling author of *School of Greatness* and host of the *School of Greatness* Podcast

❋

I've known Mark Sisson personally for many years and watched him shape and inspire the burgeoning primal/paleo/evolutionary health movement. Unlike many health and fitness leaders, Mark is open, approachable, and focused on the community instead of being dogmatic. He has the respect of everyone from those first encounters at speaking events to the leading scientists, medical experts, and elite athletes in the health world. *The Primal Blueprint* is a great way to get an easy-to-read comprehensive education on primal living.

> — **Ben Greenfield**, BenGreenfieldFitness.com

Library of Congress Cataloging-in-Publication Data

Names: Sisson, Mark, 1953- author.
Title: The primal blueprint / by Mark Sisson.
Description: 4th edition. | Oxnard, CA : Primal Blueprint Publishing, [2019]
  | Includes index.
Identifiers: LCCN 2018044691 (print) | LCCN 2018045565 (ebook) | ISBN
  9781939563521 (ebook) | ISBN 9781939563477 (pbk.)
Subjects: LCSH: Health. | Nutrition. | Human evolution. | Human genetics.
Classification: LCC RA776 (ebook) | LCC RA776 .S6387 2019 (print) | DDC
  613--dc23
LC record available at https://lccn.loc.gov/2018044691

Managing Editor: Brad Kearns
Research/Consulting/Editing: Lindsay Shaw Taylor, P.h.D, Tracy Dunigan Kearns, Aaron Fox
Design and Layout: Caroline De Vita
Illustrations & Cartoons: Caroline De Vita
Cover Design: Janée Meadows
Front and Back Cover Photos of Mark: Doug Ellis Photography
Index and Copyediting: Tim Tate
Consultants: Greg Brown, Siena Colombier, Rudy Dressendorfer, Ph.D., R.P.T, Catherine Fisse, Laura Gabler, Penelope Jackson, Walter Kearns, M.D., Doug McGuff, M.D., Amy Lucas, Phil Maffetone, D.C., Denise Minger, Timothy Noakes, Ph.D., Ronesh Sinha, M.D., Stacy Sims, Ph.D., Cate Shanahan, M.D., Kelly Starrett, DPT
Other photos used by permission and courtesy of: Wade Baker, Larry Diamond, Malika Duke, Deanna Eberlin, Doug Ellis, Faye Geiss, Brad Kearns, Steven "E" Kobrine, Nick Laszlo, Michelle Matangi, Janée Meadows, Dave Parsons, Eric Roseberg, Stephen Sankarsingh, Carrie Sisson, Mark Sisson

Primal Blueprint Publishing, 1641 S. Rose Ave., Oxnard, CA 93033
For information on quantity discounts, please call 888-774-6259 or 310-317-4414,
email: info@primalblueprintpublishing.com, or visit PrimalBlueprintPublishing.com.

Printed in the U.S.A.

TABLE OF CONTENTS

*The doctor of the future will give no medicine,
but instead will interest his patients in the care
of human frame, in diet, and in the cause and
prevention of disease.*

—Thomas Edison

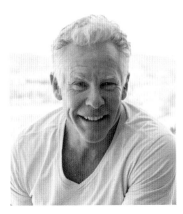

WELCOME

When I began the journey to produce this book way back in 2009, it felt like David versus Goliath redux. Yes, I had readers of my MarksDailyApple.com blog encouraging me to produce a primal manifesto attacking *conventional wisdom* (a recurring term throughout the book, akin to a yellow highway hazard sign), and I had a few fitness books under my belt from years past, but this endeavor was a call to battle against the mighty opponent of the collective status quos in the fields of medicine, fitness, weight loss, Big Pharma, and Big Agra… not to mention the staid publishing industry.

After I presented my ideas for a radically different and highly controversial diet (along with a bunch of other crazy notions—like slowing down your workout pace if you want to go faster, or ditching cushy shoes and going barefoot to prevent injuries), I'd get feedback like, "Huh?

Mark, you're not a doctor. You have no credibility." Or, "Ditching grains? Eating more fat? Making workouts slower or shorter? This stuff will never fly with today's reader." At best it was, "Clever ideas, Mark, but you need a hot celebrity attached or it won't go anywhere." Mind you, this trash talk wasn't from agents and publishers who rejected me—they didn't even have the courtesy to answer. No, this feedback was from PR experts I was paying to pitch the book!

My vision changed course after a last-ditch effort in which I pounded the pavement, making the publisher/agent rounds in New York. At the end of my journey, I was smiling and ready for battle, for I realized that I was rewriting the rules. If the publishing world wasn't going to drop everything and engage in a frenzied bidding war for the exciting new *Primal Blueprint*, I would gladly become my own author, agent, and publisher. If my mission was to tear down the status quo, why did I need the existing powers that be in the publishing world? I was going rogue.

Ordinarily, I'm not the gloating type. But frankly, I think the primal/paleo/ancestral health community should feel good these days. The movement has grown from a grassroots scene in the early 2000s to a movement that is enjoying ever-greater acceptance as evidenced by feature stories in mainstream media like *The New York Times*, *TIME* magazine, *The Week* magazine, and the *The Huffington Post*. The medical and fitness community is now sounding a familiar theme to ours: "It looks like we were wrong about eating fat and a bunch of other flawed and outdated conventional wisdom.... Who knew?"

The original hardcover version of this book was published in 2009 by an unknown outfit out in Malibu, CA (about as far away from the publishing epicenter of Park Avenue as one can get). It sold through seven printings, climbed the charts to the hit #2 overall best seller on Amazon.com in March of 2010, and occupied the #1 spot on Amazon's Exercise & Fitness and Diet & Weight Loss lists on and off for nearly a year. Combined with the 2012 paperback edition and the digital versions, over 300,000 copies have been sold, making it one of the best-selling health and lifestyle books that Park Avenue has ever passed over.

The primal/paleo/ancestral health community now boasts hundreds of books, videos, workshops, retreats, podcasts, and blogs about the ancestral lifestyle. (Rumor has it that today there are more blogs than people in the movement.) The influence of conventional wisdom on our collective psyche has never been more tenuous, as people are sick and tired of being sick and tired, fat, and overstressed. The time has come to ditch once and for all the health advice dispensed by gimmicky best-selling diet books and return to the scientific evidence about how our species not only survived against the odds, but thrived. The experience of our hunter-gatherer ancestors is worth excavating because it contains the secrets to our long-term health and survival moving forward.

This work represents the culmination of my primal philosophy that has taken shape over the past 30 years through extensive research and life experience. I'm not a scientist or doctor; I'm an athlete, coach, and student on a lifelong quest for optimal health, happiness, and peak performance. I have an insatiable curiosity about learning what is needed to achieve such goals and a growing mistrust of the answers that have been heaped upon us by the traditional pillars of healthcare wisdom: Big Pharma, Big Agra, the AMA, the FDA, and other government agencies, not to mention the assorted Internet hucksters, multilevel marketers, and those advocating and profiting from the programs that sell short-term results at the expense of long-term health.

The Primal Blueprint is my effort to distill information from the world's leading evolutionary biologists, paleontologists, geneticists, anthropologists, physicians, nutritionists, food scientists, exercise physiologists, neuroscientists, psychologists, coaches, trainers, and athletes into a concise list of behaviors—or "laws"—that have proven to promote optimal gene expression and human survival. While the book you are holding is a product of the new millennium, the Primal Blueprint laws are as old as the dawn of mankind; they merely reinform us about the fundamentals of health that seem to have been forgotten, or misinterpreted, in the modern world. Unlocking the wisdom of these ancient laws so that we can enjoy optimal health and longevity is the goal of this book.

The content in *The Primal Blueprint* comes to you unfiltered by pretense or disingenuous decorum. I am not beholden to any employer, government agency, professional licensing board, corporate sponsor, or academic institution, nor to any power that might insist on watering down my message. I have no agenda except, I suppose, to help you change your life and experience the exceptional health that is your genetic birthright.

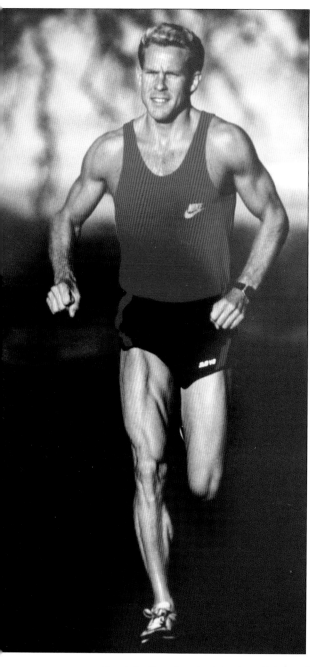

My skepticism and disappointment with conventional wisdom developed over the past 40-plus years of trying to "do the right thing" (another recurring theme) as defined by the experts of the day. For over a decade of my youth, I ran in excess of 100 miles a week with a single-minded focus toward competing in the 1980 U.S. Olympic Marathon Trials. At my peak, I was considered by many to be a picture of health: 6-percent body fat, a resting heart rate of 38 beats per minute, a marathon time of 2 hours, 18 minutes that placed me fifth in the U.S. National Marathon Championships, and later a fourth place finish in the Hawaii Ironman World Triathlon Championships.

While I reached some notable heights during my endurance career, I also experienced some devastating lows. The monumental physical stress of my training regimen and the high-carb, "high-energy" diet that fueled it resulted in a succession of serious overuse injuries, illnesses, and burnout. While I looked like a picture of health, I was really an example of overstress and inflammation. I was the fittest guy my friends knew, yet I suffered

Back in the day: Inside the slick outfit was a body falling apart from chronic inflammation, carbohydrate dependency, and suppressed immune function caused by my chronic training patterns.

from recurring bouts of fatigue, osteoarthritis in my feet, severe tendonitis in my hips, stress-related gastrointestinal maladies, and six or more upper respiratory tract infections a year.

Most people have traveled a less extreme path than I, yet nearly all of us have had similar experiences. Following the conventional wisdom of our time, weight-loss efforts doomed us to a 96 percent long-term failure rate. Chronic workout programs led to fatigue and increased our appetite for sugar. Medications and their attendant side effects too often exacerbated the underlying reasons for our pain without offering much relief.

> *The Primal Blueprint is the centerpiece of a vibrant community of people committed to living their lives to the fullest potential, challenging the status quo, and not being afraid to try something **old**.*

I applaud your effort to do the right thing, and I deeply empathize with your frustration over the whirlwind of conflicting and confusing advice. My goal with *The Primal Blueprint* is to expose much of the lucrative health and fitness industry as ethically and scientifically bankrupt; to peel back the many layers of marketing dogma and to replace it with ten simple Primal Blueprint laws which I've modeled after the evolutionary progress and ultimate survival of our ancestors.

Pause and reflect on the following simple statement for a moment, for it is the most powerful and compelling rationale for living according to the Primal Blueprint: Human beings prevailed despite incalculable odds by adapting to the life-or-death selection pressures in their environment over thousands of generations. Our primal ancestors were lean, strong, smart, and productive, which enabled them to survive, reproduce, and ultimately rule over more physically imposing members of the animal kingdom. This is no mean feat, yet conventional wisdom has essentially dismissed the legacy of our ancestors in favor of easy, quick-fix "solutions" to ill health that sell regardless of negligible long-term results.

Today at the age of 63, I feel healthier, fitter, happier, and more productive than ever. No longer a marathon or triathlon champion (but nor do I care to be one), I maintain a weight of 170 pounds (77 kg) with 8-percent body fat. I eat as much delicious food as I want, unbeholden to rigid meal times. I exercise just 3 to 6 hours per week (instead of the 20 to 30 I logged back in the day), and I almost never get sick. Hundreds of thousands of readers at MarksDailyApple.com chronicle similar success stories each week from following the Primal Blueprint. Now it is your turn.

YOUR WAY OR THE HIGHWAY

My intention in this book is to show you the immense personal power you have to control your health and fitness destiny by giving you the tools to reprogram your genes, reshape your physique, and enjoy a long, healthy, energetic, and productive life. The Primal Blueprint principles are wonderfully simple, practical, and inexpensive, and they require minimal, if any, sacrifice or deprivation. Unlike many of the gimmicky diet and exercise books that have graced the best-seller shelves in recent decades, the Primal Blueprint is intuitive and easy to follow—not just for the first 21 days or the first four months, but for the rest of your life.

I have a deep understanding and empathy for real-world concerns like the lack of time, a limited budget, motivational challenges, dysfunctional social circumstances, eating disorders, ingrained habits, and numerous influences that can sabotage the best-laid plans. On numerous occasions, I've felt the disappointment of taking a plunge with my heart and soul into a new diet or athletic training regimen, only to fall well short of the ambitious goals I had envisioned. Adding insult to injury, I often discovered later that I'd been given bad advice—by my government (thanks in no small part to the tainted influence of special interests), Madison Avenue, or a less-than-knowledgeable coach, peer, or professional expert. Few things in life are more frustrating!

With the Primal Blueprint, there's no need for trepidation. This is not a regimented program; I'm not going to shove my agenda down your throat and cajole you to go against your own common sense or pleasure-seeking human nature. The philosophical positions and practical guidelines that shape the message of this book have been validated by reputable science.

Millions of primal/paleo enthusiasts across the globe have likewise scrutinized, refined, battle-tested and validated our findings. *Note*: In this edition, you will see some significant revisions and enhancements to the original Primal Blueprint stance on important topics like the consumption of alcohol, hydration, general daily movement, gut health, and in many more areas where personal experience, breaking science, and community feedback have compelled me to update the message.

I provide the framework for living an awesome life in this book, but making the pieces fit comfortably together in your life is best left up to you. I strongly support making allowances and adjustments to suit your lifestyle, as well as occasionally deviating from the Primal Blueprint. After all, our ancestors had to adjust constantly to their unpredictable environment, providing us with the tools to adapt similarly. That's one of the primal elements that still exists in all of us. The word "blueprint" in the title connects us to the familiar analogy of construction plans that provide the foundation for action but are often altered during the actual construction project. A program that gives you the foundation, but that also allows you to go with the flow, frees you to listen more deeply to your own intuitive knowledge—a resource that is far more helpful then any outside expert.

The fact that you are in control will give you the most powerful source of motivation you can imagine: instant and ongoing direct feedback that the Primal Blueprint is working. No more chronic exercising until exhaustion or obsessing about the arduous caloric restrictions of most popular weight-loss programs. The Primal Blueprint laws are an untapped resource within each one of us, attainable precisely because they made our existence sustainable in the first place. It's time to tap into that ancient wisdom and pursue your own unique peak-performance goals and live your life to the fullest. Thank you for agreeing to take this journey with me. Let's have some fun and get primal!

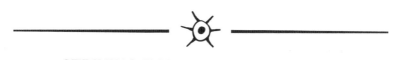

STRIVING FOR PERFECTION WITH
THE 80 PERCENT RULE

A central tenet of the Primal Blueprint is to let go of the perfectionist approach to diet and exercise and to adopt realistic lifestyle habits that fit your particular circumstances. I call it the "80 Percent Rule." It means that you can be successful without being overly strict or regimented about your diet and exercise. Programs that require strict adherence to (often questionable) guidelines end up inviting stress and anxiety and a sense of failure when we fall short of perfectionistic standards. The success and growth of the primal/paleo/ancestral health movement in recent years has unfortunately and inadvertently led a few fervent followers to develop health issues such as *orthorexia*, an eating disorder characterized by an extreme preoccupation with avoiding unhealthy foods.

As we proceed to detail the health benefits of being primal-aligned and the drawbacks of modern foods and lifestyles that conflict with your genetic programming for health, remember that if you are aligned with the Primal Blueprint 80 percent of the time, you will experience great success and likely build momentum toward becoming even more compliant, naturally and with less effort, as time proceeds.

Since this admonition is potentially controversial and easily misinterpreted ("Sisson offers a cop out!"), I'd like to further explain the spirit of the 80 Percent Rule. This is not a license to make less than a full commitment to the Primal Blueprint—that is, to strive for less than an "A" grade as your ultimate goal. Rather, I suggest that you strive for 100-percent compliance with the Primal Blueprint guidelines and zero tolerance for the unhealthy foods, exercise, and lifestyle habits that are prevalent today. With that in mind, please realize that a rigidly perfectionistic approach compromises many of the intended benefits of an otherwise disciplined "healthy" lifestyle. Your mental and emotional wellbeing are important, too. Overstriving for complete compliance may add more stress to your life, which is ultimately counterproductive. In fact, we now know that stress can disrupt some of the same hormonal processes that the primal lifestyle is designed to normalize.

The forces of our modern lifestyle (the processed food, hectic pace, sedentary work habits, and constant technological overstimulation) sometimes undermine our attempts at a more mindful, conscious, slower, primal-aligned lifestyle. That's okay. Veering off course is merely an opportunity to adjust, evolve, and regroup.

"I love your 80 Percent Rule, Mark!
I usually try to stick to it 80 percent of the time.
Will you sign my book for me?"

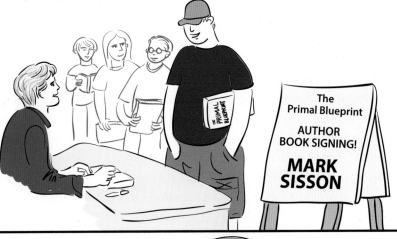

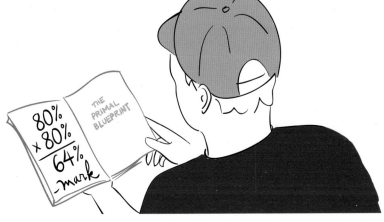

In short, shoot for the moon, leaving room to accommodate everyday reality. Stop beating yourself up when you fall short. Once clear on this philosophy, you'll realize the folly of the common dietary theme of "cheat days," something that makes me cringe every time I hear it. The Primal Blueprint eating strategy is driven by pleasure—I encourage you to strive for total satisfaction with every bite of food that you eat. A regimented program featuring cheat days implies that you are suffering on the non-cheat days! In my opinion (and those of the psychology and human behavior experts I've consulted), needing a "cheat day" is antithetical to following a health plan that is enjoyable, natural, and sustainable.

The Primal Blueprint does not endorse an overly obsessive, orthorexic approach. That said, striving for 100-percent adherence to the primal principles is important when it comes to moderating your insulin production and getting off the sugar/insulin "crash-and-burn" cycle. If you start your journey with a "try to cut back" mindset instead of a "strictly eliminate" mindset, it's likely you will linger in carbohydrate dependency and have a much greater struggle than necessary.

> *Perfection is impossible.*
> *However, striving for perfection is not. Do the best you can*
> *under the conditions that exist. That is what counts.*
> —John Wooden

The 80 Percent Rule exists because I understand how difficult lifestyle changes can be. I encourage you to make an honest and devoted effort, but I never want you to feel discouraged that you aren't measuring up. The late John Wooden, legendary UCLA basketball coach, captured the spirit of the 80 Percent Rule well when he said, "Perfection is impossible. However, *striving* for perfection is not. Do the best you can under the conditions that exist. That is what counts."

ABOUT THE 2019 VERSION OF *THE PRIMAL BLUEPRINT* COMPREHENSIVE EXPANSION AND REVISION

You are reading a comprehensive update, revision, and expansion of the original *Primal Blueprint* hardcover released in 2009, the paperback released in 2012, and the color hardcover released in 2017 (as *The New Primal Blueprint*). This paperback edition is intended to be the one and only most relevant edition of the book. (Don't stress though, the older editions will still enable you to live an awesome life!) As I mentioned in my Welcome note (originally penned in 2009), I indeed maintain a sincere commitment to having a curious, inquisitive, and open mind as I bear the responsibility of being a prominent voice in the primal/paleo/ancestral health movement.

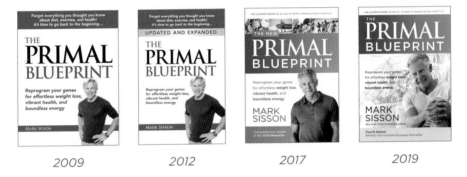

2009   2012   2017   2019

As my team and I reviewed every word and statement in *The Primal Blueprint* for this republication, we were heartened to realize that the core message of this book is timeless; it's essentially a simple, easy-to-understand guidebook for how to use the behaviors of our ancestors as models to navigate modern life in a healthy manner. However, as the evolutionary health movement has gained popularity, we have seen an escalation of criticism and naysayers, as well as assorted distortions, misinterpretations, and oversimplifications of the basic principles of the Primal Blueprint.

Considering new or alternate opinions is necessary to evolve our ideas. Indeed, questioning the status quo was my catalyst for writing *The Primal Blueprint* in the first place. Unfortunately, some of the banter is a little disturbing, as it departs from critical thinking to debating just for the sake of argument.

For example, the book *Paleofantasy* attacks the paleo diet as a farce because, as they claim, our ancestors ate all kinds of different diets, depending on where they lived on the globe and the particular environmental conditions of the day. The book *Cult Diets* asserts that because no single diet is a perfect fit for everyone, the assorted "cults" or supposed strictures of primal and paleo are ill-advised. Wait a sec! These are exactly the arguments I make as to why regimented diets are illogical, and why I insist that we must discover our own optimal eating habits *within the framework of evolutionary health principles.* We must make allowances for the enjoyment of modern life, as well as individual preferences and sensitivities. Just as we mustn't be quick to jump on the proverbial bandwagon without carefully evaluating the scientific evidence, nor should we discount something as a fad or hype simply in reaction to its relatively quick popularity.

> *Regimented diets are illogical and unsustainable; you must discover you own optimal eating habits within the framework of evolutionary health principles.*

Regarding the ancestral dietary debate, a few things are indisputable. First, it is clear what our ancestors *didn't* eat. *Hint: no processed sugars, industrial oils, or refined or even whole grains.* We also know from which categories of food they *did* choose, regardless of their environmental circumstances or location on the globe. *Hint: they ate plants and animals.* Evidence bears out that they ate—horror of horrors—a high-fat, low-carb profile, especially by comparison to the Standard American Diet (SAD). Aside from the ever-present critics of the ancestral health movement, we have also seen more scientific research validating many of the assertions and speculations that early pioneers like Dr. Boyd Eaton, Dr. Loren Cordain, and Dr. Arthur DeVany championed about the healthy examples set by our ancestors.

Today, I have a full-time editorial and research staff that assists me with the publication of a daily blog post at MarksDailyApple.com and

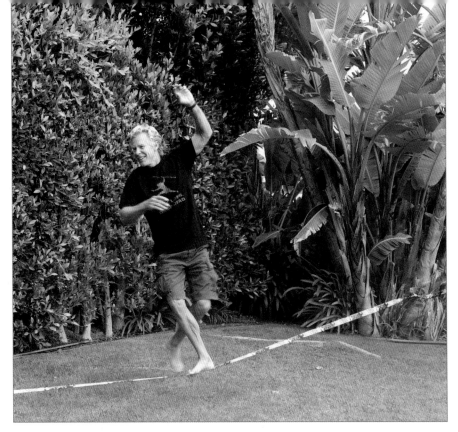

with the publishing of my own books, as well as books by numerous other authors at Primal Blueprint Publishing. (We now have dozens of titles in print. Check out primalblueprint.com/collections/books.) While certain elements of the Primal Blueprint contradict and question the conventional wisdom of some leading medical figures and agencies (not to mention challenge the ethics surrounding the billions of dollars spent and made promulgating that supposed wisdom), the research and message in *The Primal Blueprint* is unassailable.

I take great pains to clarify my positions by citing research and being open to dialogue in an effort to ensure that our words won't be taken out of context or summarily dismissed. Hopefully these efforts will calm the skeptics, as well as bolster those who already enthusiastically embrace the movement. Beyond that, I remind you again that you are in the driver's seat. You have nothing to lose by reading and deciding for yourself whether the principles of the Primal Blueprint are worth exploring and trying. Only you can decide whether your health could be better than it is right now. My main goal is for you to enjoy your life with the least amount of pain, suffering, and sacrifice possible.

The overriding principle I want you to embrace as you read this book is that of *choice*. I encourage you to take responsibility for your own health by educating yourself and choosing the path that works best for you. If you want to reject some of the concepts out of hand "just because," I understand that going to battle with you is an exercise in futility. I'm not asking you for blind faith in our message. I'm not a politician running for president on the Primal ticket. Nor am I trying to win a popularity contest. I'm simply presenting you with the latest evidence I have found about how we evolved and survived as a species thanks to evolutionary biology, genetic science, and health science, and then offering suggestions about how some of this knowledge might better inform your dietary and lifestyle choices. If you choose to smoke cigarettes or pump out excessive amounts of insulin from eating a high-sugar or grain-heavy diet, it's still possible that you will live to a ripe old age. However, statistically and scientifically speaking, it's more likely that you will suffer and struggle as a consequence of these lifestyle choices.

I've been asked the following question many times by primal enthusiasts: "How can I get my family, friends, and loved ones to go primal?" The answer is: you can't. They have to make the decision themselves, and they will only take action when the time is right for them. My best advice is to walk your talk. On that note, I must thank you from the bottom of my heart for your interest and initiative in picking up this book and giving it a shot. I hope you enjoy your experience and look forward to connecting with you.

If you have any questions, comments, or feedback, please reach out and communicate with me. I promise that your words and thoughts will be carefully considered by my staff and I as we constantly strive to build an inclusive and respectful primal community.

Mark Sisson

INTRODUCTION

CONVENTIONAL WISDOM VS. THE PRIMAL BLUEPRINT

In the Primal Blueprint (PB), we reframe these major elements of conventional wisdom (CW). Consider these alternatives with an open mind; we will discuss each in detail throughout the text.

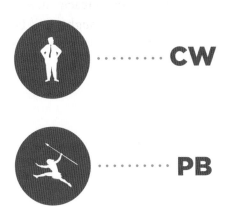

CW

PB

GRAINS: BREAD, PASTA, CEREAL, RICE, CORN, WHEAT, ETC.

 Whole grains are the foundation of a healthy diet. Eat 6-11 servings a day. Main energy source for brain and working muscles. Whole grains provide extra nutrition and fiber.

 "Worst mistake in the history of the human race" (UCLA evolutionary biologist Jared Diamond). Grains drive excess insulin production, fat storage, chronic inflammation, leaky gut syndrome, and heart disease. Allergenic and immunosuppressing. Nutritional value is inferior to plants and animals. Whole grains contain "anti-nutrients" (gluten and other lectins) that compromise immune and digestive function and promote systemic inflammation.

SATURATED ANIMAL FAT

Eating fat makes you fat, increases risk of cancer and heart disease. Replace saturated fats (meat, dairy) with polyunsaturated vegetable oils.

Excellent dietary calorie source, supports healthy hormone and cellular function, stable energy and appetite, and fat-adaptation. No evidence that saturated fat is unhealthy to eat. Drove human evolution/complex brain development for 2.5 million years.

CHOLESTEROL

 Cut cholesterol to prevent heart disease. Take statin drugs if total cholesterol is 200 or higher or if you have a family history of heart disease.

 Essential metabolic nutrient, no direct correlation with heart disease risk. Only dangerous when oxidation and inflammation are present (from high-carbohydrate, pro-inflammatory diet, chronic or lack of any exercise, and stressful lifestyle habits). Statins have considerable negative side effects and minimal, if any, direct benefit.

EGGS

 Minimize consumption due to high cholesterol content of yolk. Try processed egg white products instead!

 No correlation between egg intake and blood cholesterol levels. No correlation between egg intake and heart disease risk. Yolk among the planet's most nutritious foods.

FIBER

 Important dietary component, derived mostly from grains. Improves gastrointestinal function, lowers cholesterol, speeds elimination, and helps control weight by minimizing caloric intake.

 Incidental fiber from vegetables, fruit, nuts, and seeds is adequate for health benefits. Grain consumption promotes excess fiber intake, leading to digestive problems, nutrient deficiencies, and increased appetite.

MEAL HABITS

 Three squares (or six small meals) daily to stabilize blood sugar and to "keep the flame burning" (metabolically speaking). Skipped meals = slowed metabolism, lower energy levels, muscle breakdown, sugar cravings, and risk of binging.

 Moderating insulin and becoming fat-adapted eliminates need for regular meals and enables stable energy, mood, and appetite. Intermittent Fasting becomes effective weight management, immune boosting, anti-aging strategy. Eat when hungry, not on a fixed schedule, to fine-tune insulin sensitivity.

STRENGTH TRAINING

 Conduct prolonged workouts where you lift to "failure" through numerous muscle isolation stations or repeated sets of low weight and high reps.

 Go hard or go home! Conduct brief, high-intensity resistance workouts of 10 to 30 minutes or less a couple times a week, max. Emphasize explosive, full-body exercises to develop broad athletic competency and to stimulate a potent anti-aging hormonal response. Prolonged sub-maximal strength workouts leave you fatigued and depleted, and promote carb dependency.

CARDIO WORKOUTS

 More is better. Be consistent. Burn calories to control weight. The U.S. Surgeon General recommends getting 150 minutes of moderate-to-intense cardio exercise per week.

 *In*consistency is key! Slow down the pace if you want to improve and go faster over time and to avoid the prevailing "chronic cardio" pattern of slightly-too-difficult, overly-regimented, overly-stressful workouts that lead to burnout, carbohydrate dependency, and accelerated aging. It's not about the calories burned, it's about the health benefits of moving consistently and slowly throughout the day.

EVERYDAY MOVEMENT

 Just get your 150 minutes of cardio per week and you'll be healthy. If you're an athlete, be sure to rest and recover between workouts.

 Scientifically validated "active couch potato syndrome" observes sedentary-related disease risk factors even in devoted exercisers. Fitness, and health, is about more than just workouts—it's about moving more in general and avoiding prolonged sedentary periods.

WEIGHT LOSS

 High-complex-carb, low-fat, grain-based diet plus consistent mealtimes plus devoted portion control plus chronic cardio exercise. It's all about "calories in/calories out," willpower, regimented meal and workout patterns... and hoping that you have lucky genetics!

 High-fat, low-to-moderate-carb intake plus personalized, intuitive, sporadic meal patterns plus a strategic blend of stress-balanced primal workouts. Don't worry about portion control, regimented meals, fanatical workouts, or even genetic predispositions to fat storage. Reprogram your genes away from carb dependency to become fat-adapted, and fat reduction happens effortlessly.

PLAY

Ah, brings back fond memories of childhood. But who has time these days?

Integral component of overall health, stress management, and development of a "cognitively fluid mind"—a genetic necessity! Spontaneous, unstructured outdoor activity is the best counterbalance for our confined, predictable modern lives.

SUN EXPOSURE

Avoid the sun to prevent skin cancer! Lather up with SPF 50 sunscreen when you do go out. Drink milk for your vitamin D.

Vitamin D needs are met primarily by the sun, not by diet (by a factor of approximately 10x). Expose large skin surface areas to sunlight frequently to maintain a slight tan (a sign of healthy vitamin D levels). Vitamin D deficiency increases cancer risk, so sun (and winter supplementation) is essential to balance indoor-dominant lifestyles. Always avoid burning, and screen/shelter face and other sensitive or thin-skinned areas from overexposure.

FOOTWEAR

 Sturdy, cushioned shoes minimize injury and improve comfort. Custom orthotics can provide additional support and protection.

 Get primal—go barefoot (or minimalist)—but do it gradually to be safe. Perpetual use of "big" shoes increases impact trauma, weakens foot muscles, and increases pain and injury rates throughout lower extremities.

PRESCRIPTION DRUGS

Normal part of modern life—who doesn't have a pill bottle or three in the cabinet? Prescription drugs relieve pain, speed healing, prevent/cure disease, and address genetic frailties. Routine use can enhance quality of life (e.g., Viagra).

Wonderful to treat acute illness and infections. Chronic or excessive use masks/exacerbates underlying causes of illness, compromises natural homeostatic forces and thus health, and often comes with disastrous side effects (e.g., statins deplete CoQ10; antibiotics can compromise gut health over time). Simple lifestyle changes can negate the need for vast majority of drug treatments.

GOALS

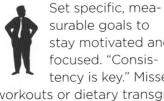 Set specific, measurable goals to stay motivated and focused. "Consistency is key." Missed workouts or dietary transgressions = guilt, weight gain, and lost fitness.

 De-emphasize specific, results-oriented goals (potential for discouragement, such as weight-loss failure or "post-marathon blues"). Stay motivated by focusing on fun, and release attachment to outcome. Rigid consistency = overstress. Vary routine to minimize stress and improve adaptive response by genes. Missed workouts allow time for recovery, drive fitness improvements, and keep exercise programs fresh.

Weight loss does not have to involve
the suffering, sacrifice, and deprivation
we've been conditioned to accept.

I'm going to ask you to forget most everything you thought you knew about diet, exercise, and health. There is a distressing amount of flawed conventional wisdom that confuses, misleads, manipulates, and complicates even the most devoted efforts to do the right things: eat healthfully, exercise effectively, control weight, and avoid common health conditions like digestive issues, arthritis, obesity, diabetes, heart disease, and cancer.

In *The Primal Blueprint*, you will learn why eating a low-fat diet rich in whole grains such as bread, pasta, and cereal can easily make you fat and malnourished. You'll learn why millions of joggers and gym-goers put in the time and effort to lose weight yet routinely compromise their health and accelerate the aging process as a direct result of their (exhausting) devotion to fitness. You'll learn why your cholesterol level and saturated fat intake are not the major risk factors for heart disease that we have been led to believe, and why a comparatively high-fat diet (of primal-approved fats that is!) promotes health, longevity, and reduction of excess body fat. I'll show how weight loss does not have to involve the suffering, sacrifice, and deprivation we've been conditioned to accept, but instead is a matter of eating the right foods (plants and animals), avoiding the wrong foods (processed carbs like sugars and grains, along with highly refined, oxidized industrial vegetable/seed oils), exercising strategically for far fewer hours than you might assume, and finding ways to move more during everyday life.

All the answers are found in a set of 10 simple, logical eating, exercise, and lifestyle practices—my Primal Blueprint "laws." Modeling your 21st-century life after our primal hunter-gatherer ancestors will help you greatly reduce or eliminate almost all of the disease risk factors that you may falsely blame on genes that you inherited from your parents. Unfortunately, too many of us narrowly define genes as largely unalterable inherited traits—height, body type, eye color, physical or intellectual traits, and a "family history" of health conditions and diseases. While some genes are indeed responsible for traits that are largely unaffected by your behavior, many more interact with lifestyle to play a bigger role in your health than you might realize. As coming chapters explain in detail, your genes—guided by what you eat, how you move, and even how you think—are the traffic cops that direct the functioning of every single cell in your body, every moment of every day.

> *Instead of falling victim to your genetic vulnerabilities, you can control how your genes express themselves in constantly rebuilding, repairing, and renewing your cells.*

Whatever you throw at them, your genes are going to respond in an effort to promote survival and, beyond that, homeostasis (the balanced and synchronistic functioning of all systems in the body). After all, this is the essence of human evolution. When you are sprawled on the couch late at night chowing down on Cheetos and Dr. Pepper, your body will still valiantly pursue homeostasis regardless of whether or not it benefits your long-term health. In the example of a junk food binge, your body will respond by releasing insulin and stress hormones into the bloodstream to remove excess glucose, which would otherwise kill you. In the short term, this is adaptive. In the long term, chronically flooding your bloodstream with these hormones will lead to a whole host of other problems.

The idea that you can reprogram your genes through your behavior is the central premise of this book. It represents a clear departure from today's fatalistic conventional wisdom, which suggests that our genes, for better or worse, determine our destiny and that we have little say in the matter... unless prescription drugs or discoveries by the Human Genome Project come to the rescue. True, you might have a genetic tendency toward alcoholism, accumulating excess body fat, or contracting type 2 diabetes like others in your family, but you'll only express these predispositions when you make poor lifestyle choices and send the wrong signals to your genes. Instead of falling victim to your (very real) genetic vulnerabilities, you can control how your genes express themselves in constantly rebuilding, repairing, and renewing your cells. Briefly, here are the most critical, life-altering elements of the Primal Blueprint:

Become a *fat-burning beast* by eliminating processed carbohydrates from your diet to minimize insulin production. This means ditching not only sugars and sweetened beverages, but also grain products, including wheat, rice, pasta, cereals, and corn. A diet that emphasizes meat, fish, fowl, eggs, nuts, seeds, and colorful natural carbs from vegetables and fruits, is the primary way to improve your general health, control your weight, and minimize the risk of heart disease, cancer, diabetes, arthritis, and other diet-influenced medical conditions.

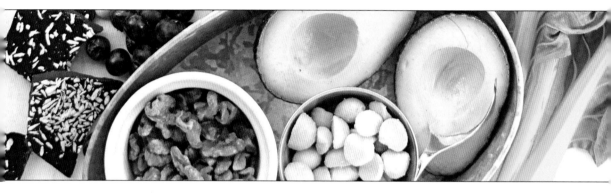

If you are carrying excess body fat, it will disappear without you having to work at it when you focus on eating the delicious, filling, nutritious foods that have nourished humans throughout the course of evolution. Seriously, it's as simple as breaking free from a lifetime of wildly excessive insulin production thanks to a Standard American Diet (SAD) rich in grains and sugar and choosing the right foods to moderate insulin production and enable your body to mobilize stored body fat and burn it for energy. You do not have to struggle and suffer with calorie restriction and exhausting exercise to shed excess body fat—you simply have to reset your appetite and the metabolic hormones that have been dysregulated by a lifetime of wildly excessive insulin production.

Optimize your exercise program by engaging in frequent, low-intensity, energizing movement (such as walking, hiking, structured cardio workouts conducted at low-level aerobic heart rates, and complementary

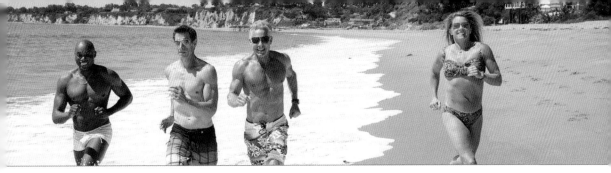

fitness activities like Pilates, yoga, tai chi, dancing, and dynamic rolling/stretching/therapy work). Avoid prolonged periods of inactivity by making a general effort to move more and take regular movement breaks throughout the day. Include regular brief, intense strength-training sessions (one to two times a week max) and occasional all-out sprints (once every seven to ten days) to improve body composition and delay the aging process.

This strategy is far superior to the conventional wisdom advocating for a regimented schedule of frequent medium-to-difficult-intensity sustained workouts, such as running, cycling, cardio machines, or group classes. This workout strategy, which I refer to as "chronic cardio," places excessive and prolonged physical stress on your body—because workout intensity is slightly too difficult, making it stressful rather than energizing—and leads to fatigue, injuries, compromised immune function, and burnout. Furthermore, the hype surrounding the fitness craze disregards the importance of general everyday movement. Even a devoted fitness regimen, with daily visits to the gym or miles on the road, is not enough to be truly fit and healthy—especially with the many sedentary forces present in modern life (commuting, office work, digital leisure time, etc.)

Manage stress with plenty of sleep, play, sunlight, and fresh air. Pursue creative, intellectual pursuits, and avoid making stupid mistakes. Rebel against the modern cultural tendency toward a sedentary life and excessive artificial light. Opt for more sleep by reducing digital stimulation after dark. In short, honor your primal genes by slowing down and simpli-

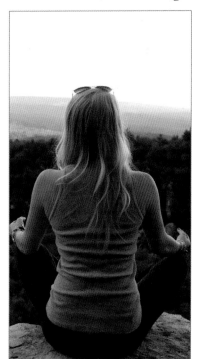

fying your life. Your ancestors worked hard to survive, but their regular respites from stress gave them the peace of mind and body that are so highly coveted today.

IS DYING OF OLD AGE GETTING OLD, OR WHAT?

As you will soon discover, our genes are designed through evolution to keep us healthy. The biological mechanisms that work synchronistically to maintain a state of homeostasis within each of us are imperative to our survival. Thanks to the hectic pace of our high-tech, modern world, many of us struggle to maintain our health. The confusion and often-repeated failure that results from our efforts to do the right thing by conventional wisdom leads many of us, whether overtly or deep down inside, to simply give up. Experience has taught us how difficult, if not impossible, it is to be lean, fit, energetic, and healthy by following conventional wisdom. Instead, we succumb to the forces of consumerism that are designed to placate our pain with silly shortcuts, comforts, conveniences, and indulgences. Consequently, the popular "Hey man, life is short!" rationalization becomes a self-fulfilling prophecy.

> *Seventy percent of today's health care expenditures are for lifestyle-related chronic diseases, such as obesity, diabetes, and heart disease.*

Eating processed foods, exercising excessively (or, conversely, being inactive), and making other poor lifestyle decisions undermines your genetic mandate for health. At the very least, you can expect adverse lifestyle practices to very quickly lead to excess body fat, subpar fitness results, aching joints, gastrointestinal problems, frequent minor illnesses, sugar cravings, energy level swings, and recurring fatigue.

That sounds bad enough as it is, but continuing to misdirect your genes with bad choices over years and decades will likely result in life-long insidious weight gain or obesity (depending on how lucky you are with genetic predispositions), diabetes, heart disease, cancer, and/or one or more of the degenerative conditions that require a doctor's care or medication. A huge percentage of all doctor visits today are a direct consequence of lifestyle choices that are misaligned with the environmental and survival conditions that shaped our primal genetic makeup.

These consequences are painfully obvious to most everyone, and our collective interest in doing the right thing has driven a booming fitness industry, incredible advancements in medicine, much greater awareness of healthy foods and lifestyle choices, sharp declines in smoking, and sharp increases in healthy restaurants and food stores. Ironically, though, Americans' collective health—and that of people in other countries that match our fast-paced culture—is worse than ever. A study released in 2008 by Johns Hopkins University predicts that by the year 2030, 86 percent of all adults in the United States will be overweight or obese (up from the estimated 65 percent of Americans who are overweight or obese today). What's more, some researchers predict that by the year 2230, *all* Americans will be obese.

We reluctantly accept as fact that a normal human life span consists of growing up to reach a physical peak in our twenties, followed by an inevitable steady decline caused by the aging process. Under this faulty belief, we allow ourselves to gain an average of one-and-a-half-pounds of fat (two-thirds of a kilo) per year starting at age 25 and continuing through age 55.[1] We also lose half a pound of muscle per year, resulting in adding an extra pound of weight per year as we age. Our last decade or two (until we reach the average American life span of 76 for men and 81 for women)[2] is commonly characterized by inactivity, diminished muscle mass, excess body fat, assorted medical conditions, and a host of prescription drugs to alleviate the pain and symptoms of chronic disease. Twenty-three percent of us will die from cardiovascular disease, and another 23 percent will die from cancer.[3] I know that 100 percent of us will die from something, but personally, I'd prefer to actualize a motto I crafted in honor of our hunter-gatherer ancestors: *Live Long, Drop Dead!*

Yes, many primal humans succumbed to primitive hazards (e.g., death by predator or infection from a minor wound) before they hit today's voting age, but many of those who avoided misfortune could live six or seven decades in exceptional health and fitness. In almost all cases, primal humans were healthy and strong for their entire lives, until they met

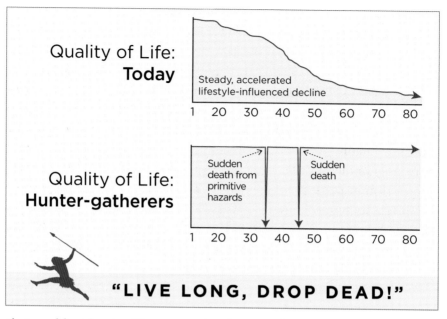

Quality of Life:
Today

Steady, accelerated lifestyle-influenced decline

1 20 30 40 50 60 70 80

Quality of Life:
Hunter-gatherers

Sudden death from primitive hazards

Sudden death

1 20 30 40 50 60 70 80

"LIVE LONG, DROP DEAD!"

their sudden demise. There was simply no such thing as today's abysmal decline into old age. In general, every individual hunter-gatherer was required to make a contribution to the clan, and there was no ability to support those who, for whatever reason or misfortune, were unable to support themselves. By any modern measure this is pretty harsh, but this was the reality of life-or-death selection pressure in primal life.

While 21st-century longevity stats are vastly superior to those of any other time in human history, these increases are largely attributable to science, not healthier lifestyle behaviors. Furthermore, modern longevity is often undesirably inflated by scientific advancements that keep us alive but do not improve quality of life: hospital machinery, pharmaceuticals, and the ability to reel in the years doing little more than putting spoon to mouth and thumb to remote control.

Of the 2.5 trillion dollars America spends annually on health care, the Centers for Disease Control and Prevention (CDC) estimates that more than 75 percent is spent on lifestyle-related chronic diseases, such as obesity, diabetes, and heart disease. A surprising number of people accept all this as a normal part of life, believing that some of us are just fortunate to have "good genes," and the rest must cross their fingers against bad luck.

Sure, millions of modern citizens contributing to these woeful statistics are completely ignorant about what is required to be healthy. It might be hard for you even to relate to this segment of humanity that hasn't a clue or a care about this stuff. However, even the most health conscious among us often struggle. Despite a sincere commitment to do the right thing by conventional wisdom, we have collectively failed to lose that last 5, 10, or 50 pounds. Injuries, fatigue, and burnout plague exercisers ranging from weekend warriors to elite competitors. We have been programmed by the health care establishment to reflexively turn to prescription drugs to treat symptoms of distress, even though most conditions are minor and easily corrected by simple dietary and lifestyle changes. In the process, we interfere with normal gene-driven metabolic processes and thwart our innate ability to heal naturally—paving our way to joining the masses on the wrong side of the stats.

The story is sad, but the good news is that your destiny for the most part is in your hands. By the time you complete this book, you will understand the big picture and all the necessary details of how to eat, exercise, and live in order to reprogram many of your genes for lifelong health. In the process, you will take control of your own body and your own life. This is really the only sensible way to counter the tremendous momentum pushing us away from health, balance, and wellbeing in our hectic modern world.

CHAPTER ENDNOTES

[1] *Physiology of Sport and Exercise*, by Drs. W. Larry Kenney, Jack H. Wilmore, and David L. Costill.

[2] These data are from a Centers for Disease Control 2013 report, which can be found at cdc.gov/nchs/data/nvsr/nvsr64/nvsr64_02.pdf. The Central Intelligence Agency's World Factbook estimates that in 2015, average American life expectancy was 79.7 years (77 for men, 82 for women).

[3] The American Heart Association reports that heart disease is the leading cause of death worldwide. In 2013, cardiovascular-related deaths accounted for 31 percent of all deaths (worldwide), and over 800,000 Americans died from heart disease, cardiovascular disease, or stroke. Data released by Centers for Disease Control confirms that heart disease was the number one cause of death for Americans in 2014 (the most recent data available), followed by cancer.

CHAPTER ONE

THE TEN PRIMAL BLUEPRINT LAWS

("Commandments" Was Already Taken)

IN THIS CHAPTER

I introduce the "re-evolutionary" premise that we should model our diet, exercise, and lifestyle behaviors after our primal ancestors from 10,000 years ago, adapting those behaviors strategically to the realities of high-tech modern life. The inexorable technological progress of civilization has diverted us from the healthy dietary habits and active, stress-balanced lifestyles that allowed primal humans to prevail under the harsh competitive pressures of evolution. However, we are almost genetically identical (in nearly all areas relevant to human health) to our hunter-gatherer ancestors, owing to the fact that evolution lost its main catalyst when the major selection pressures of starvation and predator danger (eat or get eaten!) were eliminated with the gradual advent of civilization across the globe.

Genes are much more than the narrow conventional understanding of them as fixed heritable traits (e.g., hair, skin, and eye color). Genes are the "traffic cops" that direct the function of every cell in your body at all times. Genes are activated or deactivated by the signals they receive from the environment. Drink a soda, and your genes direct the flood of insulin into your bloodstream to counteract the high glucose levels, returning you to a state of homeostasis that ensures your short-term survival. By following the Primal Blueprint laws, you can reprogram your genes in the direction of health and longevity. Even if you have strong familial genetic predispositions to disease, excess body fat, and other adverse health conditions, you can honor your *Homo sapiens* genes and render these dispositions virtually irrelevant.

The 10 Primal Blueprint laws are:

1. Eat Plants and Animals
2. Avoid Poisonous Things
3. Move Frequently
4. Lift Heavy Things
5. Sprint Once in a While
6. Get Plenty of Sleep
7. Play
8. Get Plenty of Sunlight
9. Avoid Stupid Mistakes
10. Use Your Brain

Nothing in biology makes sense except in the light of evolution.

—Theodosius Dobzhansky

The quote by Dobzhansky was also the title of his famous 1973 essay in which the noted evolutionary biologist and devout Russian Orthodox Christian acknowledged that, whether or not you believed in the existence of a higher power, you could not begin to understand even the simplest concepts in biology unless you accepted how evolution had worked to shape and differentiate the genes of every single one of the several million species on the planet.

Within the past hundred years, tens of thousands of anthropologists, evolutionary biologists, paleontologists, epigeneticists, and other scientists have worked diligently to piece together a fairly detailed interpretation of the environmental and behavioral factors that directly influenced our development as a species. As a result, we now have a very good picture of the conditions under which we emerged as *Homo sapiens*.

Some seven million years ago, hominids (our prehuman ancestors) split from apes and branched out into various new species and subspecies. Then, about 2.5 million years ago, the humanlike species *Homo erectus*, with its large brain, upright stature, skilled use of tools, eventual mastery of fire (around 400,000 years ago), and organized hunter-gatherer societies, began to take charge of the food chain. Over time, *Homo erectus* branched into various species and subspecies (*Homo neanderthalensis*, *Homo habilis*, and *Homo sapiens*, among others). Most researchers believe that modern *Homo sapiens* first appeared in East Africa around 160,000 years ago. Then, about 60,000 years ago, a very small number of *Homo sapiens* left Africa and began their great migration across the planet.

Recent archeological findings strongly support this "Out of Africa" theory[1]: that the entire human population of the planet, amazingly, can trace their origins to a small pool of intrepid *Homo sapiens* in East Africa. There were only an estimated 2,000 to 5,000 African humans at that time; and some scientists believe that only about 150 people crossed the Red Sea to begin the migration. Despite our disparate physical appearances today, and our layman's misconception of race as distinct parallel tracks of ancestry, the truth is that all humans descend from a very small clan of globetrotters, making us extremely similar from a genetic perspective.

••••••••••• GROK 🏃 TALK •••••••••••

Evolving Without Evolution

When the advent of civilization freed humans from constant selection pressure (because predator danger and the threat of starvation were greatly reduced), evolution nearly ground to a halt. This means that we are nearly genetically identical to our primal ancestors, at least in relation to those aspects that dictate how we should eat, exercise, and live in order to promote the ultimate goal of evolution: **to survive long enough to reproduce.** *Yet the essence of the Primal Blueprint is to leverage what we know of the evolutionary model far beyond the modest goal of reproducing. Our goal is to replicate as many of our ancestors' dietary and lifestyle choices as possible to promote optimal health, peak physical and cognitive performance, and longevity.*

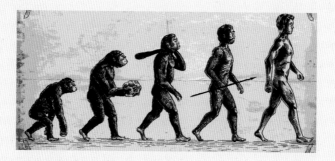

While a slender, six-foot-four, blond, fair-skinned Scandinavian might seem highly disparate from a stout, five-foot-seven, dark-skinned Indian, these physical variations are relatively superficial from a DNA perspective. As a species, we tend to inflate the significance of differences between ethnic groups. But humans are much more alike than not, genetically speaking. For example, David Epstein's brilliant book, *The Sports Gene*, references the work of Yale genetics professor Kenneth Kidd, who asserts that there is greater genetic diversity between two members of the same pygmy tribe in Africa (or any two individuals whose ancestry has been contained within the African continent since primal times) than there is among the rest of the *entire human race combined!*

Today's phenotypic differences in appearance around the globe obscure the larger truth that when it comes to DNA, we are all fundamentally human. You may have heard how we share more than 98 percent of our DNA with chimps and bonobos, so you can imagine how trying to split hairs to differentiate humans is irrelevant. One implication this genetic similarity has for your health is that you don't need to go looking for the latest fad diet that's linked to your blood type or even your ethnicity. Rather, the blueprint for healthy living comes from our shared evolutionary history as hunter-gatherers.

This is not to say that there are no meaningful differences between individuals—obviously there are. The set of genes we receive from our parents have distinct features that predispose us to being athletic, a math genius (like my friend Big George), obese, or suffer from arthritis if we nurture such positive or negative outcomes with accordant lifestyle behaviors.

It is also true there are some relatively recent examples of genetic mutations, aka *genetic drift*, that make recent ancestry potentially more relevant to your healthy eating and lifestyle choices. For example, your skin pigmentation strongly influences your vitamin D health. (Our ancestors had dark skin for over a million years; researchers believe the lightening of skin color among some peoples happened perhaps 40,000 or as recently as 10,000 years ago in conjunction with colonizing the higher latitudes.) Darker-skinned people require longer sun exposure to optimize vitamin D production and are much more susceptible to vitamin D deficiency in today's indoor-dominant lifestyle.

Another interesting example is the prevalence of lactase persistence (continuing to make the enzyme lactase, enabling one to digest lactose—the sugar in milk—throughout life) amongst those of distinct herding ancestry, such as Northern Europeans and Scandinavians. While most adults (~75 percent) across the globe become lactose intolerant after childhood, those with strong herding ancestry are nearly all (~90 percent) lactase persistent.

Thirdly, as you might discern from looking at the disparate success rates in maintaining ideal body composition despite devoted efforts, one's ability to successfully tolerate carbohydrate ingestion without getting fat has strong genetic influences. Recent science has promoted the idea that those with more copies of the AMY1 gene (a salivary enzyme involved in the breakdown of starches) can better manage carbohydrate intake without getting fat than those with fewer copies. Some scientists cite these and other examples to argue that evolution is still occurring. At a certain point, we are just arguing semantics about the effects of population expansion, genetic drift, and modern science being increasingly able to identify variations (that were likely always there) in the human genome, versus traditional conceptualizations of evolution driven by random mutations and survival of the fittest. For now, let's stay focused on the big picture: discovering the most important evolution-tested behaviors that promote optimal gene expression—behaviors that have not changed in 10,000 years. These are really all you need to know to achieve optimal health.

CIVILIZATION CUTS BOTH WAYS

I hope you are sitting down to absorb one of the most critical—and quite possibly mind-blowing—tenets of the Primal Blueprint:

Our primal ancestors were likely stronger
and healthier than we are today.

"How can this be?" you ask. It's all about survival of the fittest. The human body is the miraculous result of millions of years of painstaking design by evolution. Through natural selection—countless small genetic mutations and adaptations in response to a hostile environment—our ancestors were able to prevail over unimaginably difficult conditions and opponents and to populate all corners of the earth.

On the other hand, the development of agriculture and civilization caused humans to become smaller and sicker, leading to a dramatic decline in life expectancy. Many anthropologists suggest that the human species reached its physical evolutionary pinnacle (in terms of average muscularity, bone density, and brain size) about 10,000 years ago. After that, we started to take it easy and get soft. Our physical decline was a natural consequence of a couple of things. First, we had already spent thousands of generations leveraging our increasingly proficient brain function to manipulate and tame the natural environment (with tools, weapons, fire, and shelter) to our advantage. Doing so made life easier and survival more likely.

The second factor is perhaps the most significant lifestyle change in the history of humanity: the gradual advent of agriculture. When humans began to domesticate and harvest wheat, rice, corn, and other crops, as well as livestock, they gained the ability to store food, divide and specialize labor, and live in close civilized quarters. This virtually eliminated the main selection pressures that had driven human evolution for 2.5 million years—the threats of starvation and predator danger. Our transition from hunter-gatherer existence to agricultural societies happened independently around the globe, becoming prominent about 7,000 years ago in modern-day Egypt. North America was one of the last areas to implement agriculture, about 4,500 years ago.[2]

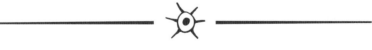

FEELIN' SOME PRESSURE TO EXPLAIN SELECTION PRESSURE

"Selection pressure" is the Darwinian-inspired term to describe life-or-death environmental circumstances that drive the evolution of all species. The evolutionary process we know as "survival of the fittest" might be more accurately expressed as "survival of the luckiest"—that is, survival of those who were lucky enough to be born with features that conferred a reproductive advantage. Consider the example of Darwin's famous Galapagos finches: a bird born with a long, pointy beak (by random genetic mutation) discovered that he was better adapted to picking seeds out of cactus fruits on his island. Consequently, he enjoyed a reproductive advantage over less well-endowed finches in that habitat, and long, pointy beaks soon proliferated on that particular island. Meanwhile, short, stout beaks (better for collecting seeds off the ground) were selected for and proliferated on a different island.

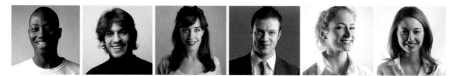

The lightening of skin pigmentation to afford better vitamin D production away from the equator is an example of Darwin's mutation and natural selection process.

Similarly, over thousands of years of human evolution, genetic mutations that promoted our survival (higher-functioning brains, explosive fast-twitch muscle fibers, etc.) appeared in the gene pool by luck through random genetic mutations in individuals and were then selected for and proliferated through reproduction. For example, as humans migrated north from the equator into the higher latitudes, getting enough sun exposure to produce ample vitamin D became a big problem with potentially fatal consequences. The first human born with lighter skin at the higher latitudes (from darker skinned parents who had emigrated there) was bestowed a significant survival advantage. Hence, the lightening of skin color spread like wildfire among humans living at higher latitudes. Conversely, unfavorable genetic mutations that compromised chances for survival and reproduction were eliminated from the gene pool with ruthless efficiency.

The idea that human DNA—the genetic "recipe" for building a healthy, lean, thriving human that resides in each of our 60 trillion cells—is almost exactly the same today as it was 10,000 years ago was first notably promoted by the work of Dr. Boyd Eaton, chief anthropologist at Emory University in Atlanta and author of *The Paleolithic Prescription* (1988) and a landmark paper published in the *New England Journal of Medicine* in 1985, "Paleolithic Nutrition." Other researchers leading the way were the late James V. Neel, founder of the University of Michigan's Department of Genetics, and Dr. Loren Cordain, professor of exercise physiology at Colorado State University, who was a pioneer in talking about eating in accordance with our hunter-gatherer ancestors in *The Paleo Diet* (2002). Today, with the evolutionary health movement exploding in popularity, more and more research is being published by anthropologists, evolutionary biologists, and genetic researchers validating the early arguments set forth by these paleo pioneers.

While our primal ancestors made the most of their genes (remember, this was not a conscious choice; the alternative was to starve or become some other creature's dinner!), most of us today fall far short. The development of agriculture and civilization caused humans to become smaller (including in brain size) and sicker (originally due to contagious diseases, but now due mostly to vastly inferior diets, exercise, and lifestyle patterns).

Human life expectancy 10,000 years ago was about 33 years. While not too impressive by 21st-century standards, and somewhat misleading due to high rates of infant mortality at the time, primal man actually lived longer relative to his civilized descendants all the way into the early 20th century! Average life expectancy reached a low of 18 during the Bronze Age (~3300-1200 B.C., Ancient Egypt), rose only slightly to

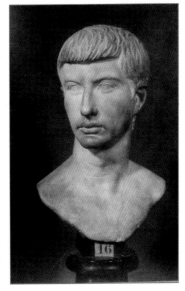

Life expectancy was brutal during the time of Brutus—under 30 years. Brutus lived to 43 (long enough to knock off Caesar), but Grok and his pre-civilized pals often bested that.

a range of 20 to 30 years through Classical Greek times (~500-300 B.C.), the Roman Empire (~0-500 A.D.), and the Middle Ages (~700-1500), and was still only between 30 and 40 years as recently as the early 20th century. Around that time, medical advancements (antibiotics, hospital and community sanitation, better infant survival, and so on) helped life expectancy skyrocket.

Fossil records show that primal humans who steered clear of fatal misfortune could routinely live six or seven decades in excellent health. The records also show a "maximum observed life span" of an astonishing 94 years![3] Among present-day hunter-gatherers (e.g., Aché, Hadza, Hiwi, and !Kung—groups with almost no modern conveniences or access to medical care), it is not uncommon to see strong, healthy folks living well into their 80s. More than a quarter of the Aché (Ah-CHAY) people of Paraguay make it to 70. Moreover, 73 percent of Ache adults die from accidents and only 17 percent from illness. Think about the extraordinary implications of hunter-gatherer longevity: with no modern medications or medical care of any kind, a massive lifelong struggle for food, clothing, and shelter, and lives completely devoid of modern comforts, primal humans (and modern humans living primally) can still live to what even we softies consider old age.

> *The Ultimate Human award*
> *goes to Grok, my nickname for*
> *the prototypical pre-agricultural*
> *human being.*

Of course, the decline in life expectancy with the onset of civilization didn't matter in a purely evolutionary context. As long as civilized humans made it to reproductive age and had children, they could pass their genes along to the next generation without penalty. While progressing beyond primal humans' harsh survival of the fittest conditions is definitely a good thing, the sober reality is that today's technological age is populated with the fattest, most sedentary humans in the history of humanity. Hence, the Ultimate Human award goes to Grok,[4] my nickname for the prototypical pre-agricultural human being. Grok is a lean, smart, healthy character, the primal representative of sorts of both this book and my blog at MarksDailyApple.com.

Unlike Grok, who ruled the planet with little more than a spear and a thatched hut in his portfolio, even the most impoverished humans of the last several thousand years, extending up to the present day's most socioeconomically stressed persons, have not really "competed" genetically. The presence of the most rudimentary modern advantages, such as the availability and storage of basic food stuffs like grains, permanent shelters, and basic defenses to nullify predator danger, all suppress the true Darwinian survival of the fittest playing field that allowed Grok to thrive.

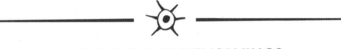

ARE WE REALLY DEVOLVING?

You might have heard that humans are actually *devolving*. Proponents of this idea argue that modern lifestyles—rife with too much sugar and too little exercise, obesity, metabolic disease, and so on—are causing unfavorable genetic changes that actually make our (long-term) survival less likely, and that we are now passing those changes on to our children. So is that true? Is the evolutionary clock actually spinning backward?

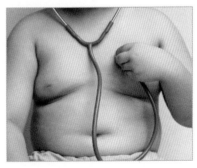

For the first time in recorded history, today's youth have a lower life expectancy than their parents.

Not exactly. True evolution in the Darwinian sense requires that genomic changes—changes to our DNA—are passed from generation to generation. There is no evidence that modern lifestyles, problematic though they are, are affecting our DNA. However, something is most definitely afoot, and that something is *epigenetic transgenerational inheritance.*

In addition to the genome with which you are undoubtedly familiar (the DNA, organized into genes, residing in each of our cells) we also have an *epi*genome. The epigenome resides outside or "on top of" (the literal meaning of *epi-*) the DNA and is comprised of chemical tags known as epigenetic marks. These marks attach to the genome and direct the expression of the genes, turning them on or off, up or down. Whereas our genome is fixed, our epigenome is malleable; it responds to internal and external stimuli. Scientists now believe we can change our epigenome through our behaviors, and this is the very essence of the Primal Blueprint: providing the kind of input and environment for our epigenome to direct favorable gene expression to promote health and longevity.

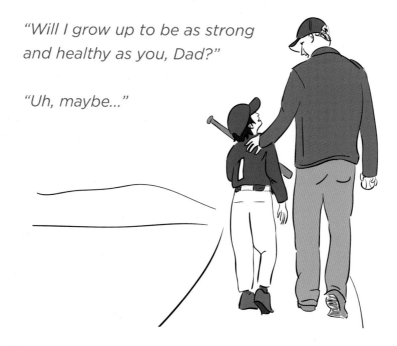

"Will I grow up to be as strong and healthy as you, Dad?"

"Uh, maybe..."

It turns out that there are even bigger stakes than our own health and longevity, though. A growing body of research shows that epigenetic changes can be passed to offspring. If individuals behave in ways or are in environments that promote unfavorable gene expression—if they overeat or eat a poor diet, are highly stressed, smoke, or are exposed to high levels of lead, for example—their offspring can inherit epigenetic markers that direct unfavorable gene expression. Studies have linked epigenetic inheritance to offspring's risk of metabolic and cardiovascular disease, abnormal stress response, mental health issues, memory problems, and asthma, among others. In studies on animals with short life spans and high generational turnover such as fruit flies, there are examples of these changes persisting for many generations. (Many studies of transgenerational epigenetic inheritance have been conducted with mice or other animals, but there are ones that demonstrate epigenetic inheritance in humans as well.)

What does this all mean? First, it means that humans are not devolving in a literal sense. Although modern lifestyles have serious negative health consequences, the most life-threatening problems mostly arise after our reproductive years are behind us, so there is no selection pressure leading to survival of the fittest. Humans won't be sprouting gills (this would definitely count as a change to our DNA!) any time soon unless the world floods over for thousands of years and we need to sink or swim. However, our genes can be literally "marked" for misfortune and those marks passed to offspring as a consequence of adverse lifestyle practices.

It's becoming increasingly clear that the choices we make affect not only ourselves but our children, our grandchildren, and maybe even further down the ancestral line. That's scary stuff, but don't get overwhelmed. It also means that we have more control over our health and our children's health than we would if genes were the be-all and end-all. And if you already had children (perhaps when you weren't as healthy as before you went primal), know that by modeling good behavior for them going forward, you are encouraging them to make choices in their own lives that direct favorable epigenetic changes. Just consider this a wake-up call and use it to motivate your own good choices in the future!

Sure, being a math whiz or a natural athlete may significantly influence your path through life and give you a competitive edge in pursuits to which you are inclined, but these genetic attributes no longer provide a survival advantage in the evolutionary sense. Candy-chomping, video-gaming slackers can reproduce just as successfully as Olympic athletes and Ph.D. candidates due to lack of selection pressure for physical or cognitive peak performance attributes in the modern world. Obviously, the elimination of ruthless selection pressure represents progress for humanity. (Consider how most of us have suffered illnesses or traumas over the course of our lives that would have killed us a century ago, let alone 1,000 or 10,000 years ago.) However, we must be vigilant not to let the advantages of modern life compromise our health (for example, by hitting the pharmacy instead of the gym to combat back pain), or worse, lead to unfavorable epigenetic transgenerational inheritance to our offspring.

The challenge is in applying the Primal Blueprint laws to modern life. How do we leverage the lessons and benefits of natural selection against the pressures of a complex modern society bent on promoting consumerism and quick fixes over the pursuit of health? How do we reprogram our ancient genes to recapture excellent health? We simply have to ask ourselves, "What would Grok do?"

YOU HAVE TO FIT YOUR GENES TO FIT INTO YOUR JEANS

In order to begin to understand the concept of "reprogramming" your genes, it will help to understand what they actually are and how they work. Each of your 50 or 60 trillion cells contains a nucleus with a complete set of DNA instructions divided into handy subsets called genes. There are approximately 20,000 different genes located on the long strands of DNA in each cell, organized into 23 pairs of chromosomes. In any given cell, only a small fraction of the total number of genes is actively involved in carrying out the main "business" of that particular type of cell. Depending on the environmental signals that cells get from their cellular environments within the body (which can be influenced by external factors), genes trigger the manufacture of specific proteins and enzymes to perform the various tasks required of them. For example, the beta cells in your pancreas manufacture insulin, but they don't grow bigger when you lift weights. Liver cells can synthesize nutrients, but they don't grow new bone tissue. And yet each cell has the entire "recipe" for a human residing in the DNA.

Genes are not self-determining; they do not turn on or off by themselves, but rather they respond to signals they receive from their immediate environment.

Genes don't know—or care—whether these environmental signals promote or compromise your health; they simply react to each stimulus in an effort to ensure your immediate survival. The most important thing to understand here is that most genes are not self-determining; they do not turn on or off by themselves, but rather they respond to signals they receive from their immediate environment. You have the power to switch on or turn off certain genes that have a profound influence on your health. You may not be able to reprogram your eyes from blue to brown, but you can certainly avoid becoming obese, even if your dad, grandpa, and brothers (who eat a grain-based, high-carbohydrate diet) all happen to be obese.

• • • • • • • • • • • **GROK** 🎿 **TALK** • • • • • • • • • • •

Genes Are All About Instant Gratification —How About You?

Genes are programmed to support short-term survival—that's it. Pound those Cheetos and Dr. Pepper on the couch, and your genes direct a flood of insulin into the bloodstream to remove excess glucose that can otherwise quickly become life-threatening. If high-insulin-producing eating habits become a lifestyle pattern, your genes will fight valiantly to keep you alive every day, but you will likely accumulate inflammation and oxidation that will compromise your long-term health. Again, with selection pressure irrelevant (you won't get eaten by a lion if you get fat), the responsibility falls entirely on you—whether you choose to promote, or compromise, long-term health with your daily lifestyle behaviors.

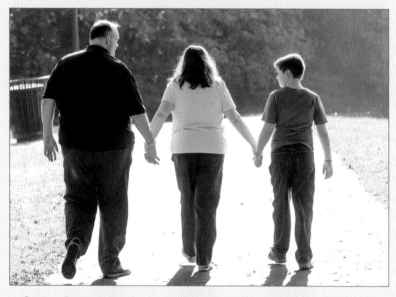

Granted, a strong familial genetic predisposition to carry excess body fat is indeed relevant and plays out routinely in many families over generations due to the driving force of high-insulin-producing diets. When you give your genes a different environmental experience (e.g., a primal-aligned diet that moderates insulin), your predisposition toward obesity will cease to be relevant. Ditto if you carry genes that predispose you to alcoholism but you don't drink.

Genes actively control cell function all the time. Your overall health is primarily dependent on which genes get turned on or off in response to their immediate environment. Sprint or lift weights, and the biochemical "byproducts" from that specific activity turn on certain genes that repair and strengthen the exercised muscles. Do too much exercise, and other genes promote excessive production of catabolic (breakdown) hormones, leading to prolonged inflammation and hindered recovery. An allergic reaction represents your body's (misdirected) genetic response to a perceived airborne or ingested threat. An autoimmune disease is often a genetic overreaction of that same system caused by pro-inflammatory foods (see Chapter 6). Type 2 diabetes typically develops after prolonged periods when your genes are trying to protect you from the dangers of eating too many processed carbohydrates.

Here's a great example of our genes' ability to switch on and off. In a 2009 report from the journal *Cancer Research*, researchers studying the link between smoking and lung cancer discovered that tobacco smoking causes hypermethylation (a complete or partial deactivation) of a single gene known as MTHFR (pronounced Mother-Fu... forget it!). MTHFR is one of many genes known to be involved with cancer and tumor growth, but among the genes included in this study, MTHFR was uniquely hypermethylated by tobacco use. This is critical because turning off MTHFR triggers global hypomethylation (systemic dysfunction) in many other genes; and global hypomethylation is known to contribute to cancer development and progression.

The idea that the environment influences whether genes are turned on or off is not a new one. In 1942, geneticist and evolutionary biologist C. H. Waddington first coined the term *epigenetics* to describe how genes might interact with their surroundings to create a unique individual. Today the study of epigenetics is one of the fastest growing subdisciplines of genetics. Moreover, the burgeoning field of nutrigenomics has identified hundreds of ways that nutrients (foods or supplements) impact gene expression. You may be familiar with the direct influence folic acid has on reducing neural tube birth defects, which is why all pregnant women are advised to take supplemental folic acid.

And it's not just about vitamins and minerals. An Australian study suggested that human genes are adversely affected by just two weeks of sugar ingestion (genetic controls designed to protect the body against diabetes and heart disease are switched off as an acute reaction to eating sugar) and that prolonged poor eating can cause genetic damage that can potentially be passed through bloodlines! On an even grander scale, research shows that certain cells within the body called mesenchymal stem cells can become bone cells, fat cells, muscle cells, or even cancer cells in adults, depending upon the environmental signals they receive.

Your lifestyle can either enhance or severely undermine many aspects of your health, and can often be far more relevant than inherited predispositions to allergies, diabetes, or even more severe conditions. Not to make light of the serious genetically influenced health challenges that many face over their lifetimes, I would argue that we are *all* predisposed to heart disease, cancer, arthritis, and today's other leading lifestyle-related health problems *if* we program our genes with diet, exercise, and behaviors that are in conflict with our genetic expectations for health and longevity.

•••••••••••• GROK ⚡ TALK ••••••••••••

What "Reprogram Your Genes" Really Means

Your genome (your complete set of DNA, including all genes) is set at birth. Your DNA is copied into every cell of your body. You cannot modify or reprogram your genome. Epigenetics expert Randy Jirtle, Ph.D., likens your genome to computer hardware, while your epigenome (the chemical compounds that direct your genome what to do) would be the software loaded onto the hard drive.

Your epigenome is what responds to environmental signals. You can manipulate chemical activity and gene expression by switching from Dr. Pepper to water, or by getting off the couch and hoisting some weights in the gym. We have immense power to turn some genes on and other genes off to generate optimal results. There are multiple possible versions of future you. It's up to you to decide which version you will become. It's up to you to make lifestyle choices that direct genes toward fat burning, muscle building, longevity, and wellness, and away from fat storing, muscle wasting, disease, and illness.

Every cell contains a complete set of genes, each with on/off switches that are largely under your control.

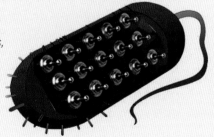

Obviously, you cannot grow your kids to seven feet tall simply by feeding them healthy food and making sure they get plenty of sleep; we all have profound limitations on how our genes can express our unique individual potential. For confirmation, just take a look at the physical marvels in the Olympic 100-meter dash or on an NFL or NBA roster, collections of the most physically gifted athletes on the planet. These athletes are one-in-a-million genetically, but they still embody optimal gene expression that has enabled them to realize their athletic potential. The choices they have made—the foods they've eaten, how they've trained, even how they've thought—have all helped them make the most of their natural-born talents to rise to the top of very competitive arenas. This is all you ought to be concerned with—making the most of your own genetic potential to enjoy a long life of excellent health and peak performance through the 10 Primal Blueprint laws.

The chapters that follow will explore the rationale behind and benefits of the 10 simple Primal Blueprint laws, and will offer practical suggestions for living accordingly. These laws represent the specific behaviors that led directly (thanks to 2.5 million years of evolution) to the genetic recipe for a healthy, lean, fit, happy human being. Almost nothing of real significance has changed in this recipe since pre-agricultural times—except the endless new ways we modern humans mismanage our genes and compromise our health.

By understanding how these behavioral "laws" shaped our genome, you can reprogram your genes to express themselves in the direction of health. And when I say "simple laws," I really mean it. If you read just this chapter and never open the book again, you'll have all the information you need to live a long, healthy, disease-free life. Here, then, is a brief description of the laws of living 10,000 years ago and a quick overview of how to adapt them to a healthy 21st-century lifestyle.

PRIMAL BLUEPRINT LAW #1:
EAT PLANTS AND ANIMALS

Plants and animals encompass everything our ancestors ate to get the protein, fats, carbohydrates, vitamins, minerals, antioxidants, phenols, fiber, water, and other nutrients necessary to sustain life, increase brain size, improve physical fitness, and support immune function. The pre-civilization human diet differs greatly from the Standard American Diet (SAD) today. Because the various diet camps passionately argue conflicting positions to a confused public, it's essential to reflect on how profoundly important and logically sound it is to model our diets after the diets of our ancestors, whose bodies evolved to survive, reproduce, and thrive on these foods. Talk about a lengthy and severely scrutinized (as in "life or death") scientific research protocol!

For one, primal humans across the globe ate widely varied diets due to environmental circumstances such as climate, geography, seasons, and activity level. There is no single regimented diet of narrowly defined foods that trumps all. Once you subscribe to the broad guidelines of the Primal Blueprint (eat plants and animals, avoid modern foods foreign to your genes), personal preference and self-experimentation—that is, discovering your body's own unique responses—will be the driving force behind your food choices each day.

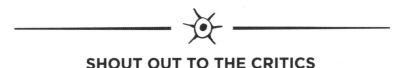

SHOUT OUT TO THE CRITICS AND THE MISINTERPRETERS

Many critics of primal/paleo argue that a Paleolithic diet is not easily definable and not sensible to follow since we don't know exactly what our ancestors ate. Other naysayers misunderstand the basics of evolutionary biology and argue that our 10,000-year exposure to a high-carbohydrate diet has prompted a genetic adaptation to high carb intake. This conjecture is easily refuted by genetic science and by looking at the ever-expanding waistlines and escalating type 2 diabetes rates among modern humans. Like it or not, we remain hunter-gatherers from a genetic perspective and will continue to be so unless some new selection pressures present themselves in the future.

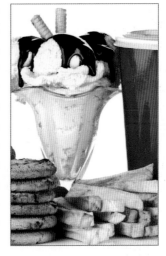

The arguments about the particulars of our ancestors' eating habits distract from the most important message, which is that we know what our ancestors *didn't* eat: sugars, sweetened beverages, grains, and refined vegetable oils, most importantly. Eliminating toxic modern foods is the most pressing issue to address, especially since they comprise the bulk of calories in the Standard American Diet. Dr. Cordain contends that 71 percent of SAD calories come from non-paleo foods.

I also want to clarify my original Primal Blueprint argument and the boilerplate paleo diet rationale that we should not consume modern foods because they are foreign to our hunter-gatherer genes. While this advice can't hurt you, and will assuredly keep you away from sodas and cotton candy, it may overshadow the most important reason to avoid certain modern foods: because they are unhealthy, pure and simple, not necessarily because we have not yet adapted to consume them. Throughout evolution, our ancestors came upon brand new food sources, consumed them, and were able to thrive because the foods offered good nutrition for the human body. Similarly, certain foods that were not eaten in hunter-gatherer times, such as dark chocolate and high-fat dairy products, offer genuine health benefits and have few or no health drawbacks.

> *We should avoid certain modern foods because they are unhealthy, not necessarily because we have not yet genetically adapted to consume them.*

When the hardcore paleo message advises against consuming grains, for example, because they weren't around 10,000 years ago and we haven't had time to adapt to them, this might obscure the more critical point that grains are unhealthy to ingest, period. The high carbohydrate content of grains contributes to wildly excessive insulin production and associated health problems like chronic inflammation and excess body fat. Furthermore, the protein molecules contained in grains (gluten and other lectins) damage the human intestinal tract. Humans are genetically adapted to digest carbohydrates (remember, all forms of carbs get converted into glucose upon ingestion), so the problem is one of quantity, concentration, and source when it comes to our modern carbohydrate consumption. It takes a lot of Grok's wild berries to equal the sugar content of a Jamba Juice smoothie!

So, while it helps to model our dietary and exercise habits after the behaviors of our ancestors, we can make adjustments and allowances for modern life and still be healthy, even if it means eating or doing modern stuff like working out with a BowFlex machine instead of hunting wild game. And we should still avoid poisonous berries or mushrooms, even if they were around 10,000 years ago!

Another notable aspect of our ancestors' diets was that they ate sporadically—mostly due to inconsistent availability of food. (Not a big issue in the developed world these days, eh?) Consequently, we became well-adapted to store caloric energy (in the form of body fat, along with a little bit of muscle and liver glycogen) and burn it when dietary calories were scarce. You may be disturbed about possessing the genetic trait to store extra food calories efficiently as fat. However, by simply eating the right kinds of foods, you can leverage this "savings and withdrawal" mechanism to your advantage, thereby maintaining ideal body-fat reserves and stabilizing daily appetite and energy levels. *Hint*: It's mostly about moderating the wildly excessive insulin production resulting from the SAD.

Focus on consuming quality sources of animal protein (local, pasture-raised, or organic sources of meat, fowl, fish, and eggs), an assortment of colorful vegetables and fresh, in-season fruits, and healthy sources of fat (animal fats, avocados, butter, coconut products, nuts and seeds, olives and olive oil). Realize that a significant amount of conventional wisdom about healthy eating is marketing fodder that grossly distorts the fundamental truth—which is that humans thrive on natural plant and animal foods—or that relies on ploys to support the dogma of flawed, manipulated research. For example, strategies such as eating at particular times (three squares or six small meals a day), combining or rotating specific food types at meals, structuring your meals according to pre-programmed phases or stages, eating foods supposedly aligned with your blood type, striving for specific macronutrient ratios, or keeping score of your portions and weekly treat allowances are all gimmicks that have no credibility in the context of evolutionary biology.

Furthermore, regimented programs are virtually impossible to enjoy and stick to over the long term because they cause eating, which should be enjoyable and gratifying, to be imbued with stress and anxiety. We humans thrive on eating a diverse array of natural foods that satisfy and nourish us, and we are designed to eat at times and in amounts and varieties that fluctuate according to personal preference, environmental circumstances, activity levels, stress levels, and many other factors. I suggest you enjoy eating as one of the pleasures of life and reject most everything you've ever heard about when and how much you should eat. Instead, eat when you are hungry and finish eating when you feel satisfied. Realize that primal foods are intrinsically the most delicious, because they satisfy your cravings and distinct tastes, stabilize mood and energy levels, and promote health and wellbeing.

PRIMAL BLUEPRINT LAW #2: AVOID POISONOUS THINGS

 The ability of humans to exploit almost every corner of the earth was partly predicated on consuming vastly different types of plant and animal life. Primal humans developed a keen sense of smell and taste, along with liver, kidney, and stomach function, to adapt to new food sources and avoid succumbing to poisonous plants that they encountered routinely when foraging and settling new areas. For example, the sweet tooth we have today is probably an evolved response to an almost universal truth in the plant world that anything sweet is safe to eat. Furthermore, gorging on sweet foods and being able to store that excess caloric intake as fat was an evolved response for surviving harsh winters with diminished food availability.

While we have little risk of ingesting poisonous plants on walkabouts today, the number of toxic agents in our food supply is worse than ever. By *toxic*, I mean human-made substances that disturb the normal, healthy function of your body when ingested. The big offenders, including sugars and sodas, chemically altered fats, and heavily processed, packaged, fried, and preserved foods, are obvious. It's not a stretch to directly compare the poisonous berries of Grok's day with much of the stuff shelved at eye level in your local supermarket.

The more insidious dietary "poisons" are the grain products that form the foundation of the SAD (wheat products like bread, crackers, muffins, pancakes, tortillas, waffles, etc., as well as pasta, breakfast cereals, rice, and corn, and also cultivated grains like oats, barley, rye, and amaranth). These global dietary staples are generally inappropriate for human consumption because our digestive systems (and our genes) are traumatized by unfamiliar protein structures that can damage the intestinal tract, causing systemic inflammation and autoimmune reactions.

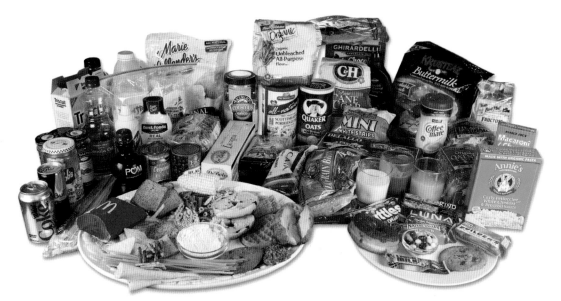

Both simple and complex carbs get converted into glucose—albeit, at differing rates—once they enter the body. Ingesting grains (yep, even whole grains, as we'll discuss in detail in Chapter 6), legumes (beans, lentils, peanuts, peas, and soy products), and other processed carbohydrates cause blood glucose levels to spike. (We use the accurate term "blood glucose" to convey what is often referred to as "blood sugar.") This spike is a shock to your genes, which are adapted to a much lower total carbohydrate intake, as well as to more complex carbohydrates that are natural, more fibrous, and much slower burning, like sweet potatoes and other starchy tubers.

When you shock your system with a glucose bomb after a well-intentioned trip to the muffin shop or smoothie bar, your pancreas rushes to the rescue by pumping out the requisite amount of insulin. After all, excess blood glucose is toxic and can quickly become life threatening, as diabetics who don't get their insulin shots on schedule can attest. While insulin is an important hormone that also delivers nutrients to muscle, liver, and fat cells for storage, there is a balance that must be carefully maintained in order to remain healthy. Modern eating habits abuse this extremely delicate hormonal process by stimulating *chronic excessive insulin production*. If I had to pick a one-liner to summarize the number one health problem facing modern society—the gateway to type 2 diabetes, obesity, heart disease, and cancer—"chronic excessive insulin production" is it.

The flood of insulin from your pancreas to counter a medium Jamba Juice Lime Colada Fruit Refresher (91 grams of carbs—you'll learn the scale to which this amount of carb intake affects your health in upcoming chapters) causes glucose to be removed so rapidly and effectively over the next hour or two that it can result in a "sugar crash." This familiar mental drain (because the brain relies heavily on glucose for fuel) and physical lethargy is followed by a strong craving for more high-carbohydrate food as a quick fix. Thus goes the vicious cycle of the ill-advised carbohydrate bomb causing a temporary high, an excessive insulin response causing a low, and cravings for more carbs to bring you back up, creating a daily energy and mood roller coaster that all starts with that All-American high-carbohydrate breakfast.

Since insulin's job is to transport nutrients out of the bloodstream and into the muscle, liver, and fat-cell storage depots, its excessive presence in the bloodstream inhibits the release of stored body fat for use as energy. This is especially true in the context of our modern lifestyles that are overabundant in food and deficient in physical movement, a combo that reduces insulin sensitivity. This means your cells become less responsive to the signals of insulin, so your pancreas must pump even more into the bloodstream to do the same amount of work.

When insulin is high, insulin's counter regulatory hormone *glucagon* is usually low. Glucagon accesses carbs, protein, and fat from your body's storage depots (muscle, liver, fat cells) and delivers them into the bloodstream for use as energy, so low glucagon means you are not able to use your stored energy efficiently. If you don't have energy in your bloodstream, your brain says, "Eat now! And make it something sweet so we can burn it immediately." The mobilization of stored body fat has been humans' preferred energy source (and weight-control device) for a couple of million years, and now we brazenly bypass that whole process with a grain- and sugar-laden diet. It's as simple as this: you cannot reduce body fat on a diet that stimulates chronically high insulin levels and low insulin sensitivity—period.

But the weight-loss frustrations associated with carbohydrate-induced insulin overload are just part of the story. The more critical reason to avoid these foods is that overstressing your insulin response system with years of eating a Standard American Diet can lead directly to devastating general system failure in the form of insulin resistance (a pathological inability of cells to respond to insulin), type 2 diabetes, obesity, cardiovascular disease (thanks to vascular inflammation, oxidative damage, and other insulin-related troubles we will learn more about later), and diet-related cancers. Furthermore, Chapter 6 will explain in detail that even whole grains (brown rice, whole wheat bread, etc.) are not particularly healthy, because they contain anti-nutrients that promote inflammation and hamper digestion and immune function (even if they have slightly more nutritional value than refined "white" grain products). Finally, a grain-based diet displaces the far more nutritious plants and animals as potential caloric centerpieces in your diet, and can lead to assorted dental problems that, as we learned in the "Are We Really Devolving?" sidebar, can be passed onto your offspring.

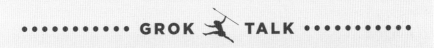

If Wisdom Teeth Are So Smart, Why Isn't There Any Room for Them?

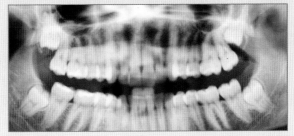

Human teeth, jaws, and faces have shrunk since primal times. Researchers believe this is due to a complex interplay between gene expression and epigenetic (environmental) influences. Because so much of today's food is "soft"—heavily processed, calorically dense (e.g., grains, sugars, sweetened beverages, and vegetable oils providing a huge percentage of total calories), we no longer need the robust chewing mechanism that we did to chew the tough foods throughout evolution. Furthermore, the nutrient-deficient modern diet is directly associated with assorted dental problems. For example, half

of all Americans require their wisdom teeth to be removed. We are hard wired to express the genes that develop wider mouths, a full set of teeth, and an extremely strong and active jaw, but we suppress these genes because we don't need them to sip apple juice from a baby bottle, and we carry on from there into a modern dietary pattern.

Dr. Mike Mew, a London orthodontist, estimates that modern humans use the masticatory system at only about 3 to 5 percent of the level that our primal ancestors did! This has led to an atrophy that has been passed to offspring for the hundreds of generations since the advent of civilization. This insight is a centerpiece of the pioneering research of Dr. Weston A. Price in the early 1900s. (You might be familiar with the Weston A. Price Foundation that does respected research, education, and activism today.) One study of Aboriginals who rapidly transitioned into a modern diet revealed elders with excellent teeth and facial structure and youth with full-blown modern soft-food-driven problems. The study abstract proposed that "the rapidity of the transition is proportional to the rapidity of urbanizational change."

PRIMAL BLUEPRINT LAW #3:
MOVE FREQUENTLY

Grok spent several hours each day moving about at what today's exercise physiologists might describe as a very low-level aerobic pace. He hunted, gathered, foraged, wandered, scouted, migrated, climbed, and crawled. This low-level activity prompted his genes to build a stronger capillary (blood vessel) network to provide oxygen and fuel to each muscle cell and readily convert stored fat into energy. (Fat is the main fuel used for low-level aerobic activity.) His daily movement also helped develop strong bones, joints, and connective tissue.

What Grok did not do was go for extended periods of time without moving, something that (as we'll soon learn in more detail) causes a host of metabolic and cognitive problems. Grok also didn't engage in a chronic pattern of sustained moderate-to-difficult-intensity efforts like today's devoted fitness enthusiasts tend to do. This counterintuitive

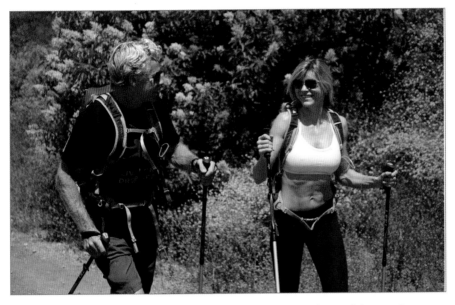

behavior would have depleted his precious muscle and liver glycogen stores and generated system-wide fatigue, leaving him vulnerable to a predator, starvation, or some other misfortune. (Plantar fasciitis anyone? Bowing out of hunting duties for six weeks probably wouldn't play too well in the clan, you know?) You may have heard the recently popularized sentiment that humans were "born to run?" More accurately, we were born with the genetic ability to perform magnificent feats of endurance now and then (with plenty of downtime in between), sprint for our lives on those rare occasions when we faced such danger, and to walk and generally move about extensively every single day. When we decide to train in chronic patterns to prepare for a 26.2-mile marathon races, this can put our health in peril.

Today most of us are either too sedentary or we conduct workouts that are too stressful and misaligned with our primal genetic requirements for optimum health. The exercise gospel for decades has been to pursue a consistent routine of aerobic exercise whether it be jogging, cycling, cardio machines, group classes, or any other sustained effort. The message was that this effort would supposedly lead to more energy, better health, and weight control. However, too many lengthy workouts at heart rates beyond a comfortable aerobic, fat-burning intensity (a pace where you can converse easily and feel absolutely no strain on your muscles or oxygen supply) can put you at risk of exhaustion, burnout, injury, and illness. The high-carbohydrate diet on which most athletes rely to fuel these workouts day in and day out only adds to the problem. At the extreme—such as with the overtrained marathon runner or ironman triathlete—a commitment to fitness can actually accelerate the aging process and elevate the risk of heart disease.

Overexercising is a common scenario—consider how modern athletes display such strong focus, dedication, and willpower to push through signs of fatigue. Our bodies are simply not adapted to benefit from chronic aerobic exercise at even mildly uncomfortable heart rates. Neither are they designed to slog through exhausting circuits on resistance machines several days a week. The mild-to-severe difficulty of these chronic cardio or chronic strength workouts overtaxes the stress response (commonly referred to as the fight or flight response) in your body, specifically from your HPA (hypothalamic-pituitary-adrenal) axis. Here, your pituitary gland tells your adrenal glands to release cortisol and other adaptive hormones into your bloodstream. Cortisol is a powerful hormone that is critical to a variety of physical functions and energy production. The spike of cortisol (and other feel-good hormones like dopamine, serotonin, epinephrine, and norepinephrine) triggered by a stressful exercise session (or other high-stimulation life event) increases respiration, heart rate, blood circulation, and mental focus, and even converts muscle tissue into glucose for quick energy.

This is a great example of how we abuse a system that was designed to ensure short-term survival, such as when Grok faced a predator. Even today, the fight or flight response is highly desirable and effective in the face of true danger or peak performance stimuli, such as an Olympic sprinter crouching in the starting blocks or an emergency worker summoning superhuman strength for a rescue effort. Unfortunately, when the stress response is triggered repeatedly (by the constant hectic pace of modern life, by a demanding boss, or by overly stressful workouts), your stress response mechanisms eventually wear out, and you produce lower-than-normal levels of cortisol and other hormones critical to many aspects of everyday health. Thyroid hormones and testosterone also become dysregulated from prolonged stress, resulting in fatigue, loss of lean muscle tissue, a suppressed immune system, and the general condition best described as burnout.

What our genes truly crave is frequent movement at a slow, comfortable pace: walking, hiking, easy cycling, or other light aerobic activities at heart rates not to exceed "180 minus your age" in beats per minute (details on this formula, championed by Dr. Phil Maffetone, in Chapter 7). These efforts are far less taxing than the typical huffing and puffing, struggling and suffering exertion level that we've been conditioned to think leads to cardiovascular fitness. In addition to structured low-level cardio workouts, it's imperative to find ways to move more often every day—taking five-minute movement breaks from your work desk, parking at the farthest edge of the parking lot instead of always trolling for the closest space, taking the stairs instead of the elevator. Finally, complementary activities in the realm of mobility and flexibility are also encouraged under the "Move Frequently" law—things like Pilates, yoga, tai chi, gymnastics, dancing, and dynamic rolling, stretching, and physical therapy work. Try as you might, it's difficult to escape the ubiquitous sedentary influences in modern life, so moving your body in assorted different ways can make a big difference in your over health and fitness.

PRIMAL BLUEPRINT LAW #4: LIFT HEAVY THINGS

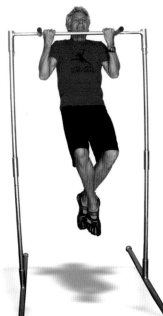

Grok's life demanded frequent bursts of intense physical effort—returning gathered items (firewood, shelter supplies, tool materials, and animal carcasses) to camp, climbing rocks and trees to scout and forage, and arranging boulders and logs to build shelter. The biochemical signals triggered by these brief but intense muscle contractions prompted improvements and adaptations in muscle tone, size, and power.

Today, conducting brief, intense workouts of full-body, functional movements (squats, pushups, pull-ups, etc.) helps you develop and maintain lean muscle mass, optimize your fat metabolism, increase bone density, prevent injuries, and enjoy balanced hormone and blood glucose levels. When it comes to lifting heavy things, there is no magic formula for the perfect workout. The specifics of the workout are less important than honoring the principles of making your workouts brief, intense, and functional. You may enjoy CrossFit, working with heavy weights in the gym, doing a machine circuit, or bending BowFlex rods at home. You can also just haul off sets of pushups, pull-ups, squats, and planks (aka the four Primal Essential Movements; see Chapter 7 for more details, or search YouTube for "Primal Essential Movements").

Conduct your strength-training sessions regularly, but without excessive regimentation, and always align them with your energy levels. This will produce results superior to a routine of going to the gym too often for workouts that last too long. The latter is a recipe for fatigue and undesirable gene expression due to excessive sympathetic nervous system activation (i.e., the fight or flight response), and the associated cortisol overproduction, that results from these overly stressful sessions. You can enjoy excellent benefits doing just a couple of brief, intense sessions per week—lasting as little as 10 minutes and no more than 30 minutes—with minimal risk of overstress.

PRIMAL BLUEPRINT LAW #5: SPRINT ONCE IN A WHILE

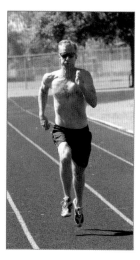 In a primal world where danger lurked around every corner, Grok's ability to run was a strong indicator of whether he would live long enough to pass down those superior genes to the next generation. Grok's occasional life-or-death sprints triggered a cascade of hormones into the bloodstream that allowed him to build the fast-twitch muscle and central nervous system resiliency to go a little faster the next time.

Today, brief, all-out sprints help increase energy levels, improve athletic performance, and minimize the effects of aging by promoting the release of testosterone, human growth hormone, and other "adaptive" (generating a health, fitness, or survival benefit) hormones into the bloodstream. Once every 7 to 10 days, when energy and motivation levels are high, choose a simple, brief sprint workout and go all out! Novices can choose low-impact options (e.g., stationary bike) and work up to actual running sprints.

An effective sprint workout could mean no more than a few minutes warmup at low intensity, some drills to promote good technique, and a series of four to five efforts lasting between 10 and 20 seconds. All told, that's only a couple minutes of max intensity performance—plenty to stimulate the hormonal adaptations that can skyrocket your fitness levels in a short time, make your mind and body more resilient for all manner of less intense exercise performance, and put the finishing touches on your transition into a fat-burning beast. Why does a little go such a long way? Well, all-out sprints require an effort level as high as 30 MET (Metabolic Equivalent of Task—30 times more metabolic activity than is required at rest). This is an extremely shocking (in a good way!) metabolic event that sends a powerful signal to your genes to upregulate fat metabolism, build or tone lean muscle, enhance mitochondrial function, and generally delay the aging process according to the "use it or lose it" maxim.

PRIMAL BLUEPRINT LAW #6: GET PLENTY OF SLEEP

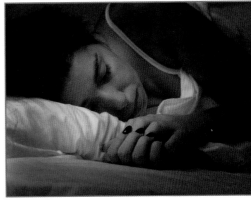

Our ancestors' activity and sleep patterns were strongly calibrated on a hormonal level by sunrise and sunset. Days started early (Grok actually caught the worm… and ate it!), and after the sun went down, it was safest to huddle together and rest. Furthermore, hunter-gatherers required plenty of downtime to repair and rejuvenate from their active lifestyles.

Today, with life exponentially more hectic and chronically stressful than at any other time in human history, adequate sleep and restoration are widely neglected. Adequate sleep promotes the release of important hormones that support immune and endocrine function, refreshes cognitive function and solidifies learning, optimizes tissue repair, and plays a major role in regulating appetite and metabolizing fat. Excess artificial light and digital stimulation after dark, along with ingestible toxins (e.g., sugar, alcohol, and prescription and over-the-counter medications), and, of course, the ubiquitous alarm clock that delivers a high-stress start to the day, all undermine healthy sleep patterns.

For optimal sleep, it's critical to minimize your exposure to artificial light after dark, to create calm, relaxing transitions into sleep time (and mellow morning routines too), and to obtain sufficient hours of sleep such that you wake up naturally (no alarm). Go to sleep at the same time each night after a tranquil, deliberate wind down—no TV, laptop, tablet or smartphone screens, no heavy exercise, and no big meals or any other high stimulation in the final couple of hours before sleep. Make sure you allow yourself enough time in bed that you are able to wake naturally, near sunrise, feeling refreshed.

You may have heard the popular maxim that eight hours per night represents an ideal amount of sleep. While this is certainly a reasonable recommendation (especially if you habitually obtain less than that!), your sleep needs are highly individualized and subject to numerous variables such as your geography and time of year (more sleep is needed when days are shorter; less during long summer days), genetic profile, exercise routine, work demands, and other life factors.

Don't be afraid to take naps when your afternoon energy levels wane. The world will not miss you while you grab a few quick winks, and science proves that you will quickly restore the optimum balance of brain chemicals to increase productivity when you get back to your day. Even a 20-minute siesta can make you feel wonderfully refreshed and can also significantly improve your cognitive performance when you are deficient in nighttime sleep.

As you pursue health and balance in the digital age, always keep in the back of your mind the reality that for millions of years, humans awakened and went to sleep in accordance with the rising and setting of the sun. The moment you flip open that laptop to catch up on emails in the evening, you introduce one of the most destructive genetic offenses in modern life: artificial light after dark. Chronic exposure to excess light and digital stimulation after dark ranks right up there with the consumption of heavily processed junk food as a major disruptor of health.

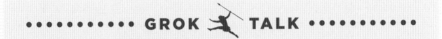

•••••••••• GROK TALK ••••••••••

For millions of years, human sleep/wake cycles were directly connected to the rising and setting of the sun. Today, we traffic in excess artificial light and digital stimulation after dark, compromising the natural hormonal processes that facilitate ideal sleep patterns. Engaging in calm, quiet, dark, mellow evenings with minimal light and screen use will help recalibrate the hormonal processes that optimize sleep.

PRIMAL BLUEPRINT LAW #7: PLAY

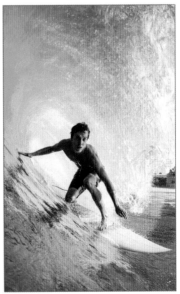

Our ancestors spent hours every day involved in various forms of social interaction not related to their core responsibilities of securing food and shelter and caring for their young. Studies of modern hunter-gatherers, such as the !Kung Bushmen of the Kalahari Desert in Africa, reveal that they generally work far fewer hours and have more leisure time than the average 40-hour-plus modern clock puncher. Anthropologist Marshall Sahlins's popular theory of the "original affluent society" argues that hunter-gatherers are able to achieve *affluence*—meaning a comfortable existence in which one's needs and wants are met—by desiring little. This enables them to satisfy their every need and desire relatively easily by doing the work of normal daily life. This is much different from the consumerism-tainted definition of affluence—being "rich" in material possessions and outward displays of wealth—with which we are most familiar.

For Grok and his clan, once the day's catch was complete, or the roots, shoots, nuts, and berries had been gathered, it was time to play. Youngsters might have chased each other around and wrestled, vying for a place higher up in the tribe's social strata. Primal humans might also have practiced throwing spears or rocks for accuracy, chased small animals just for sport, or spent time hanging out and grooming each other. The net effect of their play was to support familial and community bonding, unwind from the stresses and dangers of primal life, and to experiment, problem-solve, and process "what-if" scenarios that helped promote daily survival. Through play, our ancestors were able to increase their skills and experience free from the usual life-or-death stakes of real-life challenges.

Today *play* is a four-letter word, a fond memory from childhood, something we are too busy to even consider. After I published the first edition of *The Primal Blueprint*, one reader remarked to me, "I understand play is important, but I get to the park with my kids and realize that I don't even know *how* to play." Insufficient play is another major disconnect in modern life, causing reduced productivity, increased stress, and accelerated aging. Stuart Brown, author of *Play: How It Shapes the Brain, Opens the Imagination, and Invigorates the Soul* and one of the world's leading experts on play, calls play a "profound biological process." He explains that play, across the span of a lifetime, promotes the development and maintenance of a "cognitively fluid mind."

Cognitive fluidity—being able to go with the flow, think outside the box, process what-if scenarios, and react quickly and effectively to changes in our environment—is believed by anthropologists to represent one of the most profound breakthroughs in human evolution. This breakthrough in brain function, probably emerging 60,000 years ago, meant that humans' brains could link knowledge from different domains. The way humans understood and approached the world became both more flexible and more expansive. This enabled more creative use of technology, better transfer of knowledge between generations, and a resultant spike in human longevity. Cognitive fluidity is still essential today, helping us adapt and thrive in a complex, high-tech society. When we get stuck in patterns of overwork and overstress, we lose that important connection with our creative, intuitive, playful selves. Our work suffers and so does our happiness.

I recommend that you take some time every day to unplug from the office or daily chores and have some unstructured fun. Even a few minutes here and there makes a big difference. Particularly if you have children, you can model that play is a lifetime endeavor—and learn a few things from them while you're at it. Besides being fun, socially redeeming, and cognitively stimulating, play offers biochemical benefits in the form of endorphins released into the bloodstream, and it provides a healthy balance to the excessive stimulation thrust upon us in the digital age. If you are at a loss for how to start, I provide a few suggestions in a Chapter 8 sidebar.

PRIMAL BLUEPRINT LAW #8:
GET PLENTY OF SUNLIGHT

 Cavemen and women didn't spend their days inside caves; they were mostly outdoors pursuing various survival and leisure endeavors. Regular sun exposure allowed Grok to manufacture plenty of vitamin D (technically a precursor hormone, not a vitamin), which is critical to healthy cell function and cancer prevention. Adequate vitamin D is nearly impossible to obtain from diet alone; we must manufacture it internally via the exposure of large skin surface areas to sufficient amounts of sunlight during daily and seasonal periods of peak solar intensity. Developing and maintaining a slight tan during the summer months is a good sign that you are making and storing enough vitamin D to thrive all year long.

Our original *Homo sapiens* ancestors coming of age in East Africa had no problem getting sufficient vitamin D and even developed dark skin pigmentation and thick hair to prevent overexposure. The importance of

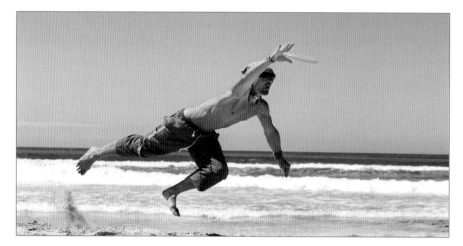

vitamin D is confirmed by the remarkable and relatively rapid evolutionary adaptation of the lightening of skin pigmentation among populations who colonized ever farther away from the equator. The straight truth is that humans would not have survived in Europe and other less sun-kissed locales without lighter skin to enable more efficient vitamin D synthesis from sun exposure (and/or eating large quantities of oily, cold-water fish—the only dietary source of vitamin D worth mentioning).

Today, getting plenty of sunlight—and hence vitamin D—is nowhere near a given, what with our penchant for spending much of our time in confined spaces such as cars, offices, and homes, and obsessively lathering up with sunscreen when we do venture out under the big, bad sun. Many modern citizens also happen to live at latitudes discordant with their ancestral genetics, putting darker-skinned residents of higher-latitude locales at significant risk for vitamin D deficiency. Experts believe a variety of serious health problems result from these relatively abrupt changes in human lifestyle. (Sound familiar from our discussion of how the advent of agriculture compromised the healthy hunter-gatherer?)

To ensure adequate, healthy levels of vitamin D, you must make a concerted effort to spend ample time outdoors, exposing large skin surface areas to direct sunlight that's strong enough to generate a tan. You can also take supplemental vitamin D to bolster your levels when sun exposure is compromised. In today's indoor-dominant lifestyle, it is essential to adopt a progressive attitude about sun exposure instead of kowtow-ing to the distorted and oversimplified conventional wisdom that sun exposure increases cancer risk. On the contrary, science strongly suggests that *lack* of sun exposure is a leading risk factor for melanoma and other cancers. Obviously, you never want to burn, as this increases the risk of carcinoma (the less serious form of skin cancer) and also melanoma. And because you are looking to expose maximum skin surface area, screening your face and neck won't materially compromise vitamin D production, but it will protect you from overexposure and carcinoma risk.

Besides the critical vitamin D requirement, sunlight also has a pow-erful mood-elevating effect that can enhance productivity and interper-sonal relations. Taking time to enjoy direct sunlight, fresh air, and open spaces (perhaps during your daily moderate exercise sessions) balances the health- and mood-compromising effects of spending long periods of time confined in homes, offices, and cars, with their artificial light and stale air.

PRIMAL BLUEPRINT LAW #9: AVOID STUPID MISTAKES

Our ancestors required a keen sense of observation and self-preservation to avoid danger. They were always scan-ning, smelling, and listening to their surroundings, ever aware of potential trouble from saber-toothed tigers, falling rocks, poisonous snakes, or even a twisted ankle from a careless step. Keen vigilance and risk management were premium skills honed to per-fection every day. Even minor mistakes could prove disastrous, such as scraping a knee on a rock and dying from an ensuing infection gone unchecked.

Today, vicious tigers are no longer a life-threatening safety concern, but we humans carelessly find ways to invite pain and suffering of a different nature into our lives. (Can you say mul-titasking?) Buckle your seat belt; don't drink and drive, nor text and drive. Be prepared and vigilant when you go backpacking in the wilderness or descend a steep hill on your 15-pound racing bike, not to mention when using a blowtorch, chain saw, or tile cutter. Devote

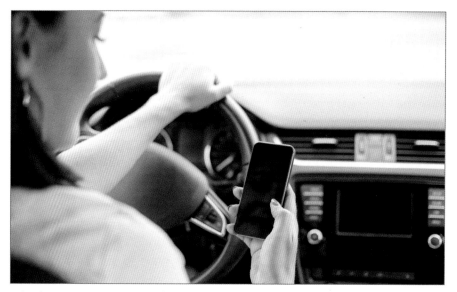

a little more attention and energy to risk management day-to-day so you can enjoy a long, happy life and pass on your own superior genes to the next generation.

I would also argue that with all the knowledge about genetics and healthy living we have today, making a less-than-stellar commitment to healthy eating, exercise, sleep, and lifestyle might be considered a stupid mistake! Thanks to the hard work of our ancestors ancient and recent, we humans in today's developed world enjoy a level of luxury, convenience, and physical ease unimaginable throughout human history. Living in a world of freedom and abundant choice, we can do what we wish with our health without the immediate penalty our ancestors faced.

Our ancestors did not have the luxury of skimping on sleep and getting lost while out foraging because their attentional systems were suffering, or of getting too fat to outrun the predator that was chasing them. The Primal Blueprint is about making informed choices and understanding the health consequences of your choices at the genetic level. I'm not here to judge what's right or wrong for you—even when it comes to stupid mistakes! But there are surely ways to have fun and be happy that do not involve becoming a victim of the modern "sick care" system, for example. Or, in my case, suffering through an athletic training regimen that compromised my health and enjoyment of life. Which leads me to the final law....

PRIMAL BLUEPRINT LAW #10:
USE YOUR BRAIN

It wasn't so long ago that *Homo sapiens* shared the planet with other hominid species. Yet, today we humans are the only ones left standing. (Pun intended.) Scientists attribute our survival not to our big brains per se (other hominids—notably the Neanderthals—had big brains, too), but to the fact that the human brain had a greater capacity for complex thought. Humans' superior capabilities for language, abstract thought, and other higher-level cognition ultimately gave us the edge in terms of adapting to an ever-changing world. And as early *Homo sapiens* used their brains to develop better tools and hunting strategies, as well as to communicate, socialize, and organize with other humans, the human brain continued to grow.

The rapid increase in the size of the human brain over just a few thousand generations was the combined result of optimum dietary choices (including high levels of healthy protein and saturated and omega-3 fats—see Law #1) and a continued reliance on complex thought—working the brain just like a muscle. The best proof of our impressive evolution in brain function is the fact that hunter-gatherers around the world developed language, tools, and superior hunting methods independently.

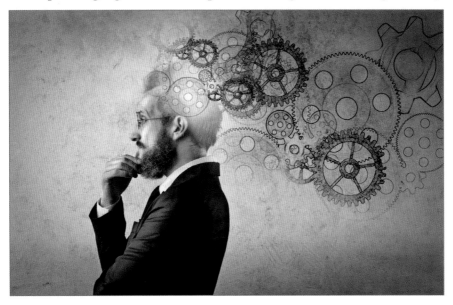

While you might argue that we use our minds plenty to navigate and make a buck in today's world, the reality is that many of us are stuck in unfulfilling or tedious jobs, or are otherwise disconnected from continued intellectual challenge and stimulation. Numerous studies of general intelligence identify *curiosity* as one of the most profound intelligence markers. Opportunities for intellectual stimulation are everywhere in daily life. Commit to some personal challenges, such as learning a new language, playing a musical instrument, or taking an evening college class. Research indicates that the risk of devastating mental conditions including depression, dementia, and Alzheimer's can be reduced by keeping your brain active as well as your body.

[My] greatest error has been not allowing
sufficient weight to the direct action of the
environments [upon evolution], i.e., food, climate, etc.,
independently of natural selection.
—Charles Darwin

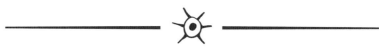

LEARN THEM, KNOW THEM, LIVE THEM!

Law #1: Eat Plants and Animals—Enjoy the nutritious, satisfying foods that fueled 2.5 million years of human evolution.

Law #2: Avoid Poisonous Things—Ditch processed modern foods laden with sugars, grains (even whole grains), and refined vegetable oils (partially hydrogenated trans fats, high polyunsaturated vegetable oils, and the new interesterified fats). These foods are foreign to our genes and make us fat, inflamed, tired, and sick.

Law #3: Move Frequently—Improve general health, cognitive function, and fat metabolism by moving more in everyday life and conducting aerobic workouts at very comfortable heart rates.

Law #4: Lift Heavy Things—Brief, intense sessions of functional, full-body movements support muscle development and delay aging.

Law #5: Sprint Once in a While—Occasional all-out sprints trigger optimal gene expression and beneficial hormone flow for a potent anti-aging effect.

Law #6: Get Plenty of Sleep—Avoid excessive artificial light and digital stimulation after dark to align your circadian rhythm with the sun and enjoy optimal immune, brain, and endocrine function.

Law #7: Play—Balance the stress of modern life with some unstructured, physical fun! Both brief breaks and grand outings are essential to mental and physical wellbeing and maintenance of a "cognitively fluid mind."

Law #8: Get Plenty of Sunlight—Don't fear the sun! Expose large skin surface areas to sun during peak times to manufacture and store enough vitamin D to ensure healthy cell function and cancer protection.

Law #9: Avoid Stupid Mistakes—Cultivate your innate abilities to be vigilant for dangers and to manage risk expertly in order to avoid the stupid mistakes that bring avoidable suffering to modern humans.

Law #10: Use Your Brain—Engage in creative and stimulating intellectual pursuits away from your core daily economic responsibilities to nurture your mental health and overall wellbeing.

THAT'S IT

Aside from—ahem—the reproductive act, I challenge you to name any other significant behavior that shaped our genes and currently plays a critical role in our health and wellbeing. Could it really be this simple? Could the prevention of and cure for obesity, diabetes, heart disease, physical decline, most cancers, and the generally overstressed existence of the modern human be contained in our genes? While you may be able to find detractors who extract bits and pieces of this blueprint and offer up a critical view, the premise is unassailable: our genes are suited for a hunter-gatherer existence, because that is how we *Homo sapiens* have spent 99-plus percent of our time on Earth.

The same genes that turn against you and promote heart disease, diabetes, atherosclerosis, high blood pressure, high cholesterol, arthritis, and most other degenerative diseases can also be reprogrammed to unlock a leaner, fitter, more energetic body, a substantially slowed aging process, and a reduced risk of illness, injury, and burnout. The secret is to do the right thing: choose behaviors that promote desirable gene expression and avoid those that promote negative outcomes.

> *The secret is to do the right thing: choose behaviors that promote desirable gene expression and avoid those that promote negative outcomes.*

That statement alone—do the right thing—is no revelation. The revelation here is how easy, natural, and fun the lifestyle and behaviors are that will help you build your ideal body. Now you can enjoy delicious, nutrient-dense foods that foster health and effortless weight management by optimizing fat metabolism. Now you have permission to back off from exhausting workouts and regimented schedules and instead enjoy an active lifestyle with regular low-intensity aerobic movement accompanied by brief, intense strength and sprint workouts. You can even lounge in the sun or take a nap in the name of health!

You will notice the benefits of the Primal Blueprint lifestyle laws in a matter of days, not weeks or months. Your genes are active all the time, either helping you build, regenerate, and maintain homeostasis or unintentionally tearing you down. It's all based on the environmental signals you provide them through your most recent meal, workout, play session, sleep session, and so forth. As we reflect on the legacy of our ancestors and the tribulations they faced to bestow good genetic fortune upon us today, it's clear that the Primal Blueprint is not about being perfect. It's about trending in the right direction, being aware of environmental hazards like junk foods or too much screen time at night, and doing the best you can under the circumstances you face each day.

Unfortunately, as you will read in Chapter 2, modern society on the whole is not doing a great job of honoring the legacy of our ancestors. So we'll go back to the beginning and learn more about Grok, contrast him sharply with his modern day antithesis, Ken Korg, and build the knowledge base and momentum to reconnect with our ancient genetic requirements for health.

CHAPTER SUMMARY

1. Evolution: The *Homo sapiens* evolutionary timeline began seven million years ago when hominids split from apes. The smart, upright, humanlike *Homo erectus* appeared 400,000 years ago. Around 160,000 years ago, the first *Homo sapiens* appeared in East Africa. Sixty thousand years ago, a small group of humans—perhaps as few as 150 individuals—ventured out to colonize the globe.

2. Grok: Survival of the fittest drove 2.5 million years of evolution and created the ultimate human being... 10,000 years ago! Grok is the nickname for our primal human role model who was bigger, stronger (on average versus modern humans—really!), and in many respects healthier than us. Soon after Grok's time, the advent of agriculture across the globe eliminated the main selection pressures on humans: starvation and predator danger. Civilization effectively resulted in a slowing of our evolution, and we have gone soft as a consequence. However, because our DNA is nearly identical to Grok's, we can adapt his evolutionary-based behaviors into our 21st-century lifestyle to pursue optimum health.

3. Genes: Your health depends upon how genes respond to signals in their immediate environment. Genes are traffic cops that direct the function of every cell in the body at all times. They respond to environmental stimuli and promote homeostasis and short-term survival. Genes don't know or care how behaviors affect long-term health. (It's up to you to care!)

4. Primal Blueprint Laws 1 and 2—Diet: Eat plants and animals! Avoid processed foods (sugary foods and beverages, grains, refined high polyunsaturated vegetable/seed oils, partially hydrogenated oils, and interesterified fats). Grains, while a global food staple long believed to be healthy, stimulate an excessive release of insulin and are less nutritious than vegetables, fruit, nuts, seeds, and animal foods. A diet emphasizing grains, even whole grains, inhibits fat metabolism and paves the way for serious disease.

5. Primal Blueprint Laws 3, 4, and 5—Exercise: Move frequently (increase general everyday movement with movement breaks, along with walking, jogging, or hiking sessions—but avoid excessive medium-to-high-intensity "chronic" cardio). Lift heavy things (conduct regular functional, full-body strength-training sessions that are brief and intense). Perform occasional all-out, short-duration sprints to stimulate growth hormone release, build muscle, turbo-charge fat metabolism, and delay the aging process.

6. Primal Blueprint Laws 6, 7, 8, 9, and 10—Lifestyle: Get plenty of sleep (mainly by minimizing artificial light and digital stimulation after dark). Find time in your busy schedule for unstructured play (relieves stress and improves emotional and mental wellbeing). Get plenty of sunlight (stimulates production of vitamin D and helps balance the negative effects of spending excessive time confined indoors). Avoid stupid mistakes by remaining vigilant and managing risk expertly when navigating potential modern hazards like texting and driving. Use your brain for creative pursuits that balance the often repetitive or intellectually rote elements of daily life.

7. Blueprint for Success: The Primal Blueprint laws are simple and intuitive, unlike many elements of conventional wisdom that suggest you have to struggle, suffer, and deprive yourself to attain your fitness and weight-loss goals. You will notice the benefits of Primal Blueprint living immediately—more even energy levels, better immune function, more enjoyable eating and exercising—as your genes direct your cells to function optimally at every moment.

CHAPTER ENDNOTES

[1] **Origin of Man:** The "Out of Africa" theory is also known as the Recent Single-Origin Hypothesis (RSOH), Replacement Hypothesis, or Recent African Origin (RAO) model. The theory, originally proposed by Charles Darwin in his *Descent of Man*, modernized by Christopher Stringer and Peter Andrews, and strongly supported by recent studies of mitochondrial DNA, says that anatomically modern humans evolved solely in Africa between 200,000 (first appearance of anatomically modern humans) and 100,000 years ago, with some *Homo sapiens* leaving Africa 60,000 years ago and replacing all earlier hominid populations including *Homo neanderthalensis* and *Homo erectus*.

[2] **Origin of Agriculture:** Dr. Jared Diamond, evolutionary biologist, physiologist, and Pulitzer Prize–winning professor of geography at UCLA, is the author of *Guns, Germs and Steel: The Fates of Human Societies* that discusses the advent of agriculture and its effects on civilization and human health. Chapter 5 of *Guns, Germs, and Steel* details agriculture's origin (including which crops were cultivated) in several locations around the globe. *The Emergence of Agriculture* by Bruce Smith also details the great transition of humanity from a hunter-gatherer lifestyle to agriculture and thus civilization.

Guns, Germs and Steel and Richard Manning's *Against the Grain* detail the negative aspects of humankind's shift to agriculture, blaming it for large-scale disease, imperialism, colonialism, slavery, and an inexorable progression to global warfare. All this thanks to the abuse of "free time" resulting from the specialization of labor and the pursuit of power over resources, humans, and geography—goals that were previously irrelevant in the largely egalitarian hunter-gatherer societies.

[3] **Primal Human Life Span:** The estimate of "maximum life span potential" from *Homo sapiens* 15,000 years ago is 94 years; this is actually higher than the prediction for modern humans, whose corresponding figure is 91 years! This material comes from the work of Dr. Richard G. Cutler, molecular gerontologist and longevity expert, who has produced more than 100 papers on the subject. Dr. Cutler was a research chemist at the Gerontology Research Center at the National Institute on Aging at the National Institutes of Health for 19 years. Dr. Cutler's estimate is derived from laboratory analysis of skeletal material, with particular emphasis on the ratio of body weight-to-brain-size. Other factors involved in making accurate life-span calculations are age-of-sexual-maturation-to-life-span ratio (a 5:1 ratio is common among humans) and rates of caloric intake and expenditure. (Of course, we know that modern humans can and do live longer than 91 years; this formula merely provides an estimate to predict relative maximum life span potential among different hominid species based on their physical characteristics, and primal humans beat us modern folk. This reinforces the notion that our relative longevity is due to technological advances, not to increasing physical robustness.)

[4] **Grok:** In Chapter 2 we talk about Grok as the patriarch of a primal family, who happens to have a wife named Grokella. However, in the interest of inclusivity and ease of reading throughout the book in general, you can view Grok as a non-gender-specific archetype for the primal ancestor(s) whom we aspire to emulate in lifestyle behaviors. For example, "Grok never ate sugar, and neither should you."

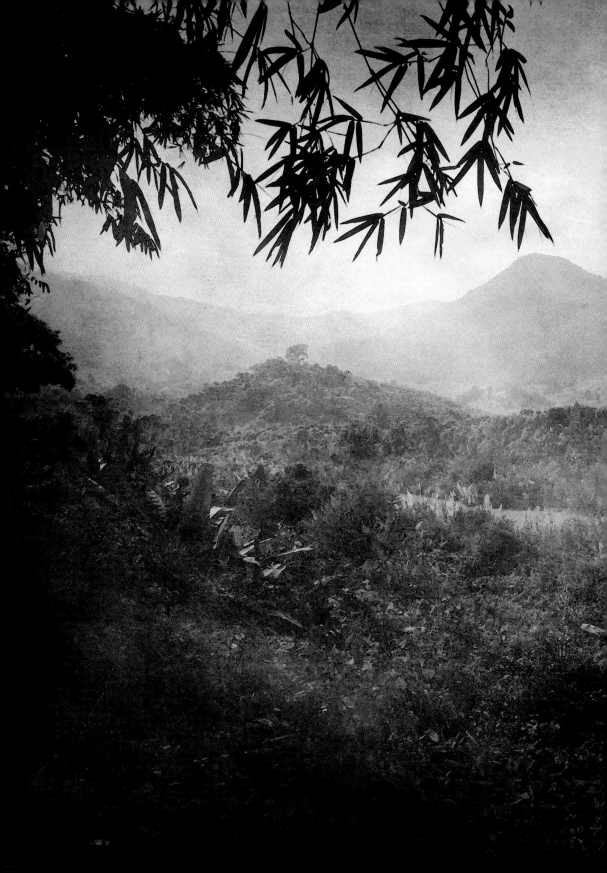

CHAPTER TWO

GROK AND KORG

From Indigenous to Digital:
One Giant Step (Backward)
for Mankind

IN THIS CHAPTER

We will contrast the daily lives of Grok and his primal family with their modern-day antithesis, the Korg family. No, not to see who can travel 20 miles more quickly (the Korgs' SUV beats Grok's bare feet with a few hours to spare... although the story might be different if it were a footrace!), but to examine the damage caused by living in conflict with our genetic predisposition to be fit, healthy, and happy, and to show the benefits of adapting primal behaviors to the modern world.

The extremely unhealthy saga of the Korgs might seem embellished, but it's actually a statistically accurate representation of many lifestyle trends today: hectic schedules that compromise quality family time, processed foods chosen in place of nutritious foods, widespread prescription drug use for assorted lifestyle-related maladies, digital entertainment replacing physical activity, and overly stressful exercise programs that cause even the most devoted to fail to achieve weight-loss and fitness goals.

While the story is distressing, the good news is that with some simple, enjoyable lifestyle modifications, the momentum can swing immediately in the direction of better health (including freedom from dependence on prescription medications), higher energy, successful long-term weight management, and a more enjoyable life for you and your family.

A man's health can be judged by which he takes two at a time—pills or stairs.

—Joan Welsh

A s we contrast Grok and Korg, we must refrain from the common knee-jerk rationalizations about the superiority of today's technological world. While infant mortality rates and death from tiger attacks are way down, it is sobering (pun intended) to consider that motor vehicle accidents (heavily influenced by alcohol use) are the leading cause of death for youths aged 15 to 24, followed by suicide and homicide. I am in no way arguing that we should discard our worldly possessions and go back in time to a life of mud huts and spears, or that we eschew the modern medicine that combats infection and disease; but we must take a hard look at our lifestyles and absorb some of the powerful lessons offered by the legacy of our ancestors.

LIVIN' LARGE 10,000 YEARS AGO

Your impression of primal human life might be negatively colored by sensationalized portrayals of pre-civilization humans as filthy, grunting savages dwelling in caves, or by the harrowing vision of a primal human potentially meeting his or her doom in the jaws of a beast or by the fangs of a snake. Unpleasant camping experiences (you know—too many mosquitoes, strange night noises, no hot showers) perhaps add to a dark vision of what it might have been like to live in hunter-gatherer times. Indeed, life was rough in many ways—much time and energy was devoted to staying safe from danger, building shelter, and obtaining food and other basic essentials that we take for granted.

Obviously, failure and misfortune abounded over the course of evolution, as only the strongest and luckiest of our ancestors survived. For purposes of our fictionalized but anthropologically accurate account of Grok's life, we'll assume he and his family have survived rudimentary setbacks and have found a bountiful area in which to settle and raise future generations (just as modern hunter-gatherers do today).

Ten thousand years ago, a time period coinciding with the end of the last major ice age, the continent of North America was populated with small bands of hunter-gatherer tribes. Many theorize that the migration into North America originated from Russia and moved very slowly eastward over dozens of generations across the Bering Land Bridge (which became submerged about 10,000 years ago) and then south into Canada and the United States. This population expansion across the continent was probably driven by the tracking of big game herds. These migrating tribes typically numbered 10 to 30 people comprising nuclear or extended families. While the average human life expectancy was about 33 in Grok's time,[1] if Grok had been able to avoid accident, predator, or illness, his life expectancy would have increased dramatically.

Shortly after Grok's time, the advent of agriculture drastically changed the nature of human life on earth and caused numerous markers of human health to steadily decline. Matt Ridley, author of *The Agile Gene*, reports that average brain size in 50,000 B.C. was 1,567 cc for males and 1,468 cc for females. Strange as it may seem, average brain sizes today are 1,248 cc for males and 1,210 cc for females, with the onset of the shrinkage closely related to the advent of agriculture.

GROK'S WALK

Grok and his longtime mate Grokella have two children, a 12-year-old boy and a 1-year-old girl. Two other children didn't make it past infancy, a traumatic yet unavoidable part of primal life. Grok and his small band totaling 25 people (including more blood relatives, such as parents and siblings and their families) live in what is now known as the Central Valley of California. It's a cool, moist climate supporting vast pine forests, owing to the lower mean temperatures of the era (mean earth temperatures have continued to rise over the last 10,000 years).

Gathered berries and other fruit, leaves, roots, nuts, and seeds provide the bulk of Grok's food supply. Grok also hunts a variety of animals and probably enjoys a fair amount of fish and mollusks, being well-positioned in the watershed of the Sierra. His band probably scores some big game occasionally (mammoth, mastodon, bison, bear, lion, saber-toothed tiger, wolf, deer, and moose), but because many of these animals were at the end of their era, more food likely came from small mammals, such as beaver, rabbit, squirrel, and mole.

Naturally, we'll start our day with Grok at sunrise. Grok and his family awaken to the sound of birds chirping. They have a simple but comfortable shelter: one of several thatched, dome-shaped huts in the clan settlement fashioned out of branches and brush. Yep, they're all the same size; there's no keeping up with the Joneses when you know you'll be moving on when the time comes, whenever that is. Grok's family begins the morning routine amidst the ageless singsong babble of a one-year-old. First things first—time to put together the morning meal. Because it's now late summer, special treats abound in the form of fat grub worms and local berries in their narrow ripening window. The current bounty is a far cry from the severe reduction in their typical food supplies the previous winter, caused by unusually heavy rains. Fortunately, Grok and the clan avoided starvation thanks to their biological ability to efficiently mobilize their stored body fat and make up for the caloric deficits in their diet. They also adapted to their winter circumstances by sleeping more and reducing their daily activity level.

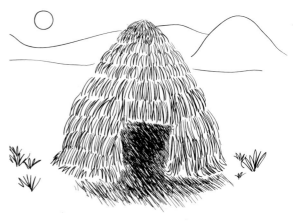

The son handles the chore of picking a basket of berries and quickly returns to camp. After breakfast, everyone turns their attention to preparing items for their daily endeavors. Working together, clan members tidy up woven storage receptacles, sharpen rudimentary weapons like spears, and pack food rations (mostly nuts and seeds) for those who will journey out in search of more bounty. Today Grok and his family and a few other companions are going for a long walk, heading east toward the Sierra foothills to gather more berries and perhaps score some small game. Everyone is eager—even though the temperature will be warm and the walk will be longer than their typical daily wanderings—because they will get to enjoy a cool dip in the river at the midpoint of their journey.

After a nutritious breakfast, the small group heads out. Arriving at the river, they feast on more berries and a few freshwater clams, sip clean water, and bathe, splash, and jump off rocks into the crystal clear and brisk river. Grok's occasional brief exposure to cold water offers more than fun.[2] He doesn't know it, but this activity is considered an "hormetic stressor" that helps boost immune function and antioxidant defense, decreases inflammation and pain, and increases blood flow and lymphatic function, something particularly therapeutic for tired muscles.

After the river splash, Grok lounges on a sunbaked rock. His eyes gradually begin to shut, and he nods off for a power nap. As soon as his eyes fully close, favorable hormonal changes occur in Grok's body.[3] Humans have adapted to obtain great benefits from even brief naps, and many modern scientists speculate that our default factory setting might be for biphasic or polyphasic sleep patterns (that is, sleeping in two or more stretches over a 24-hour period, as opposed to one long sleep at night). One reason is that the need for continued vigilance against predators and other dangers made a "good night's sleep" hard to come by until recently. Another is that the relaxed pace of primal life lent itself to afternoon shut-eye opportunities. Grok quickly drifts into the deepest, most restorative delta sleep cycle. Stress hormone levels are moderated and his brain chemicals are rebalanced, allowing him to wake up 20 minutes later refreshed and relaxed. Grok and Grokella's baby takes the opportunity to doze off for far longer, even as Grokella hoists her up into her carrying sling as the group heads off.

Clad in skirts made of plant fiber and animal skin, the group moves in bare feet over undulating terrain and makeshift animal trails. The ground is covered with rock and plant debris, including sharp burrs discarded by native plants, but they deftly cruise along for hours. Even at 12, Grok's son has already developed excellent cardiovascular endurance, muscle strength, and balance. And because a physically challenging life is routine to him, he probably doesn't moan or complain about the length of the journey or the boredom factor. ("Are we there yet?") After all, no video games await indoors. The elders pause on numerous occasions to teach their young about native plant life, point out animal markings, and dispense other environmental lessons that will serve them well and keep them safe as they grow to assume ever more challenging and valuable hunter-gatherer responsibilities.

Typical of humans 10,000 years ago, Grok and his family are of similar height and weight to a modern family, but with far more muscle and less body fat. They are agile and strong, and are capable of impressive feats of endurance when necessary. All the clan members are still lean following the hard winter, but they have been slowly packing on more adipose tissue (fat) throughout the warmer months, rebuilding their body fat "safety net." This seasonal fluctuation in body composition is normal (although they are quite resourceful about utilizing different food sources at different times of the year), but because they have to work for their food even during abundant times, they are never an unhealthy weight.

Because expectations and complexities are so minimal in primal life, the group easily goes with the flow when plans change.

While Grok's group initially had planned to return to their settlement that same evening, they change their mind after a brief chat and decide to rest for the day and camp out. Because expectations and complexities are so minimal in primal life, the group members easily go with the flow, despite being unprepared for an overnight stay. It simply means a couple hours' additional work to gather up materials and construct a temporary shelter, build a fire, and get some dinner. No worry—they are safe together.

Grok and his son head out for a quick hunt. We'd be surprised how primitive their weapons are, but the duo is able to leverage their intelligence and instinct about the natural world to procure a couple of rabbits for dinner. Walking back to camp, their celebratory banter is rudely interrupted by the appearance of a brown bear, drawn by the smell and wishing to make an unfair trade of lives for rabbits. A surge of fight or flight hormones floods the duo's bloodstreams. Grok delivers a stream

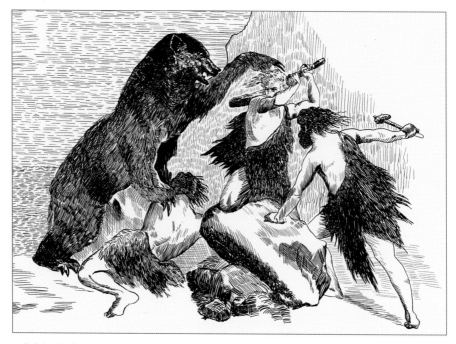

of detailed instructions to his son (back up slowly, maintain eye contact, etc.). His son nods, knowing to stifle his instinct to scream or run in the interest of survival. Grok calmly lays the rabbits down on the ground and carefully joins his son in deliberate retreat. The bear issues a couple of loud roars just to be sure everyone knows who's boss, gathers his "kill," and moseys along. For good measure, Grok and his son take off on a dead sprint for 60 seconds, until they are safely out of the predator's sight.

Twenty minutes later, the fight or flight chemicals have worn off, the father-and-son debriefing is complete, and the pair's parasympathetic ("rest and digest") nervous systems are quickly returning their bodies to their normal low-stress states. Grok arrives back at camp with empty hands and, most likely, a smile and shrug of the shoulders. This gesture epitomizes the requisite disposition for the uncertainty of primal life. It's a coping mechanism we have hardwired into our genes: "Don't worry, be happy."

Grokella has discovered some leafy green vegetation that they will eat raw or cook briefly over the campfire with a few wild potatoes. An analysis of the nutrient content of the food they consume over the course of a typical month (a sufficient time period to account for the feast-or-famine realities of primal life and humans' genetic ability to deal with it effectively) would reveal optimum levels of carbohydrates, protein, fat, vitamins, minerals, fiber, antioxidants, and other elements needed to sustain a lifetime of exceptional fitness and vibrant health. Similarly, if we were to draw Grok's blood for laboratory analysis, this primitive human would likely come up a big winner by today's health standards: free of disease markers such as high C-reactive protein levels (indicative of undesirable systemic inflammation) or elevated HbA1c values (indicative of long-term damage from excessive carbohydrate intake/blood glucose levels); possessing ideal levels of cholesterol, triglycerides, glucose, and insulin; and exempt from common modern-day nutrient deficiencies.

> *Don't bother about being modern.*
> *Unfortunately it is the one thing that,*
> *whatever you do, you cannot avoid.*
>
> —Salvador Dalí

After dinner, the group lingers around the campfire for perhaps an hour or two, relaxing, telling stories, and winding down the day as the sun sets. This routine of quality family and community time in the evening is likely more than today's average working parents spend with their children in an entire week (modern families average 19 minutes of quality time together, free from television and other distractions, per day).[4] As the sun sets, Grok and the group are ready for a good night's sleep.

THE AMERICAN DREAM—UNPLUGGED (OR SHOULD WE SAY "PLUGGED IN?")

Our modern family, the Korgs (as you've likely noticed, that's Grok spelled backward; fitting when you consider their dramatic departure from Grok's simple, healthy lifestyle and the accompanying backward steps they've taken in health), live where Grok did in California's Central Valley in what is now known as Stockton. Stockton is a medium-sized, middle-income community located on the Sacramento River delta, only an hour's drive from the metropolitan San Francisco Bay Area, which has a population of seven million. The Korgs—and thousands of other families like them in bedroom communities outside the Bay Area proper—believe they have the best of both worlds: an "easy" commute to elevated Bay Area salaries combined with affordable housing (Stockton's median home price is several hundred thousand dollars less than most comparable homes in the Bay Area), less congestion, and good recreational, educational, and cultural opportunities. Ken Korg's two hours a day in the car seem like a routine cost of living the American Dream.[5]

AN ALARMING MORNING

Waking up naturally with the sun? Not the Korgs. Ken's wife, Kelly, is up and out of the house when it's still dark, heading to the gym for a 6:00 A.M. spin class. It's a struggle for her to get to class three days a week, but Kelly knows that her only chance to get a workout—or, for that matter, to enjoy some personal time—is before the family stirs and the responsibilities pile up. Besides, Kelly has struggled all her life with her body weight and would dearly love to drop the twenty or more pounds suggested by her physician to get her body mass index (BMI) into the healthy range.

When the alarm clock emits its digital chirping bird signal (very similar to Grok's; you can also choose breaking waves or wind chimes!) in the darkness of 5:15 A.M., an immediate stress reaction initiates throughout Kelly's body. Even the benign digital birds jolt her abruptly out of restful sleep and stimulate a mini fight or flight response, causing her cortisol levels to spike. Because a variety of hormones and brain chemicals are sensitive to light and dark cycles, rising in the dark further disrupts her circadian rhythm, resulting in a physiologically stressful start to Kelly's day—ironic, since her early morning workout is part of her sincere commitment to become healthier.

The rest of the Korg family avoids Mom's cortisol spike, but due to a host of other factors, they have their own issues waking up. Ken is already awake when his alarm sounds at 7:00 A.M., but his mind and body are in no hurry to get up and out of bed. Part of his situation is psychological—he is not terribly excited to face an hour on the freeway. Other factors influencing his body's sluggish start are the medications he's taking and the previous night's late dessert—a generous slice of cheesecake made with 60 grams of processed carbohydrates, partially hydrogenated vegetable oil, and assorted unpronounceable chemical preservatives.

Ken's cheesecake spiked his blood glucose just as he was attempting to fall asleep, interfering with the release of melatonin that naturally triggers sleepiness. Instead of spending the first hour in bed drifting into ever-deeper stages of sleep, Ken was fidgeting and twitchy because of the excess blood glucose in his system. Besides the glucose coursing through his veins, Ken was jacked up from spending the final 90 minutes of his evening watching television. Even though he was exhausted and attempting to wind down after a long day, the fast-moving, flickering images on the screen (often violent or otherwise arousing) caused irregular stimulation to Ken's retina. This type of stimulus is transferred directly to the brain via the optic nerve and disturbs the normal function of the hypothalamus, the control center for many vital body functions, including the initiation of proper sleep patterns.[6]

Alas, Ken has one of the millions of sleep-aid prescriptions written for Americans every year (in 2013, more than 40 million prescriptions were written for zolpidem—generic Ambien—alone),[7] which he reaches for on occasions like these. The fast-acting sleep medication has Ken dead to the world within 20 minutes of taking the pill, but at the cost of suppressing a natural and healthy transition through the critical hormonal, organ, and muscular restoration processes that occur in the various stages of sleep, from REM to slow-wave deep sleep. Seven hours later, with the sedative effects of Ambien still trying to clear his bloodstream, Ken feels sluggish and groggy instead of naturally refreshed and energized.

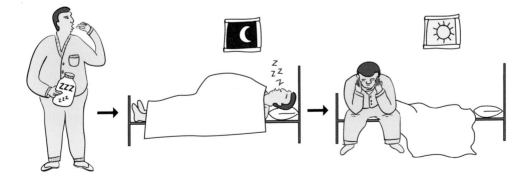

Nevertheless, it's time to get the Korg clan moving, so Ken drags himself out of bed and heads over to the bedrooms of his 14-year-old son and 6-year-old daughter. Rousing them is not an easy task. Kenny Korg is experiencing his greatest need for sleep since infancy and, like most modern teenagers, isn't getting enough.[8] Kenny is also affected by a couple of other common adolescent conditions: drowsiness during the day and a delayed circadian phase, which has him naturally wanting to stay up and wake up later. Kenny would feel much better with a regular afternoon power nap, but of course napping isn't part of the picture in teenage life, so he usually fights his fatigue by ingesting a caffeine-laced energy drink or soda. He has no problem, however, staying up late playing computer games and texting his friends. He thinks he is relaxing, but unfortunately he doesn't know that by exposing himself to the intense light emitted by digital screens long after the sun has gone down, he is preventing the natural release of melatonin that should accompany nightfall and trigger sleepiness. Because he often doesn't power down until close to midnight, the 7:00 A.M. alarm comes far too early for him to feel rested and energized.

Young Miss Cindy Korg has her own troubles waking up. The mind-numbing effects of the cherry-flavored antihistamine/decongestant/cough suppressant/analgesic over-the-counter medication her mom had given her the previous evening are still lingering after a fitful sleep. She wakes up groggy, with blocked sinuses, but must rally to get to school on time. Cindy's third upper respiratory tract infection this year was chalked up to "the bug that's going around." However, bugs are always going around; it was really her suppressed immune system—weakened by the excessive consumption of processed carbs and sugars in her diet—that prevented her from easily combating the virus after the first contact.

Kelly, always wanting to do the right thing as a mother, unknowingly prolonged little Cindy's ordeal by giving her a common cold "remedy" that was intended to ease her suffering but that interfered with her daughter's natural defenses. Pounding the cough syrup every four hours for a few days likely doubled the time required for complete recovery, quelling the low fever her body had naturally developed as a first assault (mild fever is a primary defense in helping to kill viruses), blocking the production of mucus intended to drain the virus into the stomach (where it can easily be killed by stomach acid), drying out the sinuses (thereby causing them to swell to the point that she can't breathe out of her nose at all this morning), and suppressing a productive cough that might have kept her up some at night but would have allowed her lungs to expel the virus-laden mucus. All these "symptoms" were actually Cindy's potent gene-based natural defenses—thwarted by modern medicine in the name of relief from discomfort. At any rate, Cindy finally summons the strength to get dressed and head downstairs.

Kelly bursts through the door as the family is shuffling around trying to get ready for the day. She's chipper and energized from her 50-minute class, which elevated her heart rate to 85 percent of maximum or higher for most of that time period. The intensity of the effort has released a flood of stress hormones into her bloodstream, so she's on an "exercise high" due to the effects of natural painkilling endorphins as she greets her family.

Kelly quickly sticks three whole grain waffles into the toaster for the family and dutifully cracks open a can of chocolate SlimFast meal-replacement drink for herself. Main ingredients: skim milk powder, sugar, and fructose, along with plenty of chemicals, synthetic vitamins, and vegetable oils—not much nutrition but plenty of simple carbs (38 grams) to raise blood glucose temporarily and stimulate an energy-sapping insulin surge soon after. The "good" news for Kelly: it contains only 240 calories. A minute later, the Korgs' power breakfast is ready: orange juice and waffles with a butter-like spread made from refined polyunsaturated vegetable oil (that is pro-inflammatory and immune suppressing) and "low-sugar" maple syrup made with artificial sweeteners[9] and woefully far removed from the sweet nectar that flows out of a hole drilled in a Vermont maple tree.

Kelly's second shake at lunch results in a total of only 480 calories consumed since 7:00 P.M. the previous evening—a period of 17 hours. While our bodies are adept at supplying adequate energy in periods of intermittent food consumption (such was the reality of daily life for Grok), Kelly's long-term reliance on dietary carbohydrates for energy, her high-intensity dawn workout, and the energy demands of her busy day make it the wrong time to skimp on healthy food. As a consequence, her metabolic rate will slow and the appetite center in her brain will send a strong message to consume quick-energy carbohydrates. She will end up grabbing a whole wheat bagel with light cream cheese out of desperation shortly thereafter—still, she (incorrectly) believes, being healthy while staving off the "hangry" meltdown she feels coming.

Kelly's calorie-restriction efforts will not result in the burning of stored body fat because the frequent insulin spikes after her high-carb shakes, snacks, and typical American meals inhibit fat burning and, in the long term, produce metabolic changes that make it increasingly difficult to mobilize stored fat for energy. This condition is obviously affecting Kelly, an active, disciplined person who nevertheless struggles to reduce excess body fat. The net effect of Kelly's punishing early morning workouts (surprisingly, elite athletes spend a substantially lower percentage of total exercise time at elevated heart rates than many casual fitness enthusiasts like Kelly)[10] and devoted calorie restriction is a reduction in muscle mass. This further lowers her metabolic rate, increases body fat (due to the binge eating and slowed metabolic rate), and leads to recurring fatigue and mood swings.

Frustrated, Kelly caves in and buys a weight-loss kit from her neighbor Wendy, who has dropped eight pounds (3.6 kg) in two weeks since following her new multilevel-marketing-driven diet cleanse. Those remarkable results, however, are due almost entirely to reduced water retention from the depletion of muscle glycogen (every gram of stored glycogen binds with around four grams of water in the body) and catabolized muscle tissue. The eight pounds will return in a matter of days when exhaustion causes a return to normal, or supernormal, calorie intake.

"THAT PROBLEM"... AMONG OTHERS

Ken hates these first few minutes after Kelly returns from her morning workout because her energy level is such a stark contrast to the slow-moving household. On the flip side, Kelly typically shuts down around 8:30 P.M., as the insulin begins flooding her system following her SAD dinner. With Ken's contrasting late-evening pattern, time for intimacy is virtually nonexistent. Furthermore, Ken has recently been experiencing "that problem" but is hesitant to tell anyone, let alone make an appointment with a physician to receive a prescription for Viagra.

After all, Ken is still in his forties and thinks Viagra is for old guys. Ken would be surprised to learn that about a third of all erectile dysfunction prescriptions are dispensed to men under 50 and that use by men under age 45 tripled between 1998 and 2002.

Ken has several issues that contribute to his condition. The sustained high levels of cortisol in his bloodstream from stressful lifestyle factors such as inadequate sleep and job stress suppress testosterone production, leading to diminished energy levels, weakened immune function, and, of course, reduced sex drive. His higher-than-optimum body fat levels and excessive insulin production from his high-carb diet and insufficient exercise also promote low testosterone, poor blood circulation, and other common-but-curable impotency contributors. Kelly, in turn, struggles with her body image, leading to reduced desire for intimacy. Furthermore, her stressful exercise regimen and poor nutritional habits interfere with healthy female hormone balance and contribute to the reduction of her drive.

Oh, I almost forgot Ken's Lipitor (one of the world's best-selling drugs, with total sales of over $131 billion since its release), a statin medication he takes for "high" cholesterol. Ken does not know that the medication can cause muscle and liver problems, deplete CoQ10 (coenzyme Q10, a natural antioxidant and cofactor that is critical to cellular energy metabolism—more on CoQ10 in Chapter 3), and, yes, inhibit sexual performance. He only recently (and reluctantly, to his credit) started on Lipitor, at the behest of his doctor, who was concerned about his total cholesterol count of 205. Not in the high-risk range by any means, but enough for the doc to want to bring it down some, which the statins manage to do quickly.

Unfortunately, statins also have serious side effects,[11] mainly because they block the production and flow of CoQ10 into cell mitochondria. This disturbance to mitochondrial functioning hampers the body's ability to generate normal amounts of energy (hence the common patient complaint of weakness and fatigue), as well as to fight free radicals and moderate inflammation. Furthermore, statins do not affect triglyceride (blood fat) levels or LDL (the so-called bad cholesterol) particle size, nor do they decrease risk of death in any women, in men over 65, or in men under 65 who have not had a heart attack.

Ken fills his commuter mug with coffee, hustles Cindy into the car, and they depart. The first stop is four tenths of a mile away at Cindy's elementary school.[12] It's four minutes until the tardy bell, and the front entrance is mobbed with a conga line of cars waiting to reach the drop-off zone. Ken glances in the rear-view mirror and notices his next-door neighbor and child right behind them in line! Guess we know how the morning traffic jam happens.... By the time Ken's car reaches its destination, Cindy is in a panic, as she will once again chase the tardy bell. Fear of a tardy slip may not be on par with a surprise visit from a bear, but the same fight or flight response occurs nonetheless in Cindy as it did in Grok. The parting is anything but warm and comforting—a few choice words from the first grader and a quick admonishment in return from Ken: "Fine, maybe I'll just make you walk next time!" An excellent idea, considering the short trip from home to classroom by auto has taken six minutes, whereas even a leisurely walk (say, the pace that Grok and his family maintained for several hours, while trading off carrying a small child) from home to classroom would not have taken much longer.

Ken extracts his sedan from the campus swarm and soon begins his navigation of interstate freeways. As he drives up and over the small mountain range that marks the geographic boundary of the Bay Area, Ken spends his hour of "solitude" listening to talk radio—bouncing back and forth between sports and news talk—and taking several phone calls from friends and coworkers in the office. This constant and distracted stimulation to a brain still experiencing the effects of Ambien leads to mental fatigue before he even sets foot in the office. What's more, at the 40-minute mark of Ken's journey, he is suffering from heartburn and bloating (from his regular consumption of fried foods, dairy products, alcohol, sugars and desserts, sodas and other carbonated beverages, and substantial caloric intake in the evenings) as well as from his typical recurring back pain (an affliction he shares with 60 to 80 percent of the general population).

Ken reaches into his briefcase and whips out his pill container, extracting a purple pill and a white capsule. The "healing purple pill" is Nexium (the second best-selling drug in 2013, with over $6 billion in sales that year), which is used to treat the increasingly common condition known as gastroesophageal reflux disease (GERD) and its main symptom, heartburn. Nexium, classified as a proton pump inhibitor, blocks the production of hydrochloric acid in the stomach. This provides immediate relief for Ken's pain but seriously inhibits the digestive process, which relies on hydrochloric acid and other powerful acids to break down and assimilate nutrients from food.

Next is the white capsule: Celebrex, a popular nonsteroidal anti-inflammatory (NSAID) prescription medication that reduces levels of hormone-like substances called prostaglandins that are part of a natural inflammation response occurring in Ken's body. Ken takes it to alleviate the back pain that accompanies the inflammation. He will pop another Celebrex this evening per the recommendation of his physician, who also suggested at his last visit that he schedule an appointment at a physical therapy clinic to obtain a customized back and core strengthening exercise routine. He's been meaning to schedule that but hasn't yet found the time.[13] Instead, Ken grabs some exercise here and there when the stars align and gaps open up in his schedule. Owing to his athletic youth, his competitive appetite is bigger than his physical condition. His forays into adult pickup basketball at the club usually produce more tweaks and pulls than inspiration to pursue a regular, balanced total-body fitness program.

If Ken proceeds with the typical behavior pattern, he will use these prescription NSAIDs for years and neglect sufficient regular exercise. Down the road, owing to Ken's long-term use of such a powerful systemic anti-inflammatory medication, the drug's impact will diminish (at which point his doctor will probably put him on something stronger) and his body's natural ability to control all types of inflammation will have been steadily undermined. This will set the stage for a variety of serious health conditions to potentially take root, including—owing to his poor diet and lifestyle habits—many types of cancer and heart disease. Yep, that's right, studies suggest a significant increased risk of heart attack when taking NSAIDs. Vioxx was a very popular NSAID taken by 80 million people worldwide from 1999 until 2004, when it was taken off the market due to concerns about side effects that increased heart attack risk. Celebrex sales skyrocketed as a result, until research suggested it posed similar risks. Celebrex sales then dropped sharply but nevertheless still exceeded $2.6 billion in 2014 according to parent company Pfizer.

The idea on the medical horizon is that chronic inflammation is a root cause of degenerative disease. If physicians are trained to use "food as medicine" they may not need to rely on drugs and their distressing side-effects to treat the inflammatory process.

—Dr. Andrew Weil

SPREADSHEETS AND CHOW MEIN

After an hour and eight minutes of driving from the elementary school, Ken arrives at his office. He works as an accountant for a software company. The hours are regular (unlike many of his coworkers, who are selling or developing software and routinely work 10- to 12-hour days), and he makes a third more money than he could in the same position in Stockton. Aside from the set hours and salary, the working conditions are challenging. Executives and division sales managers constantly inflict their hyperdrive mentality on the accounting team. They have a penchant for requesting ridiculously fancy presentations on short notice or strolling into Ken's office and literally breathing down his neck to obsessively review sales figures in the days counting down to quarterly close, the results of which dictate their always-fluctuating compensation.

Mind you, these high-performing folks are friendly and charming and use their extrovert personality attributes to charm Ken into performing on demand. However, Ken considers none of his coworkers a true friend. This is due not only to the artificial social circumstances in the workplace, but also to the great distance Ken lives from work and his lack of free time to socialize with work peers anyway. Meanwhile, since Ken spends so much time on the road and in the office, he is disconnected from his own neighborhood community. Neighbors who have lived a stone's throw away (how's that for a primal metaphor?) for over a decade are still just a bit more than strangers. They exchange friendly waves, maybe a greeting by name on the street, but they never set foot in one another's homes, nor have meaningful conversations besides the occasional brief discussion about neighborhood happenings and logistics.

The perk of being able to leave promptly at 6:00 P.M. each evening is muted by the mental exhaustion that overcomes Ken as soon as he opens his car door in the parking lot. In his previous job (closer to home and for significantly less pay), Ken would take a leisurely lunch hour to eat a sandwich in the park or even join a coworker for a light work-out at the gym. He'd return to work refreshed and proceed at a sensible pace through the afternoon hours, pausing often to share a laugh with coworkers. Lately, he has stayed at his desk to eat lunch, typically procured via a two-minute drive to a busy nearby intersection with numerous quick-energy, low-nutrition meal options.

Ken, inspired by Kelly's commitment, is also making a concerted effort to "do the right thing" and eat healthier. He eschews McDonald's and Burger King in favor of the Chinese buffet, which sounds healthier but is actually far from it. He returns to the office armed with chow mein noodles and sweet-and-sour chicken, trying not to spill the predominantly simple carbohydrate meal onto his spreadsheets. Laughter in the hallways has been replaced by the discernible buzz of anxiety, the unspoken fear that heads will begin to roll if Ken's spreadsheets don't impress stockholders and executives.

In contrast to the few brief moments of Grok's life-or-death encounter with a bear, Ken's workplace is essentially a daily 9-hour grind of unrelenting moderate-to-high stress. Ken and the rest of us would still choose working on spreadsheets to being surprised by a bear, but the impact of prolonged chronic stress is far more destructive to human health (and misaligned with our genes) than a pattern of brief intermittent stresses coupled with adequate downtime.

The mid-afternoon, post-high-carb-lunch sugar crash hits Ken hard, so he scarfs down one of the energy bars Kelly threw into his briefcase. (Better than a candy bar, right? Not necessarily. The PowerBar Performance Energy Citrus Burst that Ken eats has 43 grams of carbs, 29 of them sugar. Snickers has 34.5g total carbs, also with 29g sugar… whoops!) He then heads to the break room for his daily afternoon cup o' joe. Ken consumes two cups of coffee and one to two diet sodas each day, a total of about 250 milligrams of caffeine.[14] Not quite enough to classify him as an addict (that's about the daily average for Americans), but it's definitely another substance, alongside the several prescription and over-the-counter meds, which he depends on to get through his day.

LOVE, MONEY, AND INSULIN

The Korgs experience financial stresses familiar to so many, in spite of making a comfortable income.[15] After paycheck deductions for taxes, 401(k), and, of course, the incredible employee stock purchase program (which entices 5 percent of his gross income to be fed back to the monster), a third of his annual net goes to mortgage and related tax and insurance costs. Other healthy chunks go to car payments and insurance, groceries and dining out, medical expenses not covered by Ken's skimpy company policy, and the occasional whopper, such as five grand to straighten Kenny's teeth, two grand to the veterinarian for a major surgery, two grand for Kenny's school field trip to Washington, D.C., a thousand bucks for Kelly's last-minute bereavement trip to the East Coast for a family friend's funeral, and a C-note for that weight-loss "starter kit" that gung-ho neighbor Wendy foisted on them.

Kelly contributes to the family's bottom line, running her own stimulating but stressful business as a freelance graphic designer. The flexible hours are great, although the healthy boundary between work and personal life often gets blurred. One favorite ritual is picking up her daughter from school every day and taking her out for a treat—carrying on a fond family tradition she and her sisters enjoyed with their mother. As Eric Schlosser details in *Fast Food Nation*, Kelly is cooperating with the food industry's institutionalized exploitation of American families that encourages parents to replace quality time (particularly the nearly extinct family home mealtime… and also the guilty conscience that goes with being too busy for family time) with instant gratification—and therefore love—for their children.

The treat time coincides with Kelly's daily affliction of the afternoon blues. The colorful, peppy, healthy lifestyle messaging inside the local Jamba Juice franchise helps Kelly rationalize her impending insulin flash flood. She confidently orders up a 24-ounce Strawberry Surf Rider for herself and a 16-ounce Mango-A-Go-Go for her daughter. Cindy excitedly suggests adding a couple baked goods from the child-eye-level display case next to the register. Ever vigilant, Kelly scans the choices to pick the healthiest one and settles on the reduced-fat blueberry-lemon loaf. "Part of a complete breakfast—complement with a smoothie or fresh squeezed orange juice," says the Jamba Juice menu. Each loaf offers 290 calories, 73 percent of which come from processed carbohydrates (lead ingredients: sugar and flour) with virtually zero nutritional value and a guaranteed strong insulin response. Cindy finishes only half her loaf, but Kelly makes sure it doesn't go to waste.

The discipline of Kelly's "diet" of meal replacement shakes is no match for a depleted brain and body. While the 24-ounce Strawberry Surf Rider will provide Kelly with some much-deserved antioxidants and other healthy nutrients from the frozen fruit, 87 percent of its 490 calories come from sugar. Along with one-and-a-half blueberry-lemon loaves, Kelly has ingested 925 calories (make that an even thousand, counting a few long pulls on her daughter's straw to try the Mango-A-Go-Go), including 187 grams of refined carbohydrates. (That's around double the Primal Blueprint's recommended consumption for an entire day!) Her sugar/insulin roller coaster will again hamper her fat-burning efforts for hours after this onslaught and lead to fatigue and sugar cravings come dinnertime.

Studies suggest that overweight kids are highly likely to become overweight adults and consequently suffer from serious health problems and life-threatening diseases.

Young Cindy Korg's drink and half loaf send more than 100 grams of sugar into her little body, stressing her insulin system—and her immune system—yet again. The previous day, at a classmate's birthday party, she had consumed typical party fare of two slices of thin-crust cheese pizza (460 calories), a small slice of chocolate cake (235 calories) with a small scoop of vanilla ice cream (150 calories), 130 calories from some juice boxes laden with high fructose corn syrup (she opened three over the course of the party and drank only half the juice—a typical ratio, as any parent who's hosted a birthday party can confirm), and several assorted bite-sized candies from the take-home party favor bag (150 calories). Her total calories in the three-hour period came to 1,125, more than half in the form of simple sugar. That's enough to stimulate a significant insulin response in a 300-pound man, let alone a 55-pound child.

Naturally (owing to family genes, her parents rationalize), young Cindy is already somewhat overweight. Fortunately (from a psychological perspective only), unlike in past generations, her plump physique is shared by many of her fellow first graders.[16] While this protects her self-esteem somewhat, it makes it difficult to change the charted course of this young ship, sailing toward peril and an unhealthy future. Studies suggest that overweight kids are highly likely to become overweight adults and consequently suffer from serious health problems and life-threatening diseases.

KENNY'S WORLD

We haven't heard much about the Korgs' teenage son, Kenny, which is appropriate because he is already emotionally disconnected from his busy family and pulled by the powerful force of peer influence in directions that create conflict with a stable family life. In his early years, Kenny was naturally active and spent hours outside running and playing. Unfortunately, each passing preteen year saw more sedentary technological distractions commandeering his time, and innocent backyard play being exchanged for competitive organized sports.[17]

While Kenny has some innate athletic ability, he lacks the natural aggression and competitiveness that allow the most passionate young athletes to move to the front of the pack. Lacking time to connect with his son, Ken makes the common mistake of imbuing his son's athletic experience with misplaced emotion and "encouragement" that feels to his son like inflated expectations and criticism. By the time Kenny becomes a teen, he is finished with organized sports and deep into massive multiplayer online role-playing games,[18] such as Dungeon Fighter Online (400 million worldwide users), Runescape (200 million), and World of Warcraft (100 million). Here, players create digital personas and interact with many others in a virtual world, often immersed for eight or 10 hours at a time. At school, Kenny maintains grades that are decent, if below his potential, and unsurprisingly he is frequently called in for misbehaving in class. During a telephone conversation with the school counselor, the topic of attention deficit hyperactivity disorder (ADHD) is broached as a potential reason for Kenny's misbehavior.

Kenny's feelings of alienation are exacerbated at the dinner table that evening, when Ken peppers him with the exact same questions heard at the breakfast table about his son's decision to skip freshman basketball tryouts. The teen is naturally offended, unaware that one of the most common side effects of Ambien is short-term memory loss and that Ken truly has little recollection of the conversation from 12 hours prior. The exchange escalates into a blowout covering various pent-up resentments. Ken decides to make an appointment for his son to visit a psychiatrist.

At the first session, the doctor diagnoses Kenny with ADHD and promptly prescribes the amphetamine Adderall[19] despite the growing controversy surrounding its overprescription to children without a true clinical diagnosis. Nor does the potential link to serious cardiovascular side effects and the high incidence of abuse among teenagers using the stimulant recreationally receive adequate consideration in the decision to prescribe. (An estimated seven million American kids take stimulants prescribed for attention disorders, a 500-percent increase since 1991.) It's more likely that emotional factors, lack of sufficient vigorous exercise, and poor dietary habits (sugar binges, regular caffeine intake, and lack of healthy fats) are to blame for Kenny's adverse classroom behavior. Unfortunately, Kenny now has another hurdle on the path to getting his mind and body back into balance for the challenging high school years ahead: the powerful effects of stimulant medication on his growing body.

When considering the particulars of kids and their exercise, sleep, dietary habits, and school hijinks, you might think, "What's the big deal?" Kenny and millions of his peers will continue their mildly objectionable ways, but they'll get through high school just fine (provided they heed Primal Blueprint Law #9: Avoid Stupid Mistakes). They'll go off to college and pull all-nighters fueled by pizza, Red Bull, and Top Ramen, then they'll unwind after exam pressure with alcohol, more pizza, and maybe a few cupcakes at the Kappa Kappa Gamma bash. It worked for previous generations; why not for this one?

It's true that young people are incredibly resilient. Their accelerated metabolism and young endocrine system floods the bloodstream with peak levels of key growth and reproductive hormones. The raw (indeed, primal) energy of youth can often override any potential insulin-driven fatigue from a fading Red Bull buzz—at least for a while. Most can attest to the difference in energy between being at our physical peak versus the later years. At 63, I'm stoked to be able to hang (more or less… hope he doesn't read this and shake his head!) with my son Kyle when we snowboard or play Ultimate Frisbee with his crew.

However, if we consider that our genes—even young genes—are predisposed to all kinds of problems when triggered by the wrong environmental signals, we can conclude that it's just a matter of time before disease kicks in. Remember those college frat boys with six-pack abs drinking pony kegs on the weekend? A decade later, many of them sport pony keg guts and drink six-packs on the weekend. As a parent or an influential figure in a child's life, you can build a foundation of healthy lifestyle habits and a deep respect and understanding of how to get the best out of your body. Considering that many experts predict a shorter life expectancy for today's children than their parents—for the first time in recorded history—it makes sense to advocate for something different than the typical modern American family's existence.[20]

"WE HAVE MET THE ENEMY, AND HE IS US"

This quote from Walt Kelly's popular comic strip character Pogo perfectly captures the Korg family's plight. Their well-intentioned efforts to do the right thing are continually sabotaged by cultural norms and misguided conventional wisdom. We are conditioned by the powerful forces of consumerism to pursue flawed solutions to our problems and ailments. The prescription and over-the-counter drugs downed by Ken, Kenny, and Cindy; Kelly's overly stressful exercise routine and overly restrictive diet; the massive amount of unhealthy food (including unhealthy "health food") ingested by the family on a daily basis; and the lack of simple, quality family time may be disturbing to read about, yet they are absolutely the norm today.

If you felt the Korgs' tale was an appalling, melodramatic, and unrealistic example of a modern family, then perhaps your lifestyle reference points are significantly healthier and more balanced than those of the average American family. Extensive references to the Korgs' daily routine, prescription drug use, weight-loss battles, eating and exercise habits, childhood obesity, teenage behavior challenges, and digital media use are offered at the end of this chapter.

Unfortunately, the Korgs' challenges are pervasive in our modern society, and they transcend socioeconomic categories. The Korgs are among the lucky ones, for they are making ends meet (albeit in a high-stress manner), have quality health care, and can afford gym memberships, family travel, braces, therapy sessions, and so forth. They have the resources to make healthier choices, but even they struggle. Go to any Whole Foods Market and check the shopping carts of the higher-budget consumers; you might find a six-dollar tub of blueberries, organic hamburger meat, or an eight-ounce cacao dessert treat costing eight bucks, but you'll also see the excessive sugar and grain products that form the underpinnings of the Standard American Diet. (Note: organic, whole grain crackers made with recycled packaging are still converted into glucose upon ingestion.) Things are considerably more difficult for the minimum-wage worker trying to do the right thing by his or her family on a budget that is stretched to the max even before procuring many fundamentals of healthy living.

As you pursue your dream of optimal health and make the accordant consumer choices toward that goal, you contribute to a bigger shift in culture. Companies who make healthy, environmentally conscious products will thrive, and the giant industrial food manufacturers who have cavalierly peddled poison brands for decades will be forced to recalibrate when their products no longer fly off the shelves. On this topic, I will politely challenge the "everything in moderation" maxim that is bantered about with insufficient discretion. Modern life is so out of balance that extreme measures are necessary just to maintain some semblance of health. Don't forget Mark Twain's take here: "Everything in moderation, including moderation."

> *Don't forget Mark Twain's take here: "Everything in moderation, including moderation."*

As they say, your kids grow up—and you grow old—before you know it. The lack of awareness and knowledge, and sometimes, sadly, a defiant, ignorant stance toward respecting the genetic programming that informs our health and wellbeing, tragically degrades the precious time that families have together. This lost opportunity plays out every day, touching virtually every family in the modern world. It's time to stand up and take control of your health and wellbeing by honoring your genes and living according to the ancestral laws laid out by the Primal Blueprint. Question the tenets of conventional wisdom. They are too often aggressively promoted by special interests driven by a profit incentive, with little if any concern for your health or the health of the planet. They peddle outdated and scientifically flawed information that is potentially hazardous to your health. In this book, we will question this conventional wisdom, building momentum and crushing obstacles in our path as we march toward the ultimate expression of our human potential.

HOW GROK PROBABLY SPENT HIS DAY

Habitat-, shelter-, basic-human-needs–related chores....3 hours
Hunting or gathering food...5 hours
Leisure time consisting of play and family
    or group socializing..6 hours
Sleeping, napping, resting, relaxing.............................10 hours

Estimates derived from studies of the modern hunter-gatherer culture of the !Kung Bushmen in Africa.

HOW KEN KORG SPENDS HIS DAY

Commute...2 hours
Grooming, household chores, free time*....................2.3 hours
Television, computer, digital entertainment.................4 hours[21]
Sleep...6.7 hours
Workplace..9 hours

*Free time components:
   Leisure/educational reading: 24 minutes
   Meaningful conversation with child: 3.5 minutes

Estimates derived from TV Free America in Washington, D.C. and American Time Use Survey Summary (U.S. Department of Labor, Washington, D.C.).

CHAPTER SUMMARY

1. Grok's Lifestyle: Grok faced unimaginable hardships in primal life but in many ways enjoyed superior health to that of modern humans. While rates of infant mortality and death by predator or accident were far higher than they are today, if Grok were able to avoid such tragedy, he could enjoy robust health and physical fitness into his 60s or 70s.

Grok's hunter-gatherer existence involved a diet of plants and animals, hours of low-level aerobic exercise every day, and occasional short bursts of maximum strength or speed efforts. Primal existence was simpler and slower-paced. Life-or-death events occurred infrequently and were usually brief. This type of existence is more aligned with our genetic makeup than the unrelenting stress of modern life.

2. Korg Lifestyle: The lifestyle of our modern suburban family, the Korgs, diverged dramatically from that modeled by Grok's family. Today, long commutes, packed schedules, and excessive digital entertainment compromise time to develop family camaraderie. Stress caused by financial pressures, insufficient sleep or downtime, extensive use of prescription drugs, poor dietary habits, and exhausting exercise programs inevitably lead to avoidable health problems and shortened life spans.

The Korgs' diet features processed foods and insufficient natural or whole foods. In particular, they eat too many simple carbs and grains that lead to excess insulin production. These dietary mistakes lead to assorted health problems, beginning in childhood and continuing for a lifetime. Kelly Korg's well-meaning devotion to exercise and careful dieting does not lead to fat loss because the workouts are too stressful, and her diet causes excessive insulin to course through her bloodstream, inhibiting fat burning. Ken's lack of exercise, poor eating habits, work-related pressures, and reliance on prescription drugs to counter lifestyle errors make him tired and stressed and put him on the path to the eventual onset of serious disease. The Korg children are victims of disastrous cultural trends common among today's youth, such as insufficient activity, excessive digital media use, high-insulin diets, and overpressurized athletic and academic experiences that lead to poor mental and physical wellbeing.

3. Your Family: It's critical to depart from these harmful cultural trends and to create a different reality for you and your family. Modifying dietary and exercise habits to align with Primal Blueprint recommendations and placing limits on technology and jam-packed schedules in favor of relaxing family interaction will help to reverse the appalling family dynamics that so tragically characterizes the Korgs' story.

CHAPTER ENDNOTES

Grok Family References

[1] **Life Expectancy:** Life expectancy during the Paleolithic era (2.5 million years ago to 10,000 B.C.) was around 33 years, factoring in the high rates of infant mortality. If Grok reached puberty, life expectancy increased to age 39 and if he reached 39, he could expect to live until 54. And this was a ripped, energetic 54, not the 54 of a guy struggling to hang on. The fatal hazards that befell Grok during his lifetime were entirely primitive: infections, accidents, and predators—not heart disease, diabetes, or obesity.

The advent of agriculture and civilization caused life expectancy to drop significantly, reaching a low of 18 during the Bronze Age of 3,300 B.C. to 1,200 B.C. Life expectancy remained low (between 20 and 30) through 1500 A.D. and then climbed only gradually, reaching 30 in 1800 and between 40 and 50 in 1900 in the U.S.A. and Europe. The past century has seen a dramatic increase in life span in developed countries, thanks mainly to medical advances that limit infant mortality and protect against epidemic disease.

A 2004 study by Rachel Caspari at the University of Michigan and Sang-Hee Lee at the University of California at Riverside revealed a dramatic increase in human longevity that took place during the early Upper Paleolithic Period, around 30,000 years ago. The scientists studied dental information derived from molar wear patterns of Australopithecines, *Homo erectus*, and Neanderthals and discovered a five-fold increase in the number of individuals surviving to an older age (defined by doubling reproductive age—so humans could become grandparents) around that time period.

The scientists posit, "We believe this trend contributed importantly to population expansions and cultural innovations that are associated with modernity." Elders could pass on critical life knowledge to younger generations, social networks and family bonds were strengthened, and Grok could generally become a better parent by living longer, a phenomenon known as the "grandmother hypothesis." "There has been a lot of speculation about what gave modern humans their evolutionary advantage," Caspari said. "This research provides a simple explanation for which there is now concrete evidence: modern humans were older and wiser."

[2] **Cold Water Benefits:** The healing properties of water have been recognized for thousands of years. Public baths were a common feature in ancient civilizations. The Romans, Greeks, Egyptians, Turkish, Japanese, and Chinese all believed water was helpful for muscle recovery, sleep, and immune protection. In the early 1800s, Vincent Priessnitz, an Austrian farmer, pioneered the use of hydrotherapy as a medical tool. During the mid to late 1800s, a Bavarian monk named Father Sebastian Kneipp gained wide recognition for his water therapy. He cured himself of pulmonary tuberculosis (a common and typically fatal condition referred to then as "consumption") by regularly plunging into the icy Danube River to stimulate his immune system. Kneipp wrote extensively on the subject of hydrotherapy and other natural healing topics, gaining notoriety that attracted people from across the world to visit his clinic.

Several studies support the historical anecdotes that cold water offers health benefits. One study conducted by the Thrombosis Research Institute at London's Brompton Hospital found that exposure to cold baths boosted sex hormone production and improved fertility, chronic fatigue conditions, immune function, and blood circulation, reducing cardiovascular disease risk. Numerous studies indicate that the invigorating effect of cold water stimulates the release of endorphins by the autonomic nervous system.

[3] **Napping:** Data from the National Sleep Foundation suggest that "a well-timed afternoon nap may be the best way to combat sleepiness." Gregory Belenky, M.D., Research Professor and Director of the Sleep and Performance Research Center at Washington State University, says naps can help make up for insufficient sleep. "It is even possible that divided sleep is more recuperative than sleep taken in a single block," he surmises, noting the popularity of the afternoon siesta in countries across the world. Dr. Mark Rosekind's studies with NASA pilots find that pilots who napped had a 34-percent increase in performance and a 54-percent boost in alertness that lasted for two to three hours. Harvard University studies show that 60- to 90-minute naps help the brain integrate new knowledge in the same manner as nighttime sleep, while a study published in the research journal *Sleep* suggests that naps ranging from 10 to 30 minutes are optimal for improved cognitive performance and alertness.

Sleep is actually comprised of four phases (or five, according to some scientists), each of which is theorized to contribute differently to physical and cognitive growth and restoration. Leading sleep researcher Dr. Claudio Stampi has shown that naps taken in the afternoon (a common low-energy period in our circadian rhythms) are comparatively higher in the most restorative slow-wave sleep. Morning naps are proportionately higher in REM sleep and are especially useful for boosting creativity, according to nap expert Dr. Sara Mednick."

[4] **Quality Time:** The Office of National Statistics' "Time Use Survey" indicates that today's average working parent spends 19 minutes per week of quality time with his or her child/ren free of digital distractions. Likewise, the U.S. Bureau of Labor Statistics' American Time Use Survey finds that between 2010 and 2014, the average parent spent just three minutes per day talking to their children, less than three minutes per day reading to their children, and 18 minutes per day playing or doing hobbies. This is especially disturbing in light of abundant evidence that the quality of parental interactions is more important than the quantity. (And, for the record, time spent watching TV does not count as quality time.)

Korg Family References

[5] **Commuting:** The Public Policy Institute of California reports that 18 percent of Californians commute over 45 minutes each way, with 3.4 million Americans commuting 90 minutes or more each way. U.S. Census data show that the average commute time nationwide was 25.1 minutes each way in 2009, with Californians commuting 10 percent longer than the national average. Tracy, CA, a town near the Korg's home of Stockton, had one of the longest average commute times in the state in 2000: 42 minutes each way.

In a United Kingdom survey of over 400 people by the International Stress Management Association, 44 percent said that rush-hour traffic was the most stressful part of their lives. In a separate study conducted by Hewlett Packard, UK commuters' blood pressures and heart rates were "higher than those experienced by fighter pilots going into combat and police officers facing rioting mobs." According to researchers at the New York University Sleep Disorder Center, "long commuters"—those who travel 1 hour and 15 minutes, or longer—have more sleep disorders and other health problems than the general population.

There is also a significant danger of multitasking while commuting. The Harvard Center for Risk Analysis says drivers using cell phones are responsible for 2,600 traffic deaths per year and 330,000 traffic injuries. (Motorists on the road make 40 percent of all cellular telephone calls.)

[6] **Digital Media Disturbing Sleep:** Daniel Reid's *The Tao of Health, Sex, and Longevity* details how television disturbs the ocular-endocrine system. In one study, rats exposed to invisible television rays (screen was blackened) for six hours per day became hyperactive and extremely aggressive for about a week, then suddenly become totally lethargic and stopped breeding. A Columbia University study suggests that "watching late night television may put people in a state of heightened alertness and physiological arousal, preventing them from falling asleep with ease. In addition, being exposed to many hours of the bright light of the television screen may throw people off their sleep-wake cycle, while too little physical activity may cause people to become restless and struggle with sleep."

Another study published in the journal *American Academy of Pediatrics* finds children's sleep is disturbed by watching TV before bedtime, causing them to become "over-stimulated, disturbed or frightened by the content of programs... particularly those containing violence."

[7] **Sleep Medication:** Nine million people in the United States take prescription sleep medications, according to a 2013 report from the Centers for Disease Control. Many more use over-the-counter (OTC) sleep aids. One market research firm estimated the market for OTC sleep aids to be around $759 million in 2013. This is big business. Pharmaceutical company Sanofi reported sales of Ambien to be over $158 million worldwide in the first half of 2015 (more than $37 million in the United States alone). Lunesta, which claims to be the best-selling prescription non-generic sleep aid, makes hundreds of millions of dollars annually for its parent company, Sunovion.

Daniel Kripke, University of California, San Diego psychiatry professor and author of *The Dark Side of Sleeping Pills*, conducted a revealing six-year sleep study with over one million adults. Based on the results, Kripke argues that the health risk of taking sleeping pills daily is not much different than the risk of smoking a pack of cigarettes per day! A study by researchers at Beth Israel Deaconess Medical Center and Harvard Medical School demonstrates that treating insomnia with habit and attitude modification is more effective—both immediately and over the long term—than using Ambien. The sleep success techniques Kripke recommends include: don't go to bed until you're sleepy, get up at the same time each morning, avoid excessive stimulation or worry before bed, avoid caffeine for six hours before bed, avoid alcohol before bed, and spend adequate time outdoors.

[8] **Teenage Sleep:** A 2007 Mayo Clinic report asserts that teenagers require about nine hours of sleep to maintain optimal daytime alertness, but few actually get that much sleep due to jobs, homework, friends, digital media, and other distractions. According to the National Sleep Foundation, 25 percent of teens report sleeping 6.5 hours per night or less. This is partly because many teens experience a circadian phase shift in adolescence, which means they feel sleepy later, and the time they would wake naturally is also later, but school schedules do not accommodate that routine. Adolescence is also a time when individuals feel social pressure to stay up later, especially in the age of electronics and social media.

The Mayo Clinic report also notes that sleeping in or forcing an early bedtime are not adequate solutions, since they are not aligned with the teens' unique circadian rhythm. Mayo Clinic staff suggests that parents darken rooms at the desired bedtime and expose teens to bright light in the morning, discourage naps longer than 30 minutes, discourage caffeine use, and establish a consistent, quiet relaxing routine before bed—free of digital media.

[9] **Artificial Sweeteners:** According to an online review mentioned by Dr. John Briffa, "100 percent of industry funded studies proclaim aspartame to be benign; more than 90 percent of independent studies and reports in the scientific literature say otherwise." Numerous studies suggest that intense artificial sweeteners increase appetite for sweet foods, promote overeating, and may even lead to weight gain. One Purdue University study conducted with rats concludes that "consuming a food sweetened with no-calorie saccharin can lead to greater body weight gain and adiposity than would consuming the same food sweetened with higher calorie sugar." Perhaps the only evidence we need is how obesity rates continue to climb even with the advent and increased used of artificial sweeteners in the modern diet.

[10] **Cardiovascular Exercise Heart Rates:** My position that chronic cardio is harmful and that low-level aerobic work is beneficial is based on personal experience over three decades as an elite athlete, personal trainer to clients of all ability levels, and coach to elite professional triathletes. Dr. Phil Maffetone, author of *The Big Book of Endurance Training and Racing* and coach to numerous world-champion athletes, including triathletes Mark Allen and Mike Pigg, is a leading proponent of emphasizing aerobic over anaerobic exercise and protecting health in pursuit of fitness. Maffetone's "180 minus age" formula provides a simple guideline: keep your heart rate below this number to maximize aerobic benefits during workouts and avoid injury, chronic inflammation, and other risks associated with traditional chronic cardio workout patterns. The extensive work of legendary coach Arthur Lydiard is a major influence as well. Lydiard, who pioneered the concept of overdistance endurance training for track and field athletes, developed numerous Olympic gold medalists and world record holders in his home country of New Zealand and for various other national teams.

Elite athlete/authors like former professional triathletes Mark Allen (*Total Triathlete*) and Brad Kearns (*Primal Endurance, Breakthrough Triathlon Training*), former Olympic marathon runner and popular author and speaker Jeff Galloway (from the popular series of "*Training Bibles*" for various endurance sports) all echo these fundamental principles of endurance training:

- Building a base of comfortable aerobic activity is critical for success.
- High-intensity exercise should be strictly limited to a small percentage of total exercise volume and should be conducted only when a sufficient aerobic base is established.

Conversely, the American College of Sports Medicine recommends exercise intensities of 55 to 90 percent of maximum heart rate, a ridiculously disparate range that stimulates vastly different metabolic responses in the body. Sadly, this information is widely circulated by health clubs, personal trainers, group exercise programs, books, and magazines to the detriment of the average fitness enthusiast. Regularly exceeding your aerobic maximum heart rate greatly inhibits the development of a strong aerobic base and invites increased risk of injury and burnout for everyone from novice to elite athletes.

[11] **Statin Side Effects:** A Columbia University study published in the *Archives of Neurology* suggested that even short-term statin use depletes CoQ10 levels, which is a possible explanation for common statin side effects like exercise intolerance, muscle pain, and other indicators of muscle dysfunction.

The connection between cholesterol levels and disease risk commonly echoed by conventional wisdom (leading to the popularity of cholesterol-reducing statins) is increasingly being called into question. Seventeen studies on lowering dietary cholesterol were reviewed in a 2005 *Annals of Internal Medicine* report. Overall, although subjects in the studies had an average 10 percent decrease in cholesterol levels, there was no corresponding decrease in overall risk of death.

A long-term study published in the *New England Journal of Medicine* (in 1986, 1987, and 1991) showed that people taking multiple cardiac medications have a 40 percent higher risk of mortality after four years than those who take nothing. Several other large studies (one including 10,000 European men, published in the *European Heart Journal* in 1986; another including 61,000 European men, conducted by the World Health Organization and published in *Lancet*; one involving 12,000 American men, published in the *Journal of the American Medical Association*; and a study from Finland published in the *Journal of the American Medical Association* in 1991) all reached the same conclusion: medication either increases mortality or at least doesn't increase survival time.

[12] **Walking to School:** The CDC reports that the percent of children who live within a mile of school and who walk or bike to school as their primary means of transportation has declined almost 25 percent over the past 30 years (from 87 percent to 63 percent) and that children who walk or bike from any distance has declined 26 percent (from 42 percent to 16 percent).

[13] **Patient Compliance:** Poor compliance with doctor-prescribed exercise programs is a major reason for the widespread condition of lower back pain, poor recovery from surgery, and prolonged elevated risk factors for heart disease and cancer. Study after study show high rates of non-compliance with doctors' orders among patients. Typically, the rates of non-compliance are on the order of 50 percent, with variability from study to study. Some show greater rates of non-compliance when it comes to long-term lifestyle changes, compared to short-term treatments. Poor compliance is a big problem for a number of reasons. Besides leading to poor patient outcomes, non-compliance is financially burdensome for society, according to a review by Jin and colleagues in the *Journal of Therapeutics and Clinical Risk Management*. They argue that "therapeutic non-compliance has been associated with excess urgent care visits, hospitalizations and higher treatment costs.… Additionally, besides direct financial impact, therapeutic non-compliance would have indirect cost implications due to the loss of productivity, without even mentioning the substantial negative effect on patient's quality of life."

¹⁴ **Caffeine:** The average American uses about 230 milligrams of caffeine per day according to the Mayo Clinic. Side effects of consuming too much caffeine vary by individual based on body weight, levels of physical and psychological stress, and other drug use. They can include "increased heart rate and urination, anxiety, headaches, nausea and insomnia" according to the online medical encyclopedia provided by the U.S. National Library of Medicine and the National Institutes of Health. The Mayo Clinic calls caffeine the "most popular behavior-altering drug," with 9 out of 10 Americans regularly consuming some type of caffeine.

¹⁵ **Family Finances:** A 2003 book by Elizabeth Warren and Amelia Warren Tyagi called *The Two Income Trap: Why Middle Class Mothers and Fathers Are Going Broke* details the financial challenges faced even by working families who enjoy income levels far higher (even adjusting for today's dollar) than previous generations. While many blame the "affluenza" mentality (the widespread cultural ill of excessive consumption habits detailed in John De Graaf's book of the same name) for the middle class's financial challenges, Warren and Tyagi convincingly make the case that the larger, less optional expenses are the biggest culprit. Childcare, car payments, college tuition, and suburban homes prices result in millions living in financial distress. The cost of homes sold to families with children skyrocketed 79 percent in inflation-adjusted dollars from 1983 to 1998. The two income couple (comprising some three-quarters of all married couples) is a key component of the skyrocketing inflation of suburban home prices over the past 25 years. Hence, a vicious circle emerges: home prices rise because many two-income couples can afford them... because they have two incomes! This sounds like "keeping up with the Joneses" times 127 million.

The *New York Times* revealed in 2003 that a "typical household" (two income earners and one or two children—a demographic responsible for half the nation's personal consumption expenditures) making between $60,000 and $80,000 per year spent 70 to 75 percent of its take home pay on essentials such as home costs, groceries, vehicles and fuel, education, and health care. The authors of *The Two Income Trap* point out that the figure for these expenses was only 54 percent in the early 1970s. Furthermore, the remaining 25 percent of disposable income, typically categorized as "discretionary," is further eaten up by expenses that might be better defined as "essential" due to social pressures and norms: cell phones, cable or satellite TV, Internet service, high-definition TV sets, and digital entertainment like iPods. Arguably the category could extend to fashion, cosmetics, and popular diversions such as movies and vacations.

¹⁶ **Childhood Obesity:** Data from a large, nationally representative sample, published in the *Journal of the American Medical Association*, show that in 2012, 31.8 percent of youths (ages two to 19) were overweight, with 16.9 percent qualifying as obese. This number has been steadily growing; the CDC reports that childhood obesity has doubled among children and tripled among adolescents in the past three decades. Multiple research studies find that obese youth are at increased risk for cardiovascular disease, diabetes, bone and joint problems, and sleep disorders. They are also at greater risk for psychosocial problems.

¹⁷ **Children's Recreation:** There is abundant data to show that the way children spend their leisure time has changed substantially in the past several decades, and it continues to change with the ever-increasing availability of portable digital media. For example, in a longitudinal study by Juster and colleagues out of the University of Michigan, the time children (ages 6 to 17) spent engaging in sports and outdoor leisure in an average week declined by about a third between 1981 and 2002/3. Research by Sandra Hofferth shows that from the 1980s to 2000s, children have tended toward more structured activities at the expense of free, outdoor play. At the same time, media consumption continues to increase. The Kaiser Family Foundation reports, for example, that between 2004 and 2009, kids aged 8 to 18 increased their average daily consumption of music, TV, computers, and video games, but not print (reading). The average daily media exposure went from 7 hours 29 minutes in 1999 to 8 hours 33 minutes in 2004 to 10 hours 45 minutes in 2009, when including all the time kids spent multitasking.

¹⁸ **Massive Multiplayer Online Role-Playing Games:** The popularity has skyrocketed from zero in 1998 (due to poor graphics quality, slow Internet connections, and a consequent lack of interest) to an estimated 30 to 60 million active users in 2007, and to an estimated 628 million in 2013, according to Giga Omni Media, GlobalCollect, and NewZoo. Some consider this a vast underestimate, due to millions of Chinese playing in Internet cafés for four cents per hour but not registering as paid monthly subscribers. One survey published on Adpoll.com reports that 45 percent of kids play for 10 or more hours per week.

¹⁹ **ADHD Prescriptions:** Diagnosis rates of Attention Deficit Hyperactivity Disorder (ADHD) have skyrocketed 500 percent since 1991, according to the Drug Enforcement Administration. An estimated seven million schoolchildren are being treated with stimulants for ADHD, including 10 percent of all 10-year-old American boys, according to an article published in the *Journal of the American Medical Association*.

A 1998 study by researchers Adrian Angold and E. Jane Costello argued that the majority of children and adolescents who receive stimulants for ADHD do not fully meet the criteria for ADHD. The efforts of neurologist Dr. Fred Baughman, ADHD diagnosis critic, led to admissions from the FDA, DEA, Novartis (manufacturer of Ritalin), and top ADHD researchers around the country that "no objective validation of the diagnosis of ADHD exists." A Maryland Department of Education study showed that white, suburban elementary school children are using medication for ADHD at more than twice the rate of African American students.

²⁰ **Life Expectancy of Today's Child:** A 2005 report published in the *New England Journal of Medicine* suggests that the prevalence of obesity is shortening average life span by a greater rate than accidents, homicides, and suicides combined. Children today will lose some two to five years of life expectancy due to the prevalence and earlier onset of obesity-related diseases like type 2 diabetes, heart disease, kidney failure, and cancer. Dr. David S. Ludwig, director

of the obesity program at Children's Hospital in Boston, says in the report, "Obesity is such that this generation of children could be the first basically in the history of the United States to live less healthful and shorter lives than their parents. There is an unprecedented increase in prevalence of obesity at younger and younger ages without much obvious public health impact. But when they start developing heart attack, stroke, kidney failures, amputations, blindness, and ultimately death at younger ages, then that could be a huge effect on life expectancy."

[21] **American Television:** A.C. Nielsen reports that the average American watches 28 hours of TV per week and that 66 percent of households have three or more televisions at home. In the aforementioned Kaiser Family Foundation study, children between the ages of 8 and 18 spent four and a half hours per day watching television in 2009, and even more watching movies, playing video games, and using the computer.

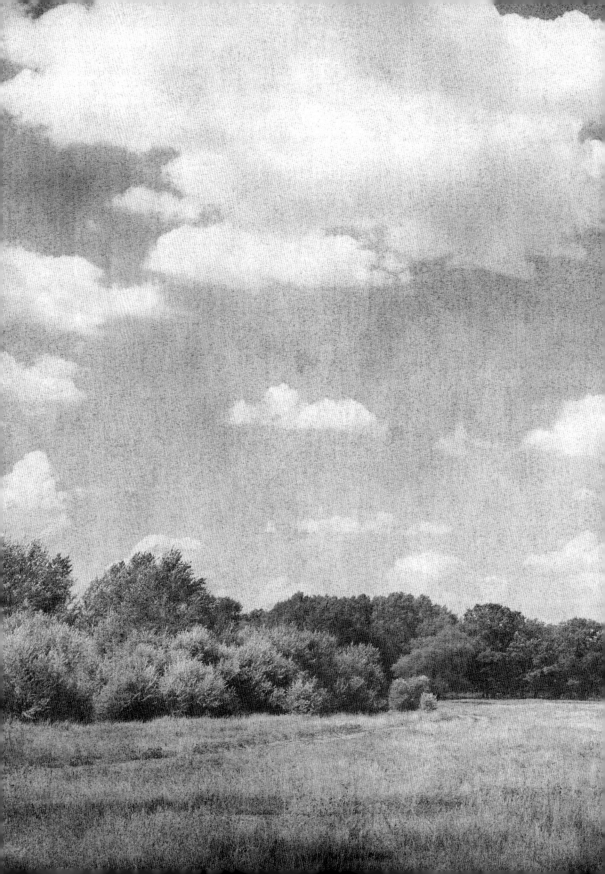

CHAPTER THREE

THE PRIMAL BLUEPRINT EATING PHILOSOPHY

"Do These Genes Make Me Look Fat?"

IN THIS CHAPTER

I present the philosophy, rationale, and benefits of eating Primal Blueprint style, emphasizing the importance of moderating insulin production and improving insulin sensitivity by limiting the intake of processed carbohydrates, which means not only sugars, but also cultivated grains (yep, even whole grains). This simple dietary modification—perhaps the single most critical takeaway action item from the Primal Blueprint—will allow you to avoid the unpleasant physical and mental effects of modern high-carbohydrate eating, succeed with long-term weight-loss goals, and prevent the most common lifestyle-related health problems and diseases.

You will learn why the conventional wisdom assertion that cholesterol is a direct heart disease risk factor is deeply flawed. The true culprits that trigger the development of atherosclerosis are oxidation and inflammation, created largely by the Standard American Diet of processed carbohydrates and refined industrial vegetable/seed oils and partially hydrogenated oils. I detail the dietary steps you can take to prevent systemic inflammation and virtually eliminate your risk of heart disease.

The concept of "eating well" means more than just making healthy food choices; it means eating sensibly and intuitively, in a relaxed environment conducive to maximum appreciation of food, and it means avoiding regimented, restrictive diets that lead to negativity, guilt, rebellion, and usually failure. Finally, I offer tips on how to succeed in converting to Primal Blueprint-style eating without causing the stress or disappointment that are so common with unrealistic diet programs.

Primal Blueprint-style eating offers many health benefits, which served Grok and his ancestors well for 2.5 million years. The most important goal of eating like Grok is to minimize the wildly excessive insulin production caused by the Standard American Diet. Making this simple change will allow you to lose unwanted fat, maintain an ideal body composition for the rest of your life, and virtually eliminate the major disease risk factors that will kill more than half of all Americans. Here are some other major benefits of the Primal Blueprint eating style:

Becoming a Fat-Burning Beast: When you reduce your consumption of grains, sugars, and other simple carbohydrates in favor of plants and animals, you will optimize your level of insulin production, enabling you to utilize fatty acids from both food intake and stored fat as your preferred fuel source. Being insulin-balanced helps regulate daily energy levels, even if you skip meals. In contrast, excess insulin production from a sugar-burner diet requires that you eat every few hours to bump up blood glucose levels that have crashed.

Effortless Weight Management: Plants and animals are much more nutritionally dense than processed-carbohydrate foods and refined vegetable oils, which comprise a large percentage of calories in the Standard American Diet. Eat like Grok, and you'll meet your nutritional needs with fewer calories and dramatically boost your antioxidant intake. Moreover, the protein and fat you will be eating provide deeper and longer-lasting satisfaction levels—more satiety—than you get from a diet high in refined carbs. Finally, consuming fewer processed carbohydrates results in less insulin production, thus causing your hunger and cravings to moderate. Remember, the crash-and-burn effect is due to your body constantly cycling back and forth from consuming carbohydrates, burning it as glucose, then kicking out insulin to moderate blood glucose, which results in you feeling lethargic, hungry, and looking for a quick fix. Stopping that cycle by reducing the intake of carbs, especially simple carbs, is important to moderate your energy and hunger levels so that you can eat intuitively rather than in response to the crash-and-burn effect of the Standard American Diet.

Enhanced Cellular Function: The high-quality fats found in primal foods provide structural components for cell membranes and encourage your body to convert stored fat efficiently into energy. This includes the well-known omega-3s (mainly from oily, cold-water fish); monounsaturated fats from avocados, macadamia nuts, olives, and extra virgin olive oil; strategically-chosen polyunsaturated fats from nuts and seeds; and even the saturated fats from animal and coconut products that conventional wisdom has warned us to avoid.

Lean Muscle Development and Maintenance: The high-quality protein found in primal foods will help you build lean muscle mass, achieve healthy bone density, and control your body's day-to-day repair and renewal requirements. When you moderate insulin production, exercise sensibly, and eat adequate amounts of protein, you become more insulin sensitive. This means the receptor sites in your muscle cells can assimilate amino acids and glucose efficiently, which is the key to muscle building and recovery.

Reduced Disease Risk Factors: Ditching grains, sugars, other simple carbs, and processed foods, especially "bad fats" (refined vegetable/seed oils and trans and partially hydrogenated oils), will reduce your production of hormone-like messengers that instruct genes to make harmful pro-inflammatory protein agents. These agents increase your risk for arthritis, diabetes, cancer, heart disease, and many other inflammation-related health problems.

Obesity is really widespread.
—Joseph O. Kern II

A SEPARATE SHELF FOR THE BLUEPRINT

You may be familiar with the decades-old Atkins diet program named after Dr. Robert Atkins, the original proponent of "low-carb" dieting. Over the years, numerous other programs (e.g., South Beach and the Zone) have battled for shelf-space supremacy. Diet best-sellers have varied from mostly credible to completely ridiculous propositions. Followers of Atkins and other low-carb diets will indeed lose fat by strictly limiting carbohydrates and thus moderating insulin production. However, an obsessive ultra-low-carb strategy can be unhealthy over an extended time period because it limits your intake of some of the most nutritional foods known to humans—vegetables and fruits. Furthermore, high-calorie-burning, low-body-fat, highly insulin sensitive folks, as well as females with certain hormonal irregularities, might not respond well to one-size-fits-all carb restriction protocols.

While the Primal Blueprint also advocates eliminating the extremely harmful processed carbohydrates and sugars from your diet, vegetables and (some) fruits are central components of the Primal Blueprint eating strategy. Vegetables and fruits (which consist mainly of carbohydrates) are nutrient dense yet calorically sparse, so even generous portions of these foods will not provoke a high insulin response. What's more, the extra energy required to digest the complex carbohydrate and highly fibrous nature of vegetables is such that you need not even count the carbohydrate grams in vegetables toward your daily goals based on the Primal Blueprint Carbohydrate Curve. Fruits are a bit different and require a bit of moderation in today's world of year-round availability and excess dietary carb intake in general—

especially if you are trying to reduce excess body fat. I discuss this topic in detail in the next chapter.

One of the online *Primal Blueprint* appendices at MarksDailyApple.com compares and contrasts the Primal Blueprint with popular diets such as Atkins, Low Fat (e.g., Ornish, McDougall, Pritikin), Metabolic and Blood Typing, paleo-themed diets, South Beach, Vegetarian, and the Zone. Of all these mentioned, the paleo eating approach is the most similar to the Primal Blueprint. However, I refrain from even calling the Primal Blueprint a "diet" due to its comprehensive nature. The Primal Blueprint is a lifestyle—with some important but extremely flexible eating guidelines. I prefer to apply the eating laws in conjunction with the other eight Primal Blueprint lifestyle laws for best results.

---

80 PERCENT OF YOUR BODY COMPOSITION IS DETERMINED BY HOW YOU EAT

The Primal Blueprint eating philosophy might seem a little unusual at first for those trying to do the right thing by conventional wisdom. After all, here's a plan that suggests that healthy fat should be the centerpiece of your diet, while supposedly "healthy" whole grains should be eliminated. In fact, one might describe the Primal Blueprint as a high-fat, moderate-protein, fairly low-carb diet—particularly in comparison to the exceedingly grain-heavy diet that has been endorsed for years by the USDA Food Pyramid and Food Plate visuals, the American Heart Association, and the American Medical Association.

We now know that the outdated and unwarranted recommendation to eat 300 or more grams of (mostly grain-based) carbohydrates each day has contributed greatly to the destruction of human health. It's not unusual for an average American, and for people in other countries following a Western-style diet, to consume 500 or 600 grams of insulin-generating, fat-promoting carbohydrates daily. Furthermore, a large proportion of these carbohydrates are likely refined, meaning they have been processed in some way that increases the severity of the glucose spike and requisite insulin response. White flour and high fructose corn syrup are two prominent examples of refined carbohydrates that are rampant in the Standard American Diet. They have no real nutritional value and can promote inflammation and oxidative damage when they are consumed regularly.

Keep in mind that Grok and his clan probably worked hard to gather natural carbohydrates like fruits, vegetables, and starchy tubers—unrefined, fibrous, slow-burning food with excellent nutritional value. While intake likely fluctuated greatly by season, our ancestors rarely ate over 100 grams of carbs per day, and in some cases/locations, they were able to survive for long periods of time on extremely minimal carbohydrate intake (for unlike fat and protein, carb consumption is not required for human survival).

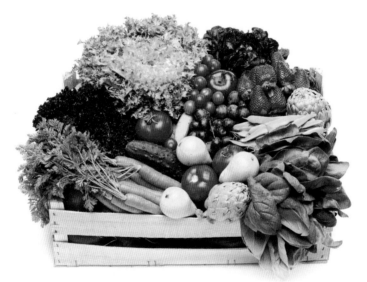

By averaging between 100 and 150 grams daily (certain folks may adjust this upward, which I'll discuss later) of vegetable- or fruit-based carbs; high-nutrient-value carbs like sweet potatoes, wild rice, and quinoa; and incidental carbs from nuts, seeds, and moderation foods such as high-fat dairy and high-cacao dark chocolate, you can achieve stable levels of insulin and other appetite and metabolic hormones, enjoy sustained energy levels, reduce excess body fat, and maintain a healthy weight. If you want to accelerate your fat loss for a period of time, lowering your average carb intake to 50 to 100 grams or less per day will allow you to easily drop an average of one to two pounds (one-half to one kilogram) of body fat per week. We will discuss this strategy in detail in Chapter 9. And you can do all this while eating until you're satisfied—no suffering!

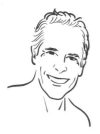

MARK TALK ——————————————————

Sitting down? Here's another zinger that will blow your mind and set you straight about the secret to weight loss and long-term body composition success: *Eighty percent of your ability to reduce excess body fat is determined by how you eat, with the other 20 percent depending on proper exercise, other healthy lifestyle habits, and genetic factors.*

It's as simple as this: if you have excess body fat, it's directly reflective of the amount of insulin you produce from your diet *combined with* your familial genetic predisposition to store fat. In plain-speak, if you eat like crap and have bad (genetic) luck, you'll get fat and sick and you'll probably die early. On the other hand, having a bad diet and good luck (carrying the "skinny gene") might allow you to avoid a plump figure, but it also might result in a physique that health experts refer to as "skinny fat"—having minimal subcutaneous fat, minimal lean body mass, and poor muscle definition, but with dangerous amounts of visceral fat surrounding the organs.

Furthermore, skinny fat folks can and do get heart disease, hypoglycemia, arthritis, sarcopenia (loss of muscle mass), chronic fatigue, compromised immune function, exhausted stress-management mechanisms, and a host of other adverse health consequences heavily attributed to diet. A slender type 2 diabetic might experience an even greater risk for serious disease because he or she is less able to activate the so-called "thrifty genes" that efficiently store excess dietary glucose in fat cells, and as a result, that glucose floats around in the bloodstream causing intense cellular damage. While the overall impact of poor lifestyle habits, including outward physique, vary widely due to luck of the draw, we all share an evolutionary genetic predisposition to suffer chronic disease when we eat foods that are misaligned with our genes.

On the positive side, if you eat right, you can look your absolute best even if you possess a genetic predisposition to store more fat than your workout partner. Your ability to reduce excess body fat and maintain desirable body composition is directly related to your ability to moderate insulin production with healthy dietary habits, to reduce inflammation (a contributor to insulin resistance), and, to a lesser extent, follow a sensible exercise program that combines extensive low-level cardio, frequent brief, intense strength-training sessions, and occasional all-out sprints. We can't all have Gisele Bündchen's or David Beckham's body, but we can all unlock the best versions of ourselves by making good—and relatively easy—lifestyle decisions. Even if you have struggled with excess body fat for your entire life, you can quickly and dramatically alter your destiny by following the simple laws of the Primal Blueprint.

I'm not talking about achieving "success" with a short-term crash program. The Primal Blueprint is based on eating as much as you want, whenever you want, choosing your favorites from a long list of delicious approved foods, and simply avoiding eating foods from a different list. When I say you will notice quick and dramatic results, I'm referring primarily to the immediate increase and stabilization of energy levels, reduced hunger and fewer mood swings related to "bonking" (running low on blood glucose), improved immune function, and a reduction in the symptoms of allergies, arthritis, and other inflammatory conditions exacerbated by the anti-nutrients in a grain-based diet.

Regarding weight loss, we must recognize that our views are so messed up on this topic that it's hard even to have a sensible conversation about it. The stories of losing massive amounts of weight in a short time are so commonplace that we seem to expect nothing less when we pursue weight-loss goals. First, the Primal Blueprint is really about optimizing body composition, instead of just reducing your weight on the scale. For most, this means a reduction in body fat percentage and an increase or maintenance of muscle or lean body mass. Clearly, gaining muscle and losing fat produces more impressive appearance changes than dropping 20 quick pounds on a crash diet that depletes muscle mass and water retention. Lean body mass (muscle, skeleton, and all the rest of you that is not fat) is also directly correlated with "organ reserve," the highly desirable ability of all your vital organs to function effectively beyond basal level (the minimum functional or effective level; for example, when your heart rate elevates during exercise). We'll discuss this critical longevity component in Chapter 7.

When you trigger your genes to stop storing body fat and start burning it, as well as to build or maintain an optimal amount of muscle mass, you can sensibly and realistically lose a pound or two of body fat per week if you are currently storing excess body fat. You can even do this with minimal exercise, but the fat loss (and the gaining, sculpting, or toning of lean muscle) will be accelerated significantly when you choose the right exercise regimen. Mostly, your success depends on how diligent you are in keeping your insulin levels moderated, thereby allowing your body to obtain more of your caloric needs from your stored body fat.

You can alter your biochemistry at each meal—to stimulate a fat-burning metabolism and maintain consistent energy levels, or to do the opposite with poor food choices.

Not a day goes by without a friend, client, or MarksDailyApple.com commenter relating to me how he or she notices improvements within days of switching to the Primal Blueprint eating style. As I will detail in this chapter, you have the chance to alter your biochemistry at each meal—to stimulate a fat-burning metabolism and maintain consistent energy levels, or to do the opposite with poor food choices. The momentum you build with good choices will make it easier to discard old habits because you experience instant gratification from satisfying meals and stable energy levels, as well as positive long-term health and metabolic consequences.

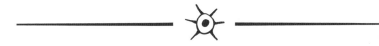

MORE THAN ONE WAY TO SKIN A CAT: THE PARADOXICAL SUCCESS OF LOW-FAT EATING

At this point in history, it's clear that the type of low-fat diet prescribed by the USDA, American Heart Association, and similar organizations has been a dismal failure. Heart disease remains a potent killer, diabetes rates continue to climb, and America—and the West at large—is no closer to beating the obesity epidemic than we were 40 years ago (actually, the population is fatter than ever), when low-fat advisories became public policy. Pushing our fat intake down to 30 percent of total calories has, it seems, done more harm than good.

Yet there remains a paradox in the nutrition community's ongoing macronutrient wars: the success of extremely low-fat diets such as those espoused by Dean Ornish, John McDougall, Rip and Caldwell Esselstyn, Nathan Pritikin, and Neal Barnard. By keeping fat intake to a rigid 10 percent of calories or lower (and emphasizing whole, unprocessed plant foods as dietary staples), these low-fat proponents claim success in treating obesity, heart disease, diabetes, and other modern chronic diseases, with a fair amount of published research supporting as much. Hold the toast! How could extremely low-fat diets yield any success when moderately low-fat diets have been so disastrous?

The answer lies in the intriguing ability for extreme fat restriction to improve insulin sensitivity and reduce the chance of post-meal fat storage. For one, in the context of a nearly fat-free meal, the insulin spikes following carbohydrate ingestion don't have any dietary fat to shove into cells, making fat gain less likely. Second, when dietary fat is combined with a hefty carbohydrate intake, the result can be that it takes more insulin to result in fat storage for that particular meal. Take away the fat in these instances, and carbohydrate metabolism improves.

Does this mean that extremely low-fat diets are a smart move for your health? Not so fast. While these diets do claim some clinical success in terms of weight loss, they're also low in (or devoid of) the important fat-soluble vitamins A, D, and K2. They can also result in essential fatty acid deficiency, are scarce in animal-based nutrients, and aren't anywhere near as satiating as a higher-fat, real-food primal diet. Likewise, their efficacy may be limited to a small number of individuals who are highly responsive to low-fat diets. And finally, a recent review of 53 published scientific studies orchestrated by researchers at Brigham and Women's Hospital and the Harvard School of Public Health found that low-fat diets were not more effective than other types of dietary interventions in terms of long-term (greater than one year) weight loss.

That being said, short-term bouts of very low-fat, high-carbohydrate eating—especially when those carbs are of the nutrient-dense primal variety—can work as a "hack" to break through weight-loss stalls, restore some insulin sensitivity, reboot hormone levels, and flood gut flora with beneficial starches and fibers. The so-called "Potato Hack," for instance, has gained popularity on Mark's Daily Apple forums. This consists of eating two to three pounds of cooked and cooled potatoes (and little else—sorry, no butter on those spuds) for several days or a week as a way to rapidly shed body fat. Along with serving as a carb refeed after periods of lower carbohydrate intake, this type of strategy can provide healthy gut microbes with an abundance of resistant starch (discussed in Chapter 5), helping rekindle the beneficial bacterial strains whose food source dwindles on a low-carb menu.

All in all, I am still convinced that a primal eating strategy containing plenty of healthy fats from both animal and plant sources is your best bet for long-term health. However, the human body is adapted to—and even expects—sporadic changes in dietary patterns. Brief windows of very low-fat eating (or its inverse, ketosis, which we'll cover in chapter 4) can be a fine component of a primal eating framework, and may even offer some benefits.

INSULIN—THE MASTER HORMONE

The insulin story is perhaps the most health-critical concept in the book, so I want you to fully understand it on both a practical and a biochemical level. A primary goal of the Primal Blueprint is to help you moderate insulin production and improve insulin sensitivity, both markers of metabolic health that will help you avoid many of the health scourges of modern society. To understand insulin, you first have to understand blood glucose. When you eat carbohydrates (starches: grains and legumes, and sugars: both processed sugars such as granulated sugar and sugars naturally occurring in fruits and vegetables), your digestive system breaks them down into their components, one of which is glucose. Glucose is delivered from your stomach and small intestine into the bloodstream, where it travels around providing fuel for your cells. When you hear the term "blood sugar," this actually refers to the amount of glucose in your blood (which is why I use the term "blood glucose" to be more accurate). Your body can burn glucose quickly and efficiently for energy, so it is the first choice for fuel when it is available. While glucose is a critical component of the body's energy system, it is toxic if it remains in the bloodstream for too long and in quantities that are too high, so it must be moved to its destination quickly. Insulin is quite literally the key to this system.

Insulin is a hormone secreted by beta cells in the pancreas in response to elevated blood glucose (as happens after a meal containing carbohydrates). Cell receptors use insulin as a key to unlock glucose channels in the membrane of each cell. With the cell "door" open, glucose can be stored inside the cell (along with other nutrients whose transport into the cell is potentiated by insulin). Any glucose that isn't needed immediately for energy is shuttled into storage for future use, first in muscle or liver cells as glycogen, or in adipose (fat) cells as triglycerides. It's an elegant way for cells to gather the fuel they need while eliminating excess glucose from the bloodstream. It's also how the body prepares itself to have sufficient energy supplies even in times of famine (which would have been inevitable for Grok, but for most of us, not so much).

In order to stay healthy and to avoid medical problems that are rampant in modern society such as heart disease, Metabolic Syndrome, obesity, type 2 diabetes, certain cancers, and hyperglycemia or hyperinsulemia, it is absolutely critical that you remain *insulin sensitive*. That simply means that insulin is able to do its job opening the figurative cell doors for glucose.

INSULIN SENSITIVITY: A LITTLE GOES A LONG WAY

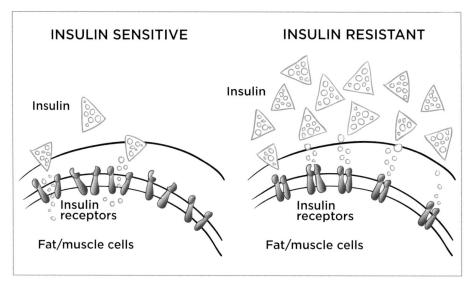

Insulin works on cell receptors to deliver precious cargo including glycogen that is frequently depleted by exercise.

To promote insulin sensitivity, the most important factor is a diet such as the one laid out in this book that helps the body maintain relatively stable, moderate insulin levels. Unfortunately, the typical modern diet is basically made up of one glucose bomb after another, in the form of breads, pastas, cereals, pastries, sweets, and even supposedly healthy foods like smoothies, trail mix, and meal replacement bars, many of which contain tons of added sugar, milk chocolate, processed corn products, and so on. Bombarding their systems in this way has many Americans on a glucose-insulin roller coaster that results in the short term in glucose spikes and crashes, increased insulin production, cravings, irritability, and weight gain, and in the long term, chronic disease.

Exercise is also instrumental for promoting insulin sensitivity, and this is another area where too many people fall short. The average person can only store a total of about 400 grams (less than one pound) of glycogen in liver and muscle tissue. (Even a highly trained athlete can only store perhaps 600 total grams.) If you frequently empty your liver and muscle cells of glycogen with brief, intense workouts, frequent low-level movement, and structured aerobic sessions, you become adept at not only burning stored energy, but also replenishing glycogen (as well as amino acids, whose metabolism is also facilitated by insulin). In this case, insulin will deliver nutrients to your liver and muscles instead of just having them go straight to fat. If you are sedentary and eat a moderate- or high-carbohydrate diet, there is no selection pressure (to borrow an apropos term from our evolution discussion) to be insulin sensitive. My foolproof prevention plan or, dare I say, cure for those with type 2 diabetes, obesity, and heart disease, no matter how overwhelming their genetic predisposition to these conditions, is to moderate dietary insulin production and exercise according to the Primal Blueprint laws.

Sadly, a grain- and sugar-heavy diet coupled with chronic inactivity has put many people on the path to *insulin resistance* instead of insulin sensitivity. The human body simply is not designed to process the amount of glucose most people dump into it day after day. For a little while, your system can cope with a poor diet and bad (or non-existent) exercise routine, although you might not like its coping strategy: converting excess ingested glucose into triglycerides in the liver and storing these triglycerides in fat cells throughout the body. Remember, although the first thing insulin wants to do with any glucose that your body doesn't immediately need is to store it as glycogen in muscle and liver cells, that has a finite capacity. Inactive folks generally have plenty of muscle and liver glycogen stored at all times, so insulin takes any carbs they ingest on an express train to their ultimate destination in fat cells. On top of that, when blood insulin levels are high, those same fat cells store not only excess glucose (as triglycerides) but also the fat you ate at your last meal.

Eventually, the strain of having chronically high glucose and insulin circulating around leads to the problem of insulin resistance, wherein cells (first muscle and liver, and then fat cells) are not receptive to insulin trying to unlock them in order to shuttle glucose out of the bloodstream. The pancreas then has to pump out even more insulin to try to get the job done, leading to a harmful cycle of insulin overproduction (resulting, eventually, in chronic hyperinsulinemia). Just as blood glucose is desirable as long as it is regulated but can be toxic if it exceeds normal levels, a moderate amount of insulin in the bloodstream is good, but a lot can be bad... very bad. The more insulin your pancreas produces to deal with excessive carbohydrate intake, the more resistant your muscle and liver cells can get. This happens because the genes responsible for these receptor sites turn themselves off, or "downregulate," in response to—and in defense against—the excessive energy that insulin is trying to shuttle into your cells. This is all part of the body's quest for balance and your genetic response to environmental signals.

Furthermore, the "do not enter" sign hanging on the liver due to insulin resistance tricks some cells in your liver into believing they are starved for glucose (which, if it were true, would be a big problem because the brain preferentially uses glucose for fuel, and a few specific types of cells, such as red blood cells, rely exclusively on glucose). In response to the liver's storage cells refusing to accept glucose, your genes signal other specialized liver cells to commence gluconeogenesis (the conversion of lean muscle tissue or ingested protein into glucose for quick energy) and dump more glucose into the bloodstream, despite the fact that there's already plenty there. Talk about a communication breakdown! Of course, your resistant muscle cells are deaf to insulin signaling as well, so the new, extra glucose your liver just made is also diverted to the eager fat cells, unless they, too, are overgorged with fat.

Taken to the extreme, as with a morbidly obese individual, even fat cells become resistant to further storage, because we only have a fixed number of fat cells. At that point, the body's last line of defense against the damage inflicted (quickly) by excess blood glucose has maxed out, in which case the glucose stays in your blood stream. Consequently, all hell breaks loose in terms of blood glucose toxicity and insulin damage, leading to even greater risk for type 2 diabetes (if it hasn't already developed, which it likely has), heart attack, blindness, the need for limb amputation, and other disasters.

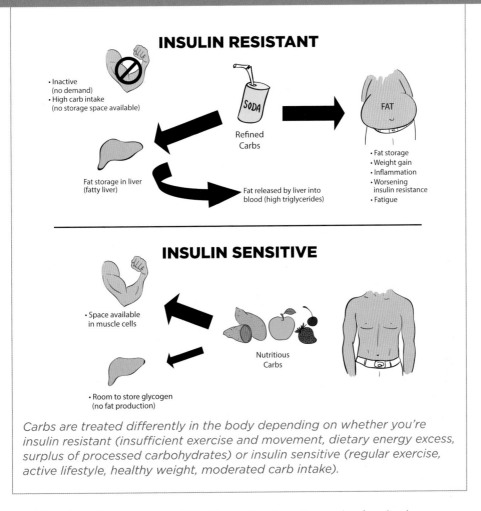

INSULIN RESISTANT

- Inactive (no demand)
- High carb intake (no storage space available)

SODA

Refined Carbs

FAT

- Fat storage
- Weight gain
- Inflammation
- Worsening insulin resistance
- Fatigue

Fat storage in liver (fatty liver)

Fat released by liver into blood (high triglycerides)

INSULIN SENSITIVE

- Space available in muscle cells

Nutritious Carbs

- Room to store glycogen (no fat production)

Carbs are treated differently in the body depending on whether you're insulin resistant (insufficient exercise and movement, dietary energy excess, surplus of processed carbohydrates) or insulin sensitive (regular exercise, active lifestyle, healthy weight, moderated carb intake).

This doesn't mean your daily PowerBar is going to lead to limb amputation any time soon, but as you gain further understanding of the insulin story, it becomes clear how the shocking statistic of the average American gaining one and a half pounds of fat (two-thirds of a kilo) a year for 30 years is achieved. It is quite easy to slide down the slippery slope of insulin resistance and end up with a host of medical problems, many of which doctors are just coming to understand are tied to insulin resistance.

In case you aren't already convinced, let's take a look at some more of the unpleasant consequences of having chronically elevated blood glucose and insulin levels and of becoming insulin resistant:

Fat cells get bigger, and you get fatter. In addition to glucose and dietary fat being delivered straightaway to adipose tissue deposits, you become less able to burn fat for energy. Insulin inhibits the fat-burning enzyme lipase, so fat cells can't release their stored energy into the bloodstream where the fatty acids could be used as fuel. So not only do you store more fat, the fat remains locked in storage.

Advanced glycation end products (AGEs) result from chemical reactions that occur when blood-borne glucose molecules bind randomly with important structural proteins used by your organs and systems, causing long-term damage. A familiar example is the wrinkling of the skin. Yes, aging and sun damage are factors, but so are AGEs. AGEs are also culprits in increased inflammation and risk of heart disease, as well as the circulation problems and neuropathies (nervous system disorders) that characterize type 2 diabetes. When glucose is not efficiently shuttled out of the blood, AGE damage can result.

Pancreatic beta cells start facing glucolipotoxicity from being overexposed to chronically high levels of glucose and free fatty acids. This leads to impaired insulin secretion, beta cell death (apoptosis), and—when other genetic and environmental factors are in place—the progression of type 2 diabetes.

Accelerated aging is associated with chronically excessive insulin production, which is dangerously pro-inflammatory and can wreak havoc throughout the body. Scientists know that within any species, those that produce the least amount of insulin over a lifetime generally live the longest and remain the healthiest.

Excessive insulin is also now believed to be a central catalyst in the development of atherosclerosis. Insulin promotes platelet adhesiveness (sticky platelets clot more readily) and the conversion of macrophages (a type of white blood cell) into foam cells, which are the cells that fill with cholesterol and accumulate in arterial walls. Eventually, a cholesterol and fat-filled "tumor" blocks circulation in the artery, a situation further aggravated by increased platelet adhesiveness and thickness of the blood. In addition, insulin and the aforementioned AGEs interfere with the production and activity of a compound called nitric oxide (NO). NO performs the critical function of keeping the endothelial cell wall—the lining of your arteries—relaxed and flexible, as well as inhibiting platelet adhesion and other mechanisms that contribute to atherosclerosis. Low NO causes your artery walls to become more rigid, which drives up blood pressure and increases the sheer force of blood against the arterial wall, further exacerbating the atherosclerotic condition. I will further detail the chain of events causing atherosclerosis and what you can do to prevent it in the cholesterol section later in this chapter.

Levels of growth hormone and other important health-enhancing hormones are also adversely affected by insulin resistance. The pituitary gland makes growth hormone, which is then sent to the liver to signal the production of insulin-like growth factors (IGFs). Many of our cells have surface receptors for IGFs. Because of its similar structure, insulin binds to IGF receptors and prevents growth-hormone-stimulated IGFs from doing their job.

High insulin levels over long periods of time also hamper sex hormone synthesis, causing levels of testosterone, DHEA, and other sex hormones to decline steeply as we age. Hormone levels naturally decline over time, but this flagship premise of the multi-billion-dollar anti-aging industry is very likely exacerbated by insulin resistance as opposed to the mere passing of the seasons. Remember, if Grok was lucky, he could enjoy dramatically better health and physical fitness into his seventies than most of today's baby boomers. Sex hormones are supposed to be transported through the bloodstream by globulin (a blood protein) to act upon target organs and tissues. When excessive insulin is present, these hormones can stay bound to globulin instead of getting dropped off at the target cells (e.g., the adrenal glands, sex organs, and brain). Even an expensive anti-aging hormone regimen cannot override this undesirable condition caused by excessive insulin.

Thyroid function is disrupted by excessive insulin. The thyroid gland produces a hormone called T4 which is converted in the liver to T3, the primary hormone that controls energy metabolism. When your liver becomes insulin resistant, conversion of T4 to T3 declines drastically.

This leads to a decrease in metabolic rate, increased fat storage, and diminished energy levels and brain function.

Hopefully by now you are convinced of the importance of insulin sensitivity and are sufficiently troubled by the possibility of becoming insulin resistant. Clearly, insulin is absolutely essential to life; it's just that chronic overproduction of insulin turns a good thing into a bad thing. Luckily, research suggests that insulin resistance can be addressed quickly by reducing carbohydrate intake and increasing activity levels. It's as simple as this: when you eat the Primal Blueprint-style foods that fit your genes, you'll be able to fit into your jeans!

But a Little Bit Won't Hurt, Right?

If these clinical details about the long-term damage from a high-insulin-producing diet are not sufficient to get you to change your breakfast order today, consider the short-term unpleasant effects of high-carbohydrate, insulin-producing meals and snacks (on otherwise healthy, non-diabetic folks).

Ingesting high-carbohydrate food (sugary foods and beverages, desserts, processed grains, etc.) generates an immediate increase in blood glucose levels, which has the short-term effect of elevating your mood, energy level, and alertness. In a matter of minutes, however, your pancreas secretes a requisite amount of insulin to quickly remove any excess glucose from the bloodstream before it becomes toxic. Depending on the type and amount of carbs you consumed and your degree of insulin sensitivity, this insulin rush can eventually cause your blood glucose levels to decline so much that your glucose-dependent brain soon becomes low on fuel. As a result, you may feel sluggish, foggy, and cranky, and have trouble focusing. While this explains the familiar post-lunch afternoon blues and grogginess, extensive data also suggest a strong link between processed carbohydrate consumption/insulin production and attention deficit/hyperactivity disorder (ADHD) and assorted other cognitive disorders.

Additionally, the ingestion of lots of carbohydrates, followed by the secretion of lots of insulin (and, subsequently, low blood glucose levels), is interpreted as a stressful event by the hypothalamic-pituitary-adrenal (HPA) axis. This homeostasis-monitoring part of your endocrine system (responsible for the fight or flight response) signals your adrenal glands to release epinephrine (adrenaline) and cortisol (the "stress hormone") into your bloodstream to cope with the perceived stress. Cortisol breaks down precious muscle tissue into amino acids, some of which are sent to the liver and converted into glucose through gluconeogenesis. The ensuing blood glucose rush gives you the boost your brain thinks you need—commonly at the expense of your muscle tissue.

Depending on your individual sensitivity to glucose and insulin, the stress response to this seesaw process may make you feel amped, jittery, edgy, or hyper, and you may experience a racing heartbeat. Others may not experience any stress-hormone buzz, likely because years of abusing this delicate life-or-death energy boosting mechanism (thanks to high-carbohydrate eating, chronic cardio, excessive artificial light/insufficient sleep, and high-stress lifestyle) have exhausted your fight or flight hormonal mechanisms. Instead, they'll just feel like taking a nap after high-carb meals. Consequently, their roller coaster ride will consist of a brief glucose high after meals, followed by a crash and carb/sugar cravings (to bring their energy levels back up) and/or a desire for a nap once insulin starts going to work. However your particular daily energy level and appetite fluctuations play out, all roads in this saga lead to burnout and elevated risk of disease and dysfunction.

Besides the unsettling energy swings and added physiological stress, sugar also seriously hampers immune function as soon as it's ingested. We know that excessive and/or prolonged production of cortisol is a potent immune suppressor (the fight or flight mechanism diverts resources to provide an immediate energy boost). Research also shows that sugar itself can impair the function of immunity-related phagocytes (immune system cells that remove bacteria or viruses from the bloodstream) for at least five hours after ingestion. This impairment happens through a process known as competitive inhibition, when excess glucose prevents all-important vitamin C from being transported inside certain immune cells. Because both molecules use the same mechanism and entry point to gain access to the inside of the immune cells, the presence of excessive glucose can overwhelm the transporter sites and block vitamin C from entering. Furthermore, your blood thickens as a response to these immune stressors, which is why heart attacks (in people predisposed to them) tend to occur after a meal.

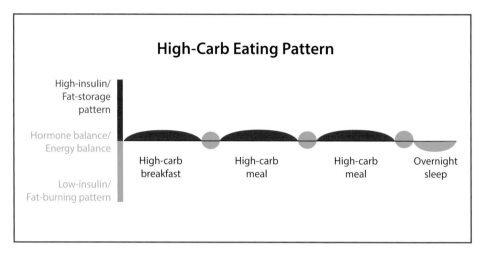

The high-carb eating pattern requiring excess insulin production causes a roller coaster of glucose spikes and dips, overstress (leading to burnout), increased appetite/caloric intake, mood/energy level swings, and lifelong insidious weight gain.

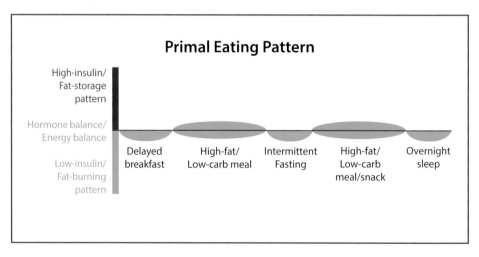

Energy balance happens from becoming fat-adapted and eating low-in-sulin-producing meals. Appetite, mood, energy, caloric intake, and blood glucose are stabilized, leading to effortless weight maintenance.

•••••••••••• GROK 🏃 TALK ••••••••••••

*Putting yourself through the roller coaster of sugar-spiking meal →
insulin response → blood glucose crash → stress-induced gluconeogenesis feels like a life-or-death matter to your primal genes. Getting
the afternoon blues and brain fog and making mistakes on spreadsheets is very bad news, but low blood sugar in primal times might
have spelled doom at the hands of the nearest predator. Fortunately,
our highly sensitive fight or flight response can turn muscle into glucose quickly when we need energy.*

*On an extreme scale, you might harness this system during times
of personal or family crisis where your appetite and food intake is
suppressed for days on end but you are still wired on nervous energy.
Cortisol will stimulate gluconeogenesis, breaking down muscle
into the sugar your brain and body need to go. On a minor scale,
a high-carbohydrate eating pattern will chip away at the stress
response by repeatedly tapping into gluconeogenesis to boost up sag-
ging blood sugar levels. When coupled with other forms of chronic
stress in modern life (including chronic exercise especially), the fight
or flight response can easily become exhausted and send you into a
state of burnout.*

Note that the chain of events described here happens routinely in a
normal, healthy person who overindulges in carbohydrates. Experiencing these high-low cycles is no fun, but it does mean you still have some
sensitivity to the negative effects of carbohydrate ingestion and insulin
production. If you don't experience significant noticeable symptoms after
eating lots of carbohydrates (particularly sugar), you are likely well on
your way to, or have already developed, the extremely problematic condition of insulin resistance. The analogy of a smoker feeling minimal ill
effects from his or her habit applies here. I'd argue that a vast majority
of the population is somewhere on this continuum, far outside of the
healthy ideal of a diet that moderates carb intake and insulin production
in line with our genetic requirements for health.

Your goal should be to maintain stable, healthy insulin levels through sensible diet and exercise choices. This does not mean cutting all carbohydrates out of your diet, but rather preferentially eating reasonable amounts of carbohydrates from vegetables and fruits that produce a much more moderate insulin response than that caused by grains or sugars. Bear in mind that while it's obviously preferable to mute insulin spikes and crashes, your diet's total insulin production is the most important element to consider. If you are routinely eating excessive carbohydrates (especially in the context of an inactive lifestyle), even if they come from "healthy" sources, you will likely gain weight and increase your risk of developing other associated health problems including the "oxidation and inflammation" syndrome that is the major culprit behind heart disease.

CHOLESTER-ALL: THE WHOLE STORY

The debate over the theory known as the lipid hypothesis of heart disease has raged for years. Big Pharma and your helpful friends at the FDA, AMA, and other respected health agencies have done a great job of vilifying cholesterol and saturated fat as the major causes of atherosclerosis and heart disease. You know their story by now. Your arteries are like pipes. Cholesterol is the fatty, sticky gunk that clogs them up if you eat too many high-cholesterol animal products (meat, eggs, butter) or saturated fats in general. According to conventional wisdom, you should eat a low-fat, low-cholesterol, high-complex-carbohydrate diet. If your diet or genetic bad luck results in a total cholesterol level of over 200, you simply take cholesterol-lowering statin medicines to "safely" reduce your risk.

In recent years, many elements of conventional wisdom's stance on cholesterol have been called into question. While there is significant dispute and uncertainty about the issue among respected experts, there is compelling evidence that freely dispensing powerful statin medications to reduce all forms of cholesterol offers minimal to no protection from heart disease and stroke. Furthermore, it's almost universally agreed that lifestyle modifications such as losing weight, reducing intake of processed carbs and refined vegetable oils, consuming omega-3 oils, exercising, and managing stress levels can do a much better job than statins in terms of eliminating the major heart disease risk factors.

Fortunately, the tide is slowly turning as the cracks in conventional wisdom's armor are beginning to show. A June 2014 cover of *TIME* bore the command "Eat Butter," with the headline "Scientists labeled fat the enemy. Why they were wrong"—a striking follow-up to the magazine's iconic 1984 cover illustrating a frowning eggs-and-bacon face with the words, "Cholesterol. And now the bad news...." In September 2015, the peer-reviewed *British Medical Journal* even published an editorial chastising the less-than-scientific underpinnings of the US Dietary Guidelines, calling for a more rigorous, less biased evaluation of the evidence (particularly that condemning saturated fat and dietary cholesterol).

Finally, in December 2015, the U.S. Department of Health and Human Services (HHS) released the new 2015–2020 Dietary Guidelines for Americans report (available on health.gov) and did away with the recommended maximum of 300 mg/day of dietary cholesterol from the 2010 guidelines. The report goes on to say that Americans should "eat as little dietary cholesterol as possible," but then states that high-cholesterol eggs and shellfish are an acceptable part of a healthy diet. So it seems that HHS doesn't know quite where it stands on cholesterol at the moment, although the report strongly implies that cholesterol probably isn't that bad, and saturated fat is the real enemy—another claim I strongly dispute. (In fairness, the report does call for more research into the relationship between dietary and serum—blood—cholesterol; but you will know by the end of this section that I'm not impressed by serum cholesterol as a health risk marker, to say the least). In an interesting behind-the-scenes look, the committee that makes recommendations to the HHS when preparing the new guidelines asserted, "[A]vailable evidence shows no appreciable relationship between consumption of dietary cholesterol and serum cholesterol.... Cholesterol is not a nutrient of concern for overconsumption." Obviously the HHS wasn't ready to make such a bold statement.

While the new guidelines are a step in the right direction, they fall short of admitting that the fearmongering around cholesterol is largely unwarranted. Moreover, there is still the hurdle of getting this accepted by medical practitioners who have been bombarded with the message that elevated cholesterol is the root of all heart disease. We may have a way to go before mainstream medicine is fully on board with evolutionarily health-aligned principles, but the trend, however slow, is at least moving in the right direction. Because I highly respect the valiant battle medical professionals are fighting with today's heart disease pandemic (after all, they often have little or nothing to do with patients until they show up in the waiting room with clogged pipes), I'd like to assert here that this is not a "Mark versus your doctor" battle of the egos. Rather, I believe this is an unbiased interpretation of cutting-edge data that extends beyond the narrow and dated "eating fat drives cholesterol drives heart disease" story that most of us are familiar with, including physicians. Remember, physicians don't necessarily have any specialized knowledge about the link between diet and heart disease from their medical training. Or if they do, it might be very outdated information. Like your plumber, their expertise is in dealing with already-clogged pipes.

For now, the best we can do is educate ourselves while the rest of the world gradually catches up. This discussion will give you a deeper understanding of exactly what causes heart disease (hint: it's oxidation and inflammation driven primarily by poor food choices, excessive insulin production, and all forms of stress in excess, including overexercising) and help you do a better job minimizing heart disease risk than just following the party line of "don't eat cholesterol—and take drugs if your numbers are high."

> *Using total cholesterol level—or even your LDL cholesterol value—is irrelevant in the absence of further context, such as Metabolic Syndrome and other accomplices to heart disease.*

Among the most notable research refuting the cholesterol story is the highly respected Framingham Heart Study. The study (which I reference often at MarksDailyApple.com) has followed the dietary habits of 15,000 participants, residents of Framingham, Massachusetts, over three generations. It is widely regarded as the longest (it began in 1948 and is still going strong!), most comprehensive study of health and illness factors on a population in medical history. It has led to the publication of more than 1,200 research articles in leading journals. Study director Dr. William Castelli summarized the issue unequivocally when he said, "Serum cholesterol is not a strong risk factor for coronary heart disease." Among the study's highlights are:

There is no correlation between dietary cholesterol and blood cholesterol levels.

Framingham residents who ate the most cholesterol, saturated fat, and total calories actually weighed the least and were the most physically active.

Luckily for us, over the past decade, hundreds of bright, clear-thinking researchers have reexamined old data, conducted new research, and written extensively on how and why the conventional wisdom lipid hypothesis of heart disease is deeply flawed. (There's even an organized group called the International Network of Cholesterol Skeptics, populated by over a hundred leading M.D.'s and Ph.D.'s from across the globe, dedicated to countering the argument that animal fat and cholesterol cause atherosclerosis and heart disease.) Their research shows that atherosclerosis is caused mainly by excessive oxidation (and the ensuing inflammation) of a certain type of cholesterol that constitutes a small fraction of the mostly good stuff flowing through your bloodstream.

Ironically, in many cases, it appears that this oxidation might be made worse by consuming the very cholesterol-free, polyunsaturated fats in vegetable and grain oils that the medical establishment led us to believe were healthier than animal fats! Furthermore, the drugs often prescribed to lower cholesterol have done little or nothing to improve the health of most of the people taking them, while the side effects and expense have been devastating to millions more.

The Lowdown on Lipoproteins

Cholesterol is a little waxy lipid (fat) molecule that happens to be one of the most important substances in the human body. (Actually, there are many types of cholesterol, but for the moment I will lump them together.) Every cell membrane has cholesterol as a critical structural and functional component. Brain cells need cholesterol to make synapses (connections) with other brain cells. Cholesterol is a precursor molecule for important hormones such as testosterone, estrogen, DHEA, cortisol, and pregnenolone. Cholesterol is needed for making the bile acids that allow us to digest and absorb fats. Cholesterol is converted by UVB energy in sunlight into the all-important vitamin D. You can't survive or thrive without cholesterol, which is why your liver actually makes up to 1,400 milligrams a day regardless of how much food-borne cholesterol you consume—or how much you avoid it like the plague—in your diet.

Because cholesterol is fat-soluble and does not dissolve in water, but must travel to and from cells in the watery environment of the bloodstream, it needs to be carried by special spherical particles called lipoproteins (the name means "part protein and part lipid [fat]"). There are several varieties of lipoproteins with different transporting functions—chylomicrons, LDLs, IDLs, HDLs, and VLDLs (as well as subfractions of those)—but the three we are concerned with here are VLDLs, LDLs, and HDLs (very low-density, low-density, and high-density lipoproteins, respectively). Each of these lipoproteins carries a certain percentage of cholesterol, triglycerides, and other minor fats. Your blood test values for triglycerides and HDL, LDL, and VLDL cholesterol represent the combined total in your bloodstream of what all the lipoproteins are transporting.

VLDLs, the largest of these cholesterol complexes, are manufactured in the liver in the presence of high levels of triglycerides. Hence, VLDLs are comprised of 80 percent triglyceride and a little cholesterol. After leaving their birthplace in the liver, these lipoproteins deliver their cargo to fat and muscle cells for energy. Once these VLDLs have deposited their triglyceride load inside a fat or muscle cell, their size decreases substantially and they convert into either large, fluffy LDLs or small, dense LDLs—in both cases bearing mostly cholesterol and a little bit of remaining triglyceride. Large, fluffy, or "buoyant" LDLs are the more innocuous form of LDL, as they go about their assigned task of delivering cholesterol to the cells that need it.

The real trouble starts when triglycerides are unusually high in the bloodstream, causing your body to convert VLDLs into small, dense LDLs. This condition can occur routinely when you eat a high-carb diet (even if it's a low-fat diet), because excessive insulin production drives the conversion of ingested carbohydrate into fat (triglycerides). Obviously, the condition can also occur when you eat a moderate-carb, high-fat diet, because insulin will see to it that both excess carbs and fat get circulated in the bloodstream and stored in fat cells.

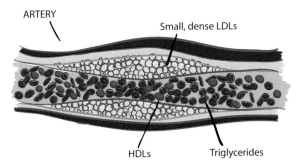

When the bloodstream is overloaded with triglycerides due to high-carb eating, VLDLs convert into the more problematic small, dense LDLs. This sets the stage for atherosclerosis.

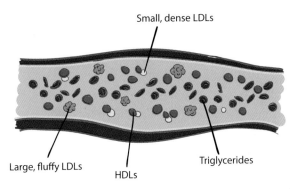

Primal eating lowers triglycerides and raises HDL. VLDLs convert into large, fluffy LDLs. HDLs—"nature's garbage trucks"—remove problematic agents from the bloodstream, keeping arteries clean.

Dr. Dean Ornish and other proponents of low-fat eating will tell you that reducing fat intake quickly reduces cholesterol and triglyceride levels. This is absolutely true, as confirmed by numerous best-selling books as well as newspaper and magazine feature stories touting quick and dramatic results (lowered cholesterol and triglyceride levels) from fat-restrictive diets. But the reason is twofold: one, triglycerides will initially drop on any diet that triggers weight loss (which extremely low-fat diets can do because they dramatically reduce food options and cause an initial reduction in energy intake—but long-term sustainability is another issue entirely); and two, your liver makes cholesterol as a raw material for the bile salts that help you digest fat, so if you aren't eating much fat, your genes will be given the signal to downregulate cholesterol production.

However, low-fat eating requires you to consume a high level of carbs, by default, to obtain your daily energy requirements. While this can work for some highly active populations that haven't been exposed to the atrocities of the Western diet and lifestyle (such as some Pacific Islander tribes and traditional Asian communities), for the rest of us, this can lead to excessive insulin production and kick-start the cycle that eventually leads to heart disease. Any way you slice it, consuming more carbs than you need sooner or later leads to high triglycerides (not to mention the other risk factors detailed in the upcoming sidebar "How to Sneeze at Heart Disease").

With high triglycerides in your blood, VLDL production skyrockets to handle the extra load, and these particles can be altered into the small, dense LDLs that appear to be a bigger factor in atherosclerosis and heart disease than large, fluffy LDLs. Being small and dense, these small, dense LDLs (why can't all medical nomenclature be this easy?) can become stuck in the spaces between cells lining the arteries and then become oxidized. This is compounded by the fact that small, dense LDLs do not bind to LDL receptors (receptors on the surface of cells, especially liver cells, that remove LDLs from the bloodstream) as easily as the larger LDL particles do. That means the small, dense LDLs stay in circulation longer, increasing the chance that they will get stuck in the arterial wall and oxidize. This oxidative damage causes inflammation and begins a process of destruction that I will detail shortly.

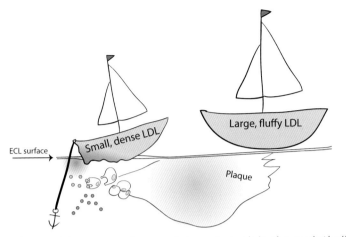

Small, dense LDLs are small enough to get stuck in the endothelial lining of the blood vessels and become oxidized, while large, fluffy LDLs sail along unscathed.

Another issue to be aware of is the difference—tragically, one rarely discussed by doctors when delivering your cholesterol results—between calculated LDL ("LDL-C") and LDL particle number ("LDL-P"). LDL-C is the value reported on most blood tests, unless you've specifically requested otherwise. It's simply a measure of the cholesterol mass within your LDL particles, calculated indirectly based on your total cholesterol, your HDL, and your triglycerides. (For people with triglyceride levels below 100, the formula used to calculate LDL-C tends to significantly overestimate LDL levels.) By contrast, LDL-P is a direct measure of the number of LDL particles in your bloodstream. As with small, dense LDL, LDL particle count is more highly correlated with heart disease than calculated LDL, since a large number of LDL particles—by sheer probability—have a greater chance of facing oxidative modification in the bloodstream and ending up embedded in artery walls.

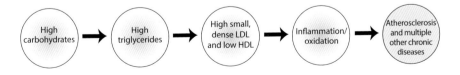

This distinction matters significantly when it comes to gauging your disease risk. If your blood is host to a party of large, fluffy LDL particles carrying plenty of cholesterol in each lipoprotein "vehicle," LDL-C will tend to be high (especially if your triglycerides are also low), even if the actual number of LDL particles is in a healthy range. Meanwhile, if your bloodstream is full of small, dense LDL packing less cholesterol in each lipoprotein, your LDL-C may appear lower, even though the number of particles is dangerously high. In other words, LDL-C can be wildly misleading; knowing your LDL particle count, and whether small or large particles predominate, is much more valuable.

The remaining cholesterol complex with which you might be familiar is the high-density lipoprotein (HDL), which takes cholesterol back to the liver for recycling. These tiny but powerful cholesterol complexes are often called the "good cholesterol" or "nature's garbage trucks" because HDLs also clean up any damaged or oxidized cholesterol that might cause problems later. They are particularly important for their role in preventing atherosclerosis, a build-up of plaque in your arteries that is often a precursor to heart attack or stroke. Atherosclerosis can occur when those small, dense LDLs get stuck in the arterial walls and oxidize, and the immune system fights back with macrophages (white blood cells) that scavenge the oxidized LDL. The macrophages end up converting into foam cells—fat-laden cells that themselves build up in the artery, causing or exacerbating atherosclerosis. HDL can remove cholesterol from these foam cells. Scientists generally agree that the more HDL you have, the lower your risk for heart disease. That's why Big Pharma has tried—so far unsuccessfully—to create an effective drug to raise HDL and address existing atherosclerosis. (Some physicians prescribe the combination of prescription fibrates and over-the-counter niacin to raise HDL, but this treatment can be problematic and is not widely used.)

Research has shown that people with Metabolic Syndrome or type 2 diabetes all have elevated levels of both triglycerides and small, dense LDL particles. As you might have imagined, they also typically have high triglycerides and low levels of beneficial HDL. Of course, these same people have substantially increased risks for heart disease and stroke. Exercise is one of the cheapest, easiest, and most effective ways to raise HDL. Consuming saturated fat is another!

TIME TO OBSESS ON SOME NEW NUMBERS

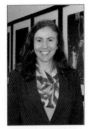

Dr. Cate Shanahan
hanging around
Lakers headquarters,
ready to plan
healthier road
trip meals.

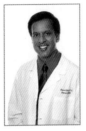

Dr. Ronesh Sinha
lectures to physician
groups about ancestral
health principles. His
success in expanding
traditional treatment
perspectives is bolstered
by the awesome results
he gets with his high-risk
patients, without drugs.

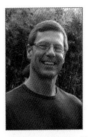

Dr. Doug McGuff
urges you to get fit
and take responsi-
bility for your own
health—so you don't
have to meet him in
the ER someday!

It follows from our discussion of the various lipoproteins that the blood value we've been obsessed with for decades—total LDL cholesterol (irrespective of particle size)—is only a small part of the heart disease risk story. A slew of other blood markers may better predict your potential for inflammation and LDL oxidation and the chronic diseases that occur as a result. Dr. Cate Shanahan—author of *Deep Nutrition* and *Food Rules*, nutrition director for the Los Angeles Lakers, Primal Blueprint Podcast recurring guest, and family physician in Denver, CO, specializing in med-ically supervised weight loss through primal-style eating—sug-gests that your **triglycerides-to-HDL ratio** is perhaps the best way of monitoring heart disease risk. It's critical to get your ratio to 3.5:1 or better, and 1:1 or better is considered superior. Remem-ber, high triglycerides suggest the body's cholesterol process-ing system is overwhelmed, and you likely have an abundance of small, dense LDL loitering around, ready to cause trouble. Meanwhile, a high level of HDL arms your vascular system for battle, while suboptimal levels of HDL leave your body vulnerable to oxidation and inflammation.

Regarding the folly of tracking total LDL without respecting particle size or looking at the bigger picture of inflammation markers, Dr. Ronesh Sinha, author of *The South Asian Health Solution* and internal medicine specialist in Silicon Valley, references a UCLA meta-analysis (which synthesizes the results of many independent studies) showing that **75 percent of patients hospitalized for a heart attack had an LDL of less than 130 mg/dl** (widely accepted as "safe"), and that half of the victims had an LDL under 100, widely considered "ideal." Unfortunately, as Dr. Sinha explains, instead of taking a holistic view of how all risk factors interplay, "[M]any physicians and drug companies are interpreting the results of the UCLA meta-study to mean we should set our LDL targets even lower."

Dr. Doug McGuff, a South Carolina emergency room physician, co-author of *The Primal Prescription* and fitness expert advocating high-intensity exercise to optimize health and delay aging, reminds us that the "beast" that is mainstream health and medicine moves very slowly, and it's up to us to think critically about the latest research and take personal responsibility for our health. "It's certain that the science will reshape conventional wisdom (to honor many of the evolutionary health-based notions presented in this book and elsewhere), but it's going to take 20 years. Personally, I don't feel like waiting that long."

It's heartening to see pioneers like Drs. Shanahan, Sinha, and McGuff making their valiant efforts to reshape culture and improve the lives of the patients they treat directly, and also to observe mainstream media beginning to investigate ideas that counter the dogma we've been fed for many decades. Indeed, it will take many more years for the masses to come around, for the random passenger next to you on the airplane to eagerly join the conversation instead of drawing a blank when you say the word "primal" (not to mention, request a gluten-free airline meal instead of mowing down on snack pretzels). When you experience stunning health and body-composition breakthroughs from primal living, it's easy to allow your enthusiasm to overwhelm others who have not yet "seen the light." I want to caution you against evangelism when it comes to any kind of lifestyle change. This area tends to be a sore spot for many people, dredging up years of weight-loss failures and frustration. The best approach is to set an example of healthy living with a willingness to think critically in the face of irresponsible or dated dogma (e.g., "I've decided to reduce my intake of carbs to get my triglycerides down and eventually go off statins. How does that sound doc?").

Murder Mystery Dinner—Oxidation and Small, Dense LDL Are Guilty!

While cholesterol in and of itself is popularly blamed for heart disease, we should really be pointing fingers at oxidative damage as the proximal cause. Because lipoproteins have a lipid surface, they are subject to oxidation. Like oils left open in your kitchen, they can go rancid when they come in contact with oxygen. When this happens, lipoproteins—and the cholesterol inside—can become damaged. As mentioned previously, small, dense LDLs are small enough that they can get trapped in the spaces between endothelial cells lining the arteries (sometimes called gap junctions). Even if they are not oxidized to begin with, once trapped, LDLs can oxidize in place because they are sitting there continually exposed to oxygen passing by that's attached to hemoglobin in the red blood cells.

Either way, this oxidation eventually causes injury and inflammation to the arterial wall, prompting the body's immune system to send macrophages (scavenging white blood cells) to gobble up the oxidized LDLs. The immune system tries hard to do its job, but the macrophages can become overwhelmed by absorbing so much oxidized LDLs. The consumption of oxidized LDLs causes certain genes to convert these macrophages into foam cells that attach to the arterial lining, laying the foundation for future trouble. The damaged area, known as a lesion, prompts more macrophages to come to the rescue. They try to gobble up more and more oxidized LDLs floating by, increasing the severity of the lesion over time. This is how plaques accumulate on the arterial wall, a saga with which you are no doubt familiar thanks to the myriad Big Pharma drug ads aimed at this problem. Arterial plaques grow and eventually compromise the inner diameter of the artery. If allowed to continue, this process can eventually occlude blood flow, or plaques can rupture and release clots into the bloodstream, preventing blood—and oxygen—from reaching a vital organ. This describes your classic heart attack or stroke. (By the way, atherosclerosis occurs in the arteries and not the veins because venous blood has very little oxygen.)

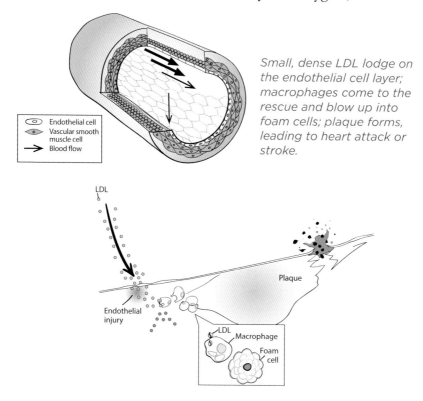

Endothelial cell
Vascular smooth muscle cell
Blood flow

Small, dense LDL lodge on the endothelial cell layer; macrophages come to the rescue and blow up into foam cells; plaque forms, leading to heart attack or stroke.

LDL

Plaque

Endothelial injury

LDL
Macrophage
Foam cell

Of course, oxidation happens all the time throughout the body, and we have evolved some effective antioxidant systems (namely catalase, superoxide dismutase, and glutathione) to prevent too much of this damage from getting out of control. Furthermore, consuming ample levels of high-antioxidant foods (vegetables, fruits, nuts and seeds, and dark chocolate) and antioxidant supplements (such as vitamin E, CoQ10, beta-carotene, and lycopene) can help mitigate some of the damage. It's also extremely convenient that HDLs can remove some of the damaged cholesterol and take it back to the liver for recycling. Your cholesterol processing system has evolved to expect a certain range and quality of dietary fat, protein, carbohydrate, and antioxidants, as well as a certain level of exercise (to help promote insulin sensitivity in the muscles and maintain high levels of HDL) to provide appropriate gene signals and avoid artery disease. The cholesterol processing system has served humans and most other mammals well for millions of years—until recently.

The oxidation of small, dense LDLs—and the concomitant inflammation and disease that are so now common—most likely happens for a variety of reasons that have to do with modern dietary habits more than anything else. A major culprit is a high intake of unstable high polyunsaturated fats from vegetable oils in the diet. (High polyunsaturated fats incorporated into the lipid layer are much more prone to oxidation than are saturated fats.) Due to vegetable/seed oils' high-temperature processing methods involving toxic chemical solvents—combined with these oils' extreme sensitivity to heat, light, and oxygen—they are essentially a bottled source of free radicals. They accelerate aging, are directly linked to assorted cancers, hamper immune and cardiovascular function, and can severely compromise your ability to remove excess body fat. Dr. Shanahan asserts that the direct and immediate damage that industrials oils inflict at the cellular level makes them "literally no different than eating radiation."

Potential damage is exacerbated by the Standard American Diet, with its focus on consuming (insulin-promoting) whole grains and reducing healthy fats from animal sources and nuts. Diets rich in processed carbs are often also low in natural antioxidants, which would otherwise mitigate oxidation. High-carb diets have also been implicated in low HDL cholesterol readings, and remember that HDL can removed oxidized lipids and combat oxidative damage.

Unfortunately for some of us, poor diet, lack of exercise, stress, certain drug therapies, and, yes, family genetic history can all contribute to the increased production of the dangerous small, dense LDL particles. Your doctor can test for them if you ask, but most common blood tests don't yet distinguish between the benign "fluffy" forms of LDL, sometimes called pattern A, and the small, dense particles, called pattern B. A comprehensive lipid blood panel such as the Berkeley HeartLab test will typically provide values for total cholesterol, HDL, LDL, VLDL, and triglycerides and indicate relative particle sizes.

It is important to remember that the oxidation and inflammation process described has little or nothing to do with your total cholesterol or even your total LDL cholesterol levels. In most cases, atherosclerosis is a result of the oxidation of a small fraction of the total amount of LDL in your blood—the small, dense LDL particles. If you have low triglycerides and high HDL (indicative of minimal small, dense LDL), your risk of heart disease drops dramatically. Also, if your HDL is high, it's very unlikely that you'll encounter a problem, because HDL does such a great job of scavenging the oxidized cholesterol from LDL in the bloodstream.

A physician will generally dispense medication if your total LDL levels exceed a certain figure (this varies by doctor and individual patient profile), knowing your body will respond to the statins with a quick overall reduction regardless of particle size. This will indeed lower all forms of LDL (including both the neutral and harmful kind), but a much more sensible—and safer—option is simply to alter dietary and exercise habits and minimize insulin production, thereby preventing excess accumulation of triglycerides in the blood and allowing the cholesterol system to work as intended. In fact, the combination of low carbs and good fats in primal foods will generally raise HDL and lower both triglycerides and small, dense LDL.

Meanwhile, compelling evidence suggests that Primal Blueprint-style eating and exercising will allow you, regardless of your genetic predisposition, to essentially have no participation in this heart disease saga whatsoever. If you feel any hesitation here, go get a "before" blood panel, eat primally for 21 days, and then get another panel. It's virtually certain you will see an impressive alteration of unfavorable numbers, giving you the motivation and clarity you need to plunge wholeheartedly into primal eating.

Statin Stats Stink!

Now that you know more about the different types of cholesterol, isn't it disappointing to discover that statins and other cholesterol-lowering meds do not have any ability to influence LDL particle size and can only lower total LDL by reducing both the neutral and harmful versions? The fact that some people taking statins experience a dramatic reduction in total cholesterol or in LDL means very little in the context of the true oxidation- and inflammation-based nature of heart disease. To be clear, statins do slightly reduce the risk of heart attacks among men under the age of 65 who have had a prior heart attack. However, many doctors now believe that these benefits are independent of their "cholesterol-lowering" properties and instead come from an anti-inflammatory effect that addresses the more proximate cause of heart disease. A cheaper and more effective anti-inflammatory effect can be achieved for most people by eating foods high in omega-3 or taking fish oil supplements, exercising sensibly instead of chronically, and getting more sleep if you are deprived.

HDL does a great job of scavenging the oxidized cholesterol from LDL in the bloodstream.... If your HDL is high, it's much less likely you'll encounter a [heart disease] problem.

By simply adopting the Primal Blueprint laws, you can enjoy superior results without the perilous side effects and huge expense of drug therapy. In the case of statins, known side effects include chronic fatigue, tendon problems, cognitive problems, impotence, blood glucose elevations, and muscle pain, weakness, and numbness. Recent data even suggests an increased risk of developing diabetes as a result of taking statins. These side effects are believed to be due in large part to statins' interference with the normal production of a critical micronutrient known as coenzyme Q10 (CoQ10). CoQ10 is essential to healthy mitochondrial function (energy production) and defending your cells against free radical damage. Statin therapy is believed to lower CoQ10 levels by up to 50 percent. Ironically, CoQ10 plays a particularly important role in the healthy function of the cardiovascular system, and heart attack patients show depressed levels of CoQ10! Some researchers suggest that statins' depletion of CoQ10 may nullify any potential benefits of statin therapy.

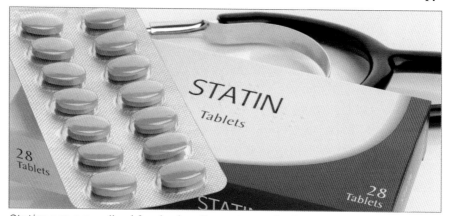

Statins are prescribed freely despite meta-study data suggesting that low LDL levels are not protective against heart attacks, and despite energy-sapping, health-compromising drug side effects.

The long and short of it is, statins offer only a small degree of protection against heart attack and stroke (and only in some segments of the population), little or even no apparent benefits in terms of life span (especially among those who don't already have heart disease), and significant side effects in a larger percentage of the patient population than they help. So why are millions being advised to take dangerous, powerful drugs when lifestyle intervention is more effective and less expensive and has no side effects? Perhaps we like to search for easy answers with quick results, and statins produce a graphic and quick decline in blood cholesterol levels. Like other elements of conventional wisdom, there are billions of dollars invested and powerful market forces pushing us in the direction of swallowing drugs and their side effects, while the full story is lost amidst the hype of "lower your numbers quickly!"

If you are currently taking statins or other medications, I realize that asking you to question conventional wisdom and the specific recommendations of your trusted physician can put you in a very uncomfortable position. I strongly urge you to engage in lifestyle modification (after all, there are no side effects or potential compromises to your drug regimen when you improve your diet), while concurrently addressing the possibility with your doctor of gradually reducing your dependence on medication based on the ensuing favorable blood test results.

HOW TO SNEEZE AT HEART DISEASE

The catchall term Metabolic Syndrome is used to describe an assortment of heart disease risk factors widely attributed to today's prevailing poor dietary and exercise habits. The highly respected Cleveland Clinic states that "the exact cause of Metabolic Syndrome is not known... [but] many features are associated with insulin resistance." The following five markers are universally used as reliable indicators of Metabolic Syndrome:

1. Elevated fasting blood glucose of **100 mg/dl** or greater.
2. Blood pressure of **130/85 mm Hg** or greater.
3. Waistline measurement of **40 inches** or more for men and **35 inches** or more for women.
4. HDL of less than **40 mg/dl** for men and less than **50 mg/dl** for women.
5. Triglycerides of **150 mg/dl** or greater.

Individuals with three or more of these markers are said to have Metabolic Syndrome. The U.S. government and other sources report that some 47 million Americans—that's one in five!—meet the conditions to be diagnosed with Metabolic Syndrome. It's a chronic condition that develops and worsens over time (with no discernible physical symptoms, except that expanding waistline...) unless you take dramatic steps to alter your lifestyle. The Cleveland Clinic and *Journal of the American Medical Association* report that more than 40 percent of Americans in their 60s and 70s have this condition.

A routine physical exam and blood panel will give you an indication of your Metabolic Syndrome status. Many experts recommend a few additional blood tests to assess overall health and risk factors, including:

C-Reactive Protein: High sensitivity C-reactive protein (hs-CRP) is produced by your liver as part of an immune system response to injury or infection. In the absence of other acute infections, high levels of hs-CRP in your blood are indicative of systemic inflammation. Because atherosclerosis is primarily a disease of inflammation, some researchers contend that hs-CRP is a strong predictor of your heart disease risk, and indeed elevated hs-CRP is associated with an increased risk of heart attack, stroke, and sudden cardiac death. Given that cholesterol tests have become less reliable in predicting risk, especially among those with normal or low cholesterol levels, hs-CRP seems to be a good alternative.

Lp2A: Another key inflammation marker associated with small, dense LDL particles.

A1c (estimated average glucose): A1c measures how much glucose is attached to a hemoglobin molecule, a reliable marker for the dangers of elevated blood glucose levels over an extended time period. This is a good companion test to the aforementioned fasting blood glucose readings (the first Metabolic Syndrome indicator above).

Fasting Blood Insulin Levels: High fasting insulin levels are indicative of prediabetic conditions.

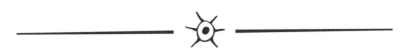

HEART DISEASE PREVENTION TIPS

If you are diagnosed with (or are on the cusp of) Metabolic Syndrome, following the Primal Blueprint for 21 days can turn four of the five Metabolic Syndrome markers around (it might take a bit longer to get your waistline back in the safe zone) and cause your heart disease risk to plummet—even if you have a family history of obesity, high cholesterol, and heart disease. Here are some specific recommendations and corresponding benefits of following the Primal Blueprint:

Ditch Industrial Oils: Eliminating consumption of processed sources of polyunsaturated fats—namely the refined vegetable/seed oils and margarines we've been told to use in lieu of butter—gives you a greater proportion of saturated (and therefore oxidation-resistant) fats in lipoprotein lipid layers and fatty membranes. Increased consumption of omega-3 oils—best sourced from oily, cold-water fish like sardines and wild salmon—helps control inflammation, the precursor for atherosclerosis and virtually all other metabolic diseases.

Exercise Primal Blueprint Style: A sensible blend of low-level cardio, regular strength training, and occasional all-out sprints helps lower LDL and raise HDL. On the flip side, chronic cardio can cause you to lose these benefits and actually increases heart disease risk factors!

Increase Antioxidant Intake: If your antioxidant intake is appreciable (eating your vegetables?), you'll help boost your natural defenses against oxidation.

Reduce Carb Intake, Especially Refined Carbs: Dr. Richard Feinman, one of the most frequently published and highly regarded researchers in the fields of nutrition and metabolism, has suggested that "Metabolic Syndrome may be defined by the response to carbohydrate restriction" (meaning that if you restrict carbs and your symptoms are improved or alleviated, carb intake is the defining variable in Metabolic Syndrome). Reducing your carb intake will help lower your production of triglycerides, raise HDL, lower LDL, and dramatically reduce your level of small, dense LDL (because it is high levels of triglycerides that prompt small, dense LDL production).

PUT INFLAMMATION AT EASE WITH OMEGA-3S

A major feature of Primal Blueprint eating is that it provides high levels of healthy saturated and unsaturated fats. While conventional wisdom generally contends that saturated fats should be diligently restricted, they are an excellent energy source and offer a variety of nutrients critical to health. Consuming ample amounts of saturated fat helps prevent direct oxidative damage to your cells. (Saturated fat is an integral part of cell membranes.) While your eyes might bug out at the following statement, it's virtually irrefutable and proven by many respected long-term studies:

Eat (healthy) fat to help prevent cancer and heart disease. Avoid fat and increase your risk of cancer, heart disease, and even obesity.

Fortunately, omega-3 polyunsaturated fatty acids don't have an image problem and are universally regarded as healthy. Adequate omega-3 consumption supports healthy cardiovascular, brain, skin, and immune function. By turning on genes that improve blood circulation, reducing inflammation, and supporting healthy cholesterol and triglyceride levels, omega-3s help reduce the risk of high blood pressure, blood clots that cause heart attacks, arthritis, autoimmune disorders, and cognitive problems such as depression, Alzheimer's, and even ADHD. The important role of omega-3s in supporting cognitive function is made even more evident by the fact that half the brain consists of fat, including concentrated levels of the omega-3 docosahexaenoic acid, or DHA.

Another form of polyunsaturated fat called omega-6 plays a vital role in our health as well, but its extreme prevalence in the Standard American Diet—from undesirable sources like vegetable oils, grain-fed animal fats, bakery items (donuts, cookies), and processed snacks that almost universally contain soybean oil or corn oil—leads to a dangerous imbalance of excessive omega-6 and deficient omega-3. The ideal omega-6:omega-3 balance (O6:O3) is 1:1 or 2:1, ratios that Grok likely met with ease. Even 4:1 is okay today, but the typical modern eater has an O6:O3 ratio of 20:1, or even 50:1! Imbalanced fatty acid intake can exacerbate the insulin resistance problem discussed earlier. Omega-6 fats (particularly arachidonic acid) suppress expression of the insulin receptor gene GLUT4 (promoting more fat storage), while omega-3 fats increase expression of GLUT4 (promoting insulin sensitivity and less fat storage).

High carbohydrate intake increases your risk of cancer, heart disease, and obesity. Cutting carbs and increasing intake of (healthy) fat lowers your disease risk and helps you maintain healthy body composition.

For years, the O6:O3 ratio has been a popular discussion topic in the primal and paleo scenes, and unfortunately, the message has become oversimplified and distorted to omega-3s are anti-inflammatory—"good"—while omega-6s are pro-inflammatory—"bad." This had led savvy enthusiasts to scale back consumption of healthy foods like nuts, most of which are predominantly omega-6. However, more recent research has shown that the concerns about O6:O3 imbalance stem mainly from the ingestion of heavily processed, high-omega-6 oils in junk foods—vegetable oils, margarine products, and processed, packaged, or frozen meals or snacks—that inflict oxidative damage on the body. (It's also possible that if you aren't eating much oily, cold-water fish, you could fall a little short of optimal omega-3 intake. More on this in Chapter 5.)

When you consume a diet laden with oxidized oils and introduce other inflammatory influences into daily life (such as insufficient sleep, overly stressful work patterns, and chronic cardio exercise habits), your genes respond by doing what they're told to do according to these signals and you experience a programmed inflammation response throughout the body. Under normal circumstances, inflammation is your body's highly desirable first line of defense against pain, injury, and infection. Inflammation processes detect and destroy toxic material in damaged tissue before it can spread to the rest of the body. Consider examples like a bee sting, taking an elbow to the face, or turning an ankle on a hiking trail. The reddened skin, black eye, and ballooned ankle help your body quarantine the damage from the trauma to the inflamed areas instead of letting toxins run wild through the bloodstream.

Unfortunately, an out-of-control inflammation response (also known as systemic inflammation)—resulting from stress and imbalanced dietary and exercise habits—confuses your body into thinking it's under assault from destructive, infectious foreign agents or that a major trauma has just occurred. That's when the disease process begins.

In my own athletic example, the extreme stress of my chronic cardio training regimen coupled with my highly inflammatory grain-based diet led to excessive and prolonged inflammation throughout my body as evidenced by repeated injuries and illnesses I couldn't shake. What I should have been seeking was a more desirable temporary state of moderate inflammation (pumped muscles, elevated heart rate, oxygenated lungs) from a Primal Blueprint-aligned training regimen and plenty of recovery time for my body to return to homeostasis. The systemic inflammation I experienced from overtraining tore down my muscles, joints, and immune system.

Interestingly, after extreme endurance events like a marathon or ironman triathlon, blood levels of CPK (creatine phosphokinase, an enzyme that leaks into the bloodstream when muscle, heart, or brain tissue is traumatized) can be elevated for weeks. In fact, if you ran a marathon and then—just for kicks—immediately headed over to a hospital emergency room for a blood draw, a doctor might think you were suffering from a heart attack! In my case, when I adjusted my diet and training habits, virtually all my inflammatory and immune-suppressing conditions vanished.

We know that most forms of systemic inflammation have a strong dietary component and can usually be resolved with a few dietary modifications. Nevertheless, conventional wisdom within the medical community has recommended fighting our widespread inflammation-related health problems with corticosteroids, COX-2 inhibitors such as Vioxx and Celebrex, and other nonsteroidal anti-inflammatories. (Asthma meds work on a similar chemical pathway.)

I have a nonscientific name for this approach: *digging a hole to install a ladder to wash the basement windows.* As you might imagine, because these medications interfere with normal hormone pathways and gene expression, they almost never address the underlying cause of inflammation. They simply mask the pain in the short term—if they mask it at all. Dietary modification (and exercise modification if you are currently overdoing it) is almost always a superior method of treatment and protection against pain and serious diseases triggered by systemic inflammation.

> *I have a nonscientific name for treating lifestyle-related health problems with pharmaceuticals:* **digging a hole to install a ladder to wash the basement windows.**

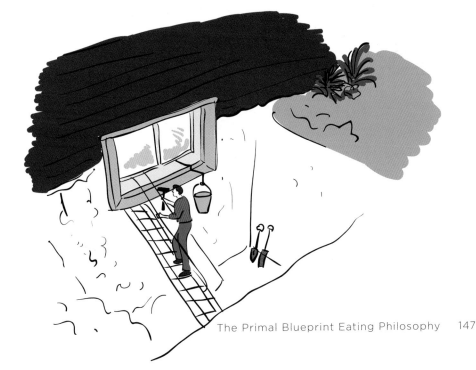

The Primal Blueprint eating style, with its emphasis on nutritious, inflammation-reducing foods and its aversion to processed, pro-inflammatory foods, will help you naturally avoid the systemic inflammation that is now believed to be the root cause of the major health problems affecting modern humans.

EATING WELL

The Primal Blueprint is about enjoying a healthy, happy, balanced lifestyle. As Dr. Andrew Weil said in describing the title of his book *Eating Well for Optimum Health*, "eating well" refers not only to choosing natural, nutritious foods, but also to enjoying the experience as one of the great pleasures of life. It's likely that Grok appreciated food much more than we do today because he had to work so hard for his meals and was never assured of success. Throughout history, food has represented a centerpiece of cultural celebration—let's not kill the momentum now! The key to eating well is to eliminate distractions and negative influences while you are eating. This will allow the physical sensations of hunger and the simple pursuit of pleasure to have predominant influence on your dietary habits.

If you wish to succeed with healthy dietary habits, it's important that you discard any negative emotions you have toward eating and embrace each meal as an opportunity to enjoy yourself. I strongly recommend that you give yourself permission to eat *as much as you want, whenever you want, for the rest of your life*. While this suggestion might scare the heck out of you, releasing yourself from restriction and deprivation enables you to become more connected with your physical nutritional needs rather than being driven by emotional triggers.

Take notice of that point in every meal where you have attained satisfaction and feel comfortable stopping—not the point at which you are stuffed full and need to take your belt out a notch, but the point at which you are no longer hungry for the next bite—knowing that you can eat again whenever you like. If you wish to enjoy a treat once in a while, choose with discretion and enjoy it with full attention and awareness to the pleasure that every single savored bite gives you. Reject feelings of anxiety, guilt, or rebellion connected to your food choices, and replace them with the idea that you deserve to eat the most delicious, nutritious foods possible.

When it comes to what to include or exclude, or how to dial in the perfect food choices for you, I prefer to let my taste buds guide me to the most enjoyable and nourishing food choices within the broad guidelines of the Primal Blueprint. Forget the scientifically unproven admonitions to eat certain macronutrient combinations at certain times, or to align your food choices with your racial heritage or blood type, for example. Despite whatever percentages your genetic heritage test from ancestry. com reveals, we are *all* East African *Homo sapiens* for purposes of eating foods that promote optimal gene expression.

There are foods that are unhealthy for all humans (e.g., refined carbohydrates and industrial oils) and other foods that are more problematic for certain humans than others (e.g., sensitivity to fat storage with carbohydrate intake). While not every primal-approved food will be healthy for every human (e.g., some have allergies or autoimmune responses to certain vegetables, nuts, or even eggs), all humans can craft an enjoyable, varied, and healthy diet from the list of primal-approved foods.

Essentially, my goal is for you to become a modern forager with a keen sense of what you need to do (or not do) to thrive day in and day out. When you eat Primal Blueprint style, there is no city to which you can't travel, no restaurant at which you can't eat, no grocery store in which you can't shop, and no family holiday you can't endure!

Eating on Grok's Clock

While those immersed in carbohydrate dependency from SAD eating patterns will become hungry and irritable when missing even a single meal, you can free yourself from dependency on regular meals when you become fat-adapted through a sustained period of primal-aligned eating. Our ancestors ate sporadically—with continually varied mealtimes and food choices. Given seasonal variables and hunting success or failure, they didn't always have enough food or a varied diet. Our genes thrive on intermittent scarcity and can even handle occasional excess. In fact, they expect it.

Our genetic ability to thrive on intermittent eating habits is an important concept to grasp, because it unburdens you of having to eat every meal on a set schedule, to balance food groups (meat with starch, grains with protein, etc.), or to align your foods with time-of-day traditions (cereal for breakfast, sandwich for lunch, etc.). Skipping meals, fasting briefly, and simply freeing yourself from an obsessive need to eat three squares or six small meals a day when the clock strikes a particular hour will most definitely benefit your body by improving your ability to tap into stored body fat for energy, optimizing cellular repair, moderating your appetite, and enhancing your appreciation for the meals you eat when you're actually a little, or a lot, hungry! Unburdened by the strict and ill-advised "rules" of conventional wisdom, eating becomes much simpler and more intuitive, relaxing, and enjoyable.

On this topic, it's interesting to note that your need to consume calories on a regular schedule will diminish substantially when blood glucose levels are moderated and you start burning fat and ketones (as discussed in Chapter 4) more efficiently through low-insulin Primal Blueprint dietary choices. By contrast, if you eat the typical Western diet of 300 to 500 grams of carbohydrates per day (instead of the 100 to 150 from high-nutrient plant sources as suggested by the Primal Blueprint), you are going to experience significant blood glucose fluctuations and corresponding cravings for quick-energy, high-carbohydrate foods. This is perhaps the single quickest and most exciting revelation for converts to the Primal Blueprint eating style. By eliminating sweetened beverages, sugars, grains, and highly refined vegetable or seed oils from your diet and emphasizing primal foods, you will experience more consistent energy levels and a comfortably diminished appetite. You'll become a fat-burning beast!

> *By eliminating sugars, grains, and legumes from your diet and emphasizing primal foods, you will experience more consistent energy levels and a comfortably diminished appetite.*

These benefits will be long lasting, but they might take a bit of time to realize. Every once in a while, people commenting on MarksDailyApple.com mention difficulties with energy level swings during the first three weeks of their transition to a primal eating style. During this transition period, your

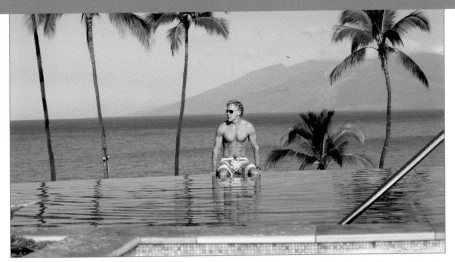

I love my morning routine as much as any breakfast enthusiast; there is just no food involved. Instead, I take a cold plunge for a brief, natural stressor and then enjoy a deliberate cup of coffee.

body expects sugar as fuel (of which it's probably getting considerably less) but hasn't rediscovered yet how to get the most out of its fat reserves. Don't worry, it will. By limiting carbs (and, hence, lowering insulin) you are sending a new series of hormonal signals to your genes. In turn, they are downregulating their sugar-burning systems and upregulating their fat- and keto-burning machinery.

While you may experience a few episodes of lightheadedness during your transition (because your body is relearning how to sustain energy without constant carb infusions), rest assured that the shift will be complete in a few weeks. Energy levels, appetite, mood, and cognitive ability will stabilize even when you eat sporadically. During your transition from carb dependency to fat-adaptation, you can do everything possible to make things smooth and comfortable. Going primal is not about struggling, suffering, starving, or fighting through cravings with willpower. Instead, you can surround yourself with satiating, high-fat foods to enjoy whenever you feel an energy dip or have a hankering for one of your old standby snacks. These primal food choices will totally satisfy you without bringing about a sugar crash later, as will happen when you reach for a bagel or energy bar. This is due to the high caloric density and slow burn rate of foods high in fat and/or protein (such as meat, fish, fowl, eggs, avocados, butter, coconut products, nuts and seeds, olives, and high-fat dairy products) and the high water and fiber content of vegetables and fruits.

Because modern life is all about schedules, we often find it convenient and enjoyable to eat regular meals. This is fine. I'm simply suggesting you pay more attention to your hunger levels than to the clock. For example, over the years of primal living I have become accustomed to skipping breakfast and eating in a compressed time window of around noon to 7 P.M. each day. I'm not doing this for weight loss or to save money on eggs; it's simply a routine I've arrived at that gives me the most pleasure. By the time lunchtime rolls around, I'm ready to enjoy my biggest meal of the day. I might even enjoy a "breakfast" offering like a world-famous MarksDailyApple.com Big Ass Omelet (three eggs, cheese, chopped mushrooms, peppers, onions, and tomatoes, and topped with some bacon and avocado), or a Big Ass Salad with assorted fresh veggies, nuts, and steak, chicken, or tuna. Other days, especially when I'm traveling, I'll just have a Primal Fuel smoothie during the day and carry on until dinner.

When your food choices and meal times are flexible, you feel less stress and more pleasure from your diet. The key is to make informed choices that minimize your exposure to toxic foods and, when you indulge or get off track, allow your body to return quickly to balance. If you enjoy a decadent dessert or a weekend away from healthy food options, simply eat a few low-insulin-producing meals in a row and return to regulated energy levels and optimal metabolic function. Even a short walk, or a quick set of squats or pushups, after a big meal and rich dessert can mitigate the insulin response by diverting glucose from the bloodstream into working muscles.

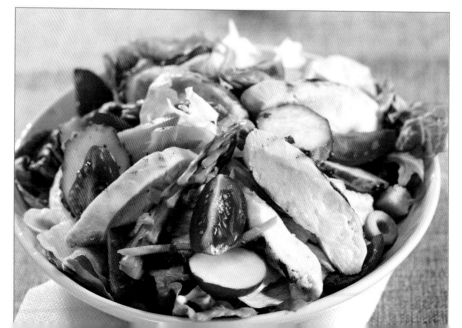

ONE SMALL SCOOP FOR MANKIND

When you eat Primal Blueprint style, the consequences of your food choices become crystal clear. Eat right and you have discernibly more energy and health. Stick with it, and altering your body composition happens with much less effort than the dated calorie-counting strategies. Slide a little bit, and you might get halfway to your goal, have a little less energy, and maybe catch an extra cold or two due to compromised immune function (due in part to insulin-driven sugar crashes and cravings).

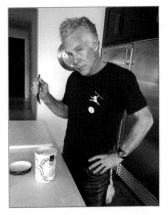

And with this goes my chances for a dairy council endorsement deal...

Every once in a while, I'll give in to temptation and indulge in something like a small scoop of gourmet ice cream. It tastes delicious for the few minutes it takes to eat it (though not quite up to par with a bowl of fresh blueberries and raspberries with homemade whipped cream), but invariably I experience bloating and gas in the ensuing hour as well as a discernible sugar crash. When I lay down at bedtime, I can detect a slightly elevated heart rate and have some difficulty falling asleep normally. Because these lapses are out of my normal pattern, I am highly sensitive to the consequences of choices like these. Heaven knows that back in the day I could polish off an entire half-gallon of ice cream over the course of a leisurely evening to no ill effects—that I was conscious of at the time.

The important point here is that I enjoy the taste of ice cream as much as anyone, but I will reassert my position that after eating primally for some time, even the occasional treat that's not Primal Blueprint approved isn't worth it for me once I weigh the fleeting pleasure against the lingering post-consumption effects on my body. You may feel like you can handle your routine of lime mojitos, strawberry daiquiris, high-carb finger foods, or occasional rich desserts on the holiday party circuit with no ill effects. But it's only when you eliminate these indulgences for a significant time period that you are truly able to compare and contrast the negative impacts on your body from these influences. Over time it becomes easier to stay the course, or to recalibrate quickly when you do decide to occasionally indulge yourself.

What's more, you'll soon learn that much of the emotional comfort related to eating comes not from the food itself, but rather from the *rituals* surrounding it. Primal enthusiasts discover how easy it is to separate an offensive food from the overall experience. Barbequing burgers can still be fun if you opt for a lettuce wrap. You can make a tasty soda with carbonated water, some vanilla, big squeezes of lemon and lime, and perhaps a pinch of stevia extract. Heck, there are entire books, like *Primal Cravings*, dedicated to recipes that replace offensive ingredients with primal-friendly alternatives so you can still enjoy your pancakes, muffins, lasagna, and gelato! There are many ways to enjoy all the pleasures we have learned to associate with food while still making optimal food choices.

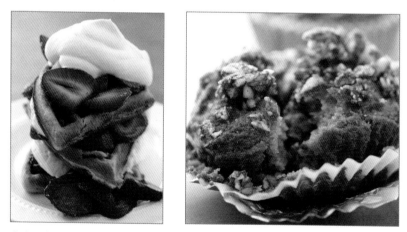

Primal Cravings' Strawberry Shortcake Waffles and Cherry Almond Streusel Muffins

Granted, major lifestyle changes and habit modifications can be a struggle, but the first step toward transformation is to clearly understand the consequences of each and every food (and lifestyle) choice that you make, whether they are aligned with your primal genes or not. It is then that you accept personal responsibility for your health instead of hiding behind rationalizations and defense mechanisms like "Everything in moderation," "You only live once," "Things are too hectic this month to worry about my diet; I'll start the program next month," or "My grandfather smoked and drank and still lived to 98, so I have good genes." When you tell yourself such stories, you gloss over the fact that the years and decades of those little ice cream outings and extra servings from the bar can literally add up to hundreds of pounds of ingested substances that are toxic to your body. Furthermore, as unhealthy food choices ingrain themselves (pun intended) into your daily life, I believe you become desensitized to the negative effects they have on your health. This concept is illustrated by the tolerance levels of heavy tobacco or caffeine users who are able to function somewhat normally (that's not saying much) with volumes of chemicals in their bloodstream that would floor the casual user or teetotaler.

The complete lack of regimentation or caloric deprivation in the Primal Blueprint eating style (I refuse to use the word diet because it implies regimentation and calorie counting) is the secret to its long-term success. You don't have to force yourself to go hungry or to feel deprived or negative about eating. Simply make sensible choices by welcoming the abundant selection of delicious foods whenever you want, and transition out of habitually consuming foods that may taste great for a brief moment but make your body feel bad or create long-term metabolic stress.

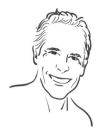

MARK TALK ─────────────────────────────

While I take great pains to emphasize a relaxed, intuitive approach to primal eating, we have to face the reality that carbohydrate dependency has serious hormonal and psychological underpinnings that require dedication to overcome. Sugar and wheat both have addictive properties, and the insulin roller coaster is difficult to dismount if you allow doses of carbs to leak into the picture here and there... and there... and here. If you adopt an extremely disciplined approach for the first 21 days to ditch sugars, grains, and bad oils, you will build momentum toward fat-adaptation. This will make it much easier over the long term to avoid the backsliding that is so common among dieters, and I fear among primal/paleo enthusiasts who "try" instead of commit. Remember, once you become fat-adapted (when you notice your energy levels stabilize throughout the day, and you can skip a meal—or two!—with no ill effects because you are burning off stored body fat for energy), minor departures from primal eating are easily handled by the body because your genes are calibrated to burn fat instead of carbohydrates.

DEALING WITH THE (MAYBE RADICAL) CHANGE TO PRIMAL BLUEPRINT EATING

If you argue that life will never be the same without your bowl of Raisin Bran or a heaping plate of pasta and garlic bread, try these suggestions:

80 Percent Rule: When you first make the switch to primal eating, I recommend following the Primal Blueprint recommendations as closely as possible for the first 21 days. That is how long it will probably take initially to break the cycle of carb addiction and to set you on the right path. That is not to say that you will never be tempted by a cupcake or a plate of pasta again—you will. Do the best you can, and relieve yourself from the pressure of perfection. If you make departures from primal-aligned choices, make sure you get back on track quickly to minimize the damage. Over time, as you experience the benefits of making healthy changes, you will naturally and comfortably become more compliant, particularly with the restriction and elimination of grains, sugars, and toxic vegetable oils.

Build Momentum: As you continue to make progress eating the way you were designed to eat, you will notice a heightened sensitivity to how food affects your body, both positively and negatively. During my years as an athlete, I thought my recurrent digestive bloating and post-meal fatigue were due to hard training or simply the end of a long day—not from subclinical allergic reactions to excessive processed carbohydrates and/or dairy products.

Can you relate to that hyper, racing-heart sensation that comes after consuming a sugary dessert? It's probably something that we've been aware of since childhood—a little annoying but no big deal, right? It was only when I started to aggressively clean up my diet a decade ago that my sensitivity went to the next level. What a pleasure it was to leave the dinner table feeling totally satisfied, yet alert and energetic! Passing on dessert took a little getting used to, but I noticed that the sacrifice of a few moments of instant gratification paled in comparison to not having to deal with sugar highs and sugar crashes. Plus, grains and sugars are confirmed to have significant addictive properties. So when you cut them out, you begin to lose your craving for them. (Really!) Hence, you escape the vicious cycle that befalls even those with tremendous willpower trying to do the right thing but eating the wrong stuff.

Five Favorite Meals Strategy: Pick your five favorite Primal Blueprint-approved meals and rotate them for the first three weeks of your transition to Primal Blueprint eating. Maybe it's broiled salmon with lemon butter and a heaping plate of steamed broccoli or Brussels sprouts loaded with butter. (Sorry Weight Watchers, but eating more fat is how you lose weight and keep it off!) Or lamb chops with grilled zucchini and summer squash (loaded with butter). Maybe rotisserie chicken (with the skin, preferably organic) and a large steamed vegetable (again, loaded with butter) is your cup of tea. Eat as many colorful, creative salads as you want, drizzled with healthy olive oil or avocado oil dressings. Snack liberally on Primal Blueprint-approved snacks. Yes, you are removing the baked potato, corn on the cob, Cheerios, baguettes, and other beige staples from the picture, but the discomfort of a habit change can be greatly minimized when you can look forward to as much as you want of your favorite primal foods during this crucial transition period to the Primal Blueprint eating lifestyle.

Never Struggle, Suffer, or Go Hungry: Surround yourself with Primal Blueprint-approved foods and enjoy them as much and as often as you like. Always have primal snacks nearby to help you through the transition period. That said, pay close attention to your hunger levels, and eliminate emotional triggers that lead to unhealthy eating. Eat because you are hungry, not because you are bored, tired, or stressed. Stop eating when you are no longer hungry, rather than when you feel full, because by then you've likely over eaten.

Substitute: Consider whether you can switch out some of your old favorite meals, snacks, and even treats for interesting new Primal Blueprint options. I used to be a big blueberry pancakes and granola guy, but whatever deprivation I might have felt at first in eliminating the "stack" from my life was more than made up for by a dozen bites of a delicious primal omelet. Consider the overall impact of your current favorite foods on your body and if they are all truly worth it. A fine Italian meal of pasta and gelato will please most any palette, but if you feel bloated, gassy, jittery, and then groggy in the hours afterward, a better strategy might be to consider some of the many other delicious, Primal Blueprint-approved items on the menu (or off it, but likely available by polite request) at the same restaurant.

CHAPTER SUMMARY

1. Primal Blueprint Benefits: Benefits of Primal Blueprint eating include becoming fat-adapted instead of carbohydrate dependent, enhancing cellular function, improved immune and antioxidant functioning, optimal development and repair of muscle tissue, reduced disease risk factors, and stabilization of daily appetite and energy levels. While primal eating is low-carb in comparison to the Standard American Diet, it advocates abundant consumption of nutritious carbs in the form of all vegetables and some fruits. For body composition goals, 80 percent of your success is dependent upon what you eat, particularly when moderating the wildly excessive carbohydrate intake of the Standard American Diet.

2. Insulin Is the Master Hormone: Perhaps the most important health benefit of eating primally is moderating the wildly excessive insulin production associated with the Standard American Diet. Eighty percent of your ability to achieve your preferred body composition is determined by what you eat, specifically the level of insulin you produce as a consequence of your carbohydrate intake and insulin-desensitizing lifestyle factors. When you moderate insulin production and maximize insulin *sensitivity*, you access and burn stored body fat for energy, preserve or build muscle, and reduce disease risk factors.

When the delicate insulin balance is abused by years of consuming too many carbs (especially heavily processed ones), havoc ensues: cells become insulin *resistant,* excess glucose is present in the bloodstream, and more fat is stored, making it increasingly difficult to mobilize that fat as an energy source. This sets the stage for the development of serious conditions such as Metabolic Syndrome, type 2 diabetes, and heart disease. Synthesis of important hormones, including thyroid hormones, testosterone, and human growth hormone is also hindered by excessive insulin production, creating an accelerated aging effect that has more to do with your breakfast choices than chronology. While the long-term effects of excess insulin production are dire, there are also serious *immediate* drawbacks to consuming high-carb snacks or meals. The sugar high/insulin release/ stress response cycle causes problems with fatigue, mental focus, mood swings, and jitters, resulting in burnout.

3. Cholesterol: Cholesterol is critical to healthy cell structure and numerous metabolic functions. Conventional wisdom's lipid hypothesis of heart disease is now widely acknowledged as a flawed and oversimplified view of the risk factors that contribute to heart disease. The lipid hypothesis has been refuted in recent years by the Framingham Heart Study and many other respected studies and experts. The true risk factors for heart disease are best characterized by the common health condition known as Metabolic Syndrome—oxidization and inflammation in the cardiovascular system—which is prompted largely by the ingestion of sugars, grains, and refined vegetable oils. When tracking heart disease risk, blood values like high triglycerides, low HDL, high glucose values, and other inflammation markers are more relevant than the oversimplified obsession with total cholesterol values and the subsequent routine dispensation of statin drugs to lower that number.

What triggers Metabolic Syndrome and other adverse blood values is excessive intake of processed carbs and easily-oxidized fats (trans and refined polyunsaturated fats such as canola, safflower, and soybean oil). Poor exercise habits (either sedentary or too chronically stressful) also promote the inflammation and oxidation symptomatic of Metabolic Syndrome. Raising HDL through consumption of saturated fat and engaging in sensible exercise can help mitigate the potential threat of small, dense LDL becoming oxidized. Conversely, the primary function of statin drugs—lowering cholesterol levels—does not directly address these risk factors. Statins' purported anti-inflammatory benefits can be easily achieved through diet, exercise, and supplementation, saving the expense and harmful side effects of prescription statin therapy.

The key to preventing heart disease is to ditch toxic vegetable fats, exercise according to the Primal Blueprint plan, increase antioxidant intake, and reduce your intake of grains and sugars.

4. Healthy Fats: Primal foods provide high levels of nutritious saturated, monounsaturated, and omega-3 fatty acids. A diet with ample amounts of these healthy fats supports cardiovascular, brain, skin, and immune functioning as well as increases dietary satiety. Unfortunately, the Standard American Diet features excessive levels of unhealthy oxidized fats and insufficient intake of nutritious fats. This leads to the condition of systemic inflammation, which is a catalyst for many disease processes.

5. Eating Well: Enjoy your meals without deprivation, restriction, emotional stress, or other negativity. Choose your favorite foods from the broad list of Primal Blueprint-approved choices and don't obsess about calories, nutrient ratios, regimented mealtimes, or food combinations. Eat until you feel satisfied instead of habitually stuffing yourself until you are full (or depriving yourself in the name of weight loss). Realize that your genes evolved to easily handle sporadic eating habits without energy lulls or metabolic slowdowns and can do so after 21 days of reprogramming, allowing you to become a fat- and keto-burning beast!

6. Transitioning to the Primal Blueprint: When adjusting to the Primal Blueprint eating style, choose primal foods that appeal to you (you can rotate them over and over if you like) and discover desirable substitutes for non-primal options to avoid feelings of deprivation from discarding old meal choices. Have plenty of Primal Blueprint-approved foods available for snacks and meals so you don't suffer, feel depleted, or "cheat" for lack of good options. Be strict in the first 21 days so you can build momentum toward fat-adaptation and make it easier to stay the course over the months, and years, ahead. In the big picture, follow the 80 Percent Rule by being compliant 80 percent of the time and not stressing about perfection. Notice your heightened sensitivity to how foods affect your body, and leverage that awareness to stay on the path of high energy, effortless weight management, and optimal gene expression with Primal Blueprint foods.

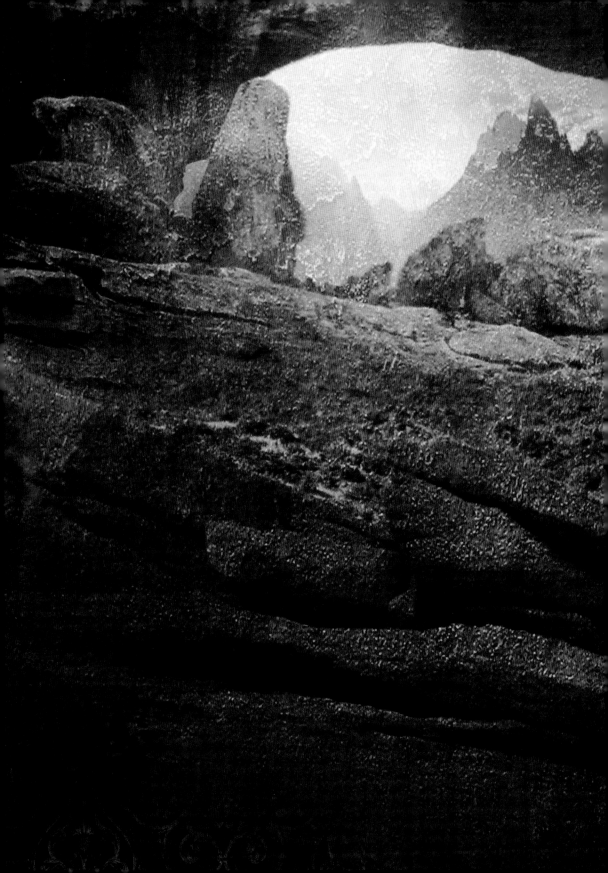

CHAPTER FOUR

UNDERSTANDING MACRONUTRIENTS

"Calories In, Calories Out" Is Out!
It's All About Content and Context

IN THIS CHAPTER

I discuss how each macronutrient (protein, carbohydrate, fat, and the "fourth fuel" ketones) affects your eating strategy, energy levels, and overall health. Protein starts the discussion because of its essential role in building and repairing body tissues. It's easy to obtain enough protein for health: you can determine how many grams you need per day, on average, with a simple calculation based on lean body mass. The wildly excessive carbohydrate intake characteristic of the Standard American Diet can largely be corrected by ditching sugars and grains in favor of choosing high-nutrient-value carbohydrates. Weight-loss goals can be targeted by honoring the ranges on the Primal Blueprint Carbohydrate Curve. With protein intake optimized and carb intake moderated, fat becomes the predominant macronutrient source, and the main variable for achieving satiety and satisfaction at meals.

"Calories In/Calories Out" is Out!
...It's all about content and context

While you likely have a basic understanding of what carbohydrate, protein, and fat do in the body, it's important to examine the role of each nutrient further from a Primal Blueprint perspective. This is particularly true in light of the massive misinformation, distortion, and confusion presented by opposing camps on the issue of the optimal macronutrient balance in the diet.

The concept of "calories in, calories out" fails to account for how different foods influence your appetite and metabolic hormones.

Most popular diets and exercise programs targeting fat loss adopt an oversimplified "calories in, calories out" approach, failing to understand the importance of hormones and other variables that influence whether your body stores or burns the calories you ingest (and whether you feel famished or satiated in the process). The macronutrients you consume are not just burned or stored for use as energy later, but also for basic health maintenance and assorted hormonal functions. Moreover, the body can store fuel (and act as a toxic "waist" site), and it has the capacity to generate its own energy, depending largely on the hormonal signals it gets from your behaviors. Since your body always seeks to achieve homeostasis (balance), the notion of you trying to zero in on a precise day-to-day or meal-to-meal eating plan is generally fruitless, not to mention incredibly frustrating and demotivating. Your body does a great job of adjusting to variations in caloric intake and energy expenditure through an assortment of hormonal and genetic processes that will always supersede your diligent efforts to calculate food and exercise calories.

To figure your true structural and functional fuel needs (and, hence, to achieve your body composition goals), it's important to understand how the major macronutrients work in the body—or should work when you eat in a manner aligned with optimal gene expression.

Protein

Protein is essential for building and repairing body tissues and for overall healthy function. Unlike the wildly varying opinions about the role of fat and carbohydrate in the diet, there has long been a general consensus among nutritionists, medical experts and fitness experts on recommended average daily protein intake. However, as I'll detail shortly, recent research has called into question whether we might be recommending more protein intake than necessary, and I have recently lowered the recommendations that I published in the original *Primal Blueprint* in 2009.

It's clear that there is a minimum protein requirement to ensure the healthy functioning of your organs, skeleton, muscles, and numerous body systems. This is believed to be in the neighborhood of .5 grams per pound (1.1 grams per kilo) of lean body mass on average. Beyond your basic needs, conventional wisdom has long promoted the idea that your protein needs escalate in tandem with your activity level, with moderately active people going for higher than 0.5, and highly active people, growing youth, and pregnant or lactating mothers encouraged to average 1 gram per pound of lean mass (2.2 grams per kilo).

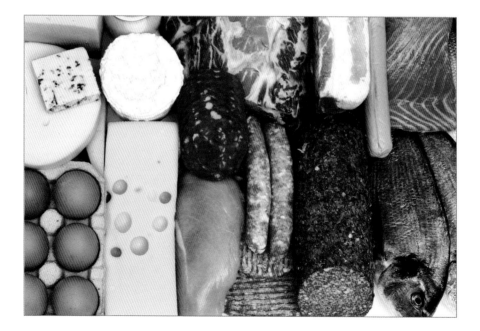

The "average" concept is important here, as the body is adept at compensating for variations in daily and even seasonal caloric intake. Our ancestors endured long periods of time with insufficient protein and low total calories and managed to survive those tough winters or fruitless hunts well enough to perpetuate the human race for hundreds of thousands of years. They also had bountiful times where they may have consumed well in excess of their minimum requirements, likely fattening up for a rough winter on the horizon. Your eating patterns will likely not have such dramatic highs and lows, of course. The point is that it's unnecessary to stress about your protein intake at every meal if you are getting an appropriate amount over the course of a week or a month.

A pattern of excess protein intake accelerates aging and increases cancer risk.

The original Primal Blueprint position was to fall in line with these scaled recommendations. New research suggests that even devoted fitness enthusiasts can easily meet their protein requirements by consuming an average of 0.7 grams per pound of lean mass daily. Surprising research reveals that strength training actually makes you more efficient with protein—you'll do more with less thanks to your fitness efforts.

On the flip side, mounting research suggests that many people may be over-consuming protein to their detriment. Consider the popularity of high-protein diets for weight loss, and the general emphasis on protein in marketing messaging to equate with healthy living. Dr. Ron Rosedale, a leading voice in the concerns about excess protein, suggests that .5 grams of protein per pound of lean mass is plenty for everyone. Functional medicine expert and evolutionary health leader Chris Kresser, author of *Your Personal Paleo Code*, suggests that most everyone meets their protein requirements, because under-consumption patterns result in fatigue, emaciation, and intense cravings for high-protein foods! I now recommend that you strive to average 0.7 grams per pound regardless of your activity level.

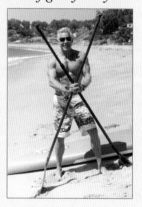

Calculating Lean Body Mass

You can calculate your lean body mass by subtracting your fat weight from your total weight. First, estimate your body fat percentage if you don't actually know it. A fit male is around 15 percent body fat and a fit female is around 22 percent; a moderately fit male is around 22 percent body fat and a moderately fit female is around 30 percent. Alternatively, you can get your body fat measured with the reliable equipment available at many gyms and health care facilities. Armed with your estimate, multiply your body fat percentage by your total weight to get your fat weight, and then subtract that figure from your total weight. What remains is your lean body mass. For example, I weigh 170 pounds (77 kilos) at 10 percent body fat. So my fat weight is 17 pounds (8 kilos), and my lean body mass is 153 pounds (70 kilos). Even at my high activity level, I thrive with a conservative average daily protein intake level of .5 grams per pound of lean mass, or 76 grams per day. See Chapter 10 for a detailed macronutrient analysis of my diet over a three-day period.

It may be more relevant to worry about getting too much protein rather than not enough. When you slam your body with excess protein—more than it needs to fulfill the growth and repair functions that are the primary uses for protein, some potential adverse consequences ensue. You will either work hard to excrete it, producing nitrogen waste products that stress the liver and kidneys; or, if you are locked into a carbohydrate dependency diet, you will convert excess protein into glucose via gluconeogenesis.

The conversion of excess protein into glucose on a high-protein, low-carb crash diet will compromise your fat-loss goals, and essentially make anything considered a high-protein diet to be a high-carbohydrate diet in reality (due to gluconeogenesis). What's more, excess protein consumption continually primes you for accelerated cellular division and growth, instead of the more natural pattern of varying between anabolic (repair, rejuvenation, growth), catabolic (breakdown from exercise and life stressors), and metabolic (normal chemical reactions producing energy). This is why athletes, especially bodybuilders looking to gain mass or athletes training in chronic patterns and struggling to recover each day, are obsessed with protein reloading to promote a continued anabolic state.

Consuming protein stimulates a kinase called mTOR (mammalian target of rapamycin), a key component of an extremely complicated signaling network that regulates cellular growth and proliferation by synthesizing information related to energy input and output, endogenous growth factors, nutrient availability, and stress. While mTOR is crucial for normal cellular growth, emerging research shows that enhanced mTOR stimulation (as happens, for example, when you follow a pattern of excess protein consumption) is associated with obesity, cancer, diabetes, insulin resistance, osteoporosis (via urinary calcium loss), kidney dysfunction (due to the stress of excreting nitrogen), and the aging process itself. On the flip side, laboratory studies on mice and observational studies of very long-lived humans suggest that decreased mTOR signaling (a great way to achieve this is through calorie restriction) is associated with longer life spans.

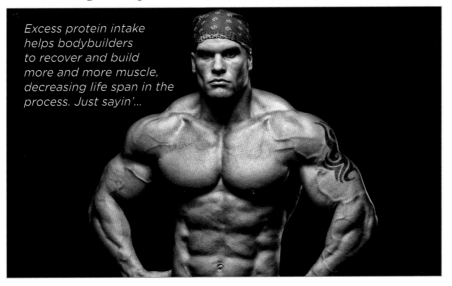

Excess protein intake helps bodybuilders to recover and build more and more muscle, decreasing life span in the process. Just sayin'...

The fact is, when you accelerate cell division, you accelerate aging. Bodybuilders might not care as they pursue ever-larger muscles, and chronic exercisers might be more concerned with muscle recovery than the adverse health consequences of their obsessive refueling, but over-fueling is simply not aligned with health or longevity. By the way, the consumption of excess carbohydrates also gives cells too much fuel over the long term, accelerating cell division and increasing the risk of cell mutation and cancer because excess glucose promotes glycation, oxidation, and inflammation. And as you know, carbohydrates also stimulate insulin release, which itself activates mTOR.

It's true that some research shows that high-protein diets have a slight advantage for weight loss. This is probably partly because eating a lot of protein makes you feel full, which can lead to eating fewer calories overall. It might also be partially due to the inefficient, energy-guzzling process of converting protein to glucose and then to fat. (Your body burns more calories to convert protein to usable energy, promoting weight loss.) Frankly, I suspect the effect is largely attributable not to the increased protein per se but to the reduction in carbohydrates, especially sugary processed foods, and the resulting increase in insulin and leptin sensitivity (which have been directly implicated in weight management).

As we will cover in more detail in Chapter 9—A Primal Approach to Weight Loss, the simple path to losing excess body fat (without harming your long-term health in the process) is to limit your carb intake in accordance with the Primal Blueprint Carbohydrate Curve, optimize protein intake by landing closer to 0.7 grams per pound of lean body mass, and finally to eat just enough dietary fat in order to feel satisfied and energized.

With your macronutrients dialed in, you will effortlessly obtain additional caloric energy from stored body fat until you attain your ideal body composition.

Carbohydrates

If you've forgotten everything you ever learned in biology, just remember this: carbohydrate controls insulin; insulin controls fat storage. (The full story is a bit more nuanced, of course, but when it comes to understand-

Humans survived for 2.5 million years on extremely minimal carbohydrate intake, until we were suddenly bombarded with massive amounts of carbs with the advent of civilization.

ing how food affects your body weight, this is the most critical take-home point.) Carbohydrates are not used as structural components in the body; instead, they are used only as a form of fuel, whether burned immediately while passing by different organs and muscles or stored for later use. All forms of carbohydrates you eat, whether simple or complex, are rapidly converted into glucose upon ingestion. For reference, a little less than one teaspoon of glucose dissolved in the entire blood volume of your body (about five quarts in the case of a 160-pound male) represents an optimal level of blood glucose.

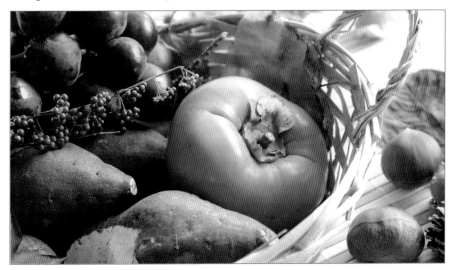

As you learned in Chapter 3, it's insulin's job to take glucose out of the bloodstream and put it somewhere fast. In most healthy people, glucose that is not burned immediately will first be stored as glycogen in muscle and liver cells. When these sites are full, glucose is converted into triglycerides and stored in fat cells. Unless you deplete lots of muscle glycogen every day, there is no physiological need for you to consume high levels of carbohydrates. In fact, carbohydrates are not required in the human diet for survival the way certain fats and protein are. The body has several backup mechanisms for generating glucose internally: from dietary fat and protein, as well as from gluconeogenesis (using either ingested protein or stripping down lean muscle tissue). Researchers have estimated that the body manufactures up to 200 grams of glucose every day from the fat and protein in our diet or in our muscles. These are all adaptive survival mechanisms for a human species that was forced to survive over the course of 2.5 million years through periods of extremely low carbohydrate availability (compared to today, anyway!)—until the advent of agriculture suddenly bombarded our ancestors with massive amounts of carbs in the form of cultivated grains.

> *There is no biological requirement for dietary carbohydrate in the human diet. The Primal Blueprint is an "eliminate bad carbs" diet.*

That said, the Primal Blueprint is not anti-carb, nor is it even rigidly low-carb, because this position might exclude certain individuals with elevated carbohydrate requirements who thrive wonderfully when they choose whole, nutrient-dense sources of carbs. Instead, the Primal Blueprint is about making informed choices based on the ancestral health model, experimenting to determine what works best for you, and being flexible instead of rigid so you can enjoy your life. So while carb intake may vary according to personal preference, it's important to recognize a couple things:

- If you are trying to lose excess body fat, the most direct path is to moderate carb intake.

- There is no call for anyone to consume grains, sugars, sweetened beverages, or other highly processed, high-carb fare, ever.

It's easy to stay in the Primal Blueprint Carbohydrate Curve's optimum range of 100 to 150 grams per day—even while eating heaping servings of colorful vegetables, or the occasional fresh seasonal fruits, and other incidental sources of carbs. For example, a huge salad, two cups of Brussels sprouts, a banana, an apple, a cup of blueberries, and a cup of cherries totals only 139 grams of carbohydrates. I don't advocate portion control or even diligently counting your macronutrient intake. You may want to journal now and then to establish benchmarks and reference points. (Visit FitDay.com or Cronometer.com and input a day or two of the food that you eat to get a breakdown of macronutrients and calories.) But you don't really need to do this unless you're struggling to reduce excess body fat and want to accelerate your progress.

Note: Perhaps you are familiar with the concept of "net carbs" when measuring macronutrient intake. This is a calculation that subtracts fiber from total carbohydrate intake because fiber is usually not digested, and it moderates the blood glucose impact of a carbohydrate food. Incidentally, some types of fiber can also be converted into short-chain fatty acids by bacteria in your gut, making fiber's role more like a fat than a carbohydrate. What's more, some experts suggest that you can omit non-starchy vegetables like leafy greens from your carb intake calculations, believing that their high fiber content and low energy yield makes them practically "carb neutral" for metabolic purposes. Personally, I don't recommend painstakingly counting and subtracting fiber grams from your daily carb count, nor discounting the carbohydrate grams in vegetables. If you decide to journal food intake and use an online calculator like FitDay.com, you'll see that even your gross intake of carbs will fall into a healthy zone if you are resolute in eliminating grains and sugars from your diet. If you are making strict efforts to get into ketosis, limiting your carb intake to 50 grams per day still allows for a healthy level of vegetable consumption.

THE CARBOHYDRATE CURVE—WHAT'LL IT BE? THE "SWEET SPOT" OR THE "DEATH SPIRAL"?

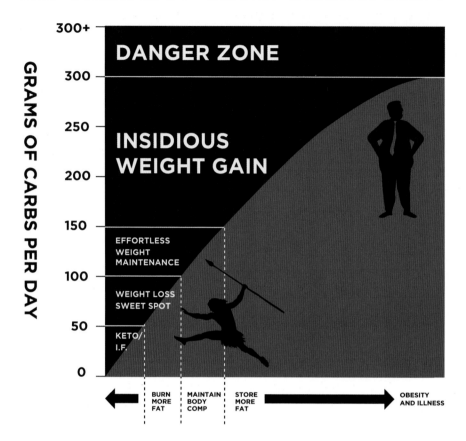

The Primal Blueprint Carbohydrate Curve provides a rough illustration of how carbohydrates impact the human body and the degree to which we need them (or don't) in our diet. It most strongly applies to those who are "metabolically damaged" from decades of suboptimal eating and lifestyle habits (which, ahem, is most of us), since those factors collectively reduce carbohydrate tolerance. (Hence the apparent paradox of why some non-industrialized populations—who don't spend the bulk of their adult lives stuck at desk jobs and eating vending machine food—can get away with a higher carb intake without suffering the waistline ravages we see in the West.) For those "damaged" individuals, carb reduction is an even more powerful tool in their weight-loss arsenals.

For most people, carb intake is a major factor in weight-loss success or failure, and excessive refined carb consumption is arguably the most destructive modern lifestyle behavior. Eliminating grains and sugars from your diet could be the most beneficial thing you ever do for your health!

0 to 50 grams per day: *Ketosis and Accelerated Fat Burning*
This benchmark is an excellent catalyst for quick, relatively comfortable fat reduction, but it requires a sustained period of primal-style eating to become fat-adapted before attempting. Ketogenic eating is an advanced strategy that has become more popular in recent years, particularly among endurance athletes who want to liberate themselves from glucose dependency during exercise with disciplined dietary carb restriction. It also shows promise for treating the global obesity/type 2 diabetes epidemic and other assorted diseases, including certain brain cancers and cognitive disorders. Because ketogenic eating is such an extreme departure from the Standard American Diet, and even from typical primal-style eating, the strategy should be used with discretion by experienced primal eaters. Note that it's acceptable to dip into and out of a ketogenic state through Intermittent Fasting.

50 to 100 grams per day: *Primal Sweet Spot for Effortless Weight Loss*
This minimizes insulin production and accelerates fat metabolism. By meeting average daily protein requirements, eating nutritious vegetables and fruits, and staying satisfied with delicious high-fat foods (meat, fish, fowl, eggs, nuts, seeds), you can lose one to two pounds of body fat per week in the "sweet spot." Delicious menu options that land in the sweet spot are detailed in Chapter 9.

100 to 150 grams per day: *Primal Blueprint Maintenance Range*
This allows for genetically optimal fat burning, muscle development, and effortless weight maintenance. The rationale is supported by the fact that humans evolved while eating in this range or below for millions of years. This rate allows an abundant intake of nutritious vegetables, sensible amount of fresh seasonal fruits, and a moderate intake of assorted other carbs such as starchy tubers, dark chocolate, high-fat dairy, and nuts and seeds. A history of heavy carb intake may result in a brief period of dis-

comfort during the transition to Primal Blueprint eating, but emphasizing high-satiety foods (e.g., animal products, nuts and seeds, avocado, olive, and coconut products) helps protect against feeling deprived or depleted.

150 to 300 grams per day: *Steady, Insidious Weight Gain*
This level of daily carb intake leads to continuous insulin-stimulating effects which prevent efficient fat metabolism and contribute to widespread health conditions—especially among those with already-reduced insulin sensitivity from modern diet and lifestyle habits. This zone is the de facto recommendation of many popular diets and "official" health authorities (including the USDA Food Pyramid!) despite the clear danger of developing or exacerbating Metabolic Syndrome. Extreme exercisers, active, growing youth, members of non-Westernized populations (whose diets and lifestyles grant a great deal of protection), and those with physically strenuous jobs may eat at this level for an extended period without gaining fat; but for many, eventual fat storage and/or metabolic problems are highly probable.

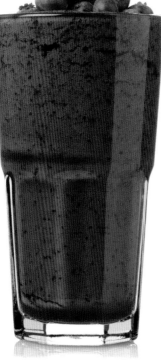

This insidious zone is easy to drift into, even for health-conscious eaters, when processed grains are a dietary centerpiece, sweetened beverages or snacks leak into the picture here and there, and excessive fruits and starchy vegetables are added to the total. Recall that Kelly Korg's trip to Jamba Juice for a "healthy" afternoon snack resulted in 187 grams of carbs ingested in *one* sitting. Starting your day off with a bowl of muesli cereal, a slice of whole wheat toast, and a glass of fresh

The image of a smoothie has become synonymous with health, vitality, and super nutrition. Yes, you are getting a good dose of antioxidants, but mainly it's a massive insulin bomb.

orange juice might seem right off the "heart-healthy" menu at the luxury spa, but the numbers start racking up (that's 97 grams of carbs!), and the disastrous insulin-spike/sugar-craving cycle is set in motion. Despite trying to do the right thing by cutting fat and calories, many frustrated people still gain a pound or two of fat per year for decades as a result of carb intake in the insidious range.

300 or more grams per day: *Danger Zone!*
This is the typical carb intake of someone eating the Standard American Diet and is in excess of official USDA dietary guidelines (which suggest you eat 45 percent to 65 percent of calories from carbs), thanks to stuff like soda tipping the scales. Extended time in the danger zone means weight gain and the beginning (or exacerbation) of Metabolic Syndrome are highly probable. Consuming carbs in the danger-zone level (especially when they're heavily processed and accompanied by a sedentary, insulin-sensitivity-reducing lifestyle) is the primary catalyst for the global obesity and type 2 diabetes epidemics, as well as numerous other significant health problems stemming from systemic inflammation and constant energy surplus. An immediate and dramatic reduction of sugars, sweetened beverages, grains, and other processed high-carb foods is critical.

Carb Curve Variables: The 50-gram/200-calorie variation within each range on the curve attempts to account for individual energy disparities: a light, moderately active female should aim for the low end of the range, while a heavy, active male will be comfortable at the high end. Certain extreme calorie burners who maintain ideal body composition can consume more high-nutrient-value carbs than these general ranges suggest and still enjoy good health and peak performance. However, chronic exercisers (and other high-stress folks who, thanks to "lucky" genes, are less predisposed to storing excess body fat) can still suffer from the inflammatory, health-compromising effects of danger zone carb intake, even if they don't show it on the outside.

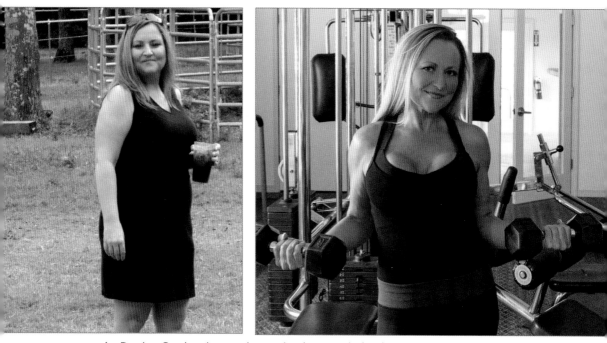

As Denise Cooke shows, dramatic changes in body composition can occur as a byproduct of eating primally; much more fun than the conventional approach of obsessive calorie counting and burning.

There is no single right answer to the question, "How many carbs should I eat?" It depends on many idiosyncratic variables, including your particular goals. If you're looking to optimize your body composition and also to obtain sufficient carbs to fuel fitness endeavors, ensure healthy hormonal function (especially for women who are sensitive to carb restriction), or to feel healthy and energetic, determining your ideal carb intake starts with asking yourself a simple question: "Do I have excess body fat or not?" If you want to drop unwanted fat, the simplest and most direct path is to dial back carb intake per the Carbohydrate Curve guidelines. Some people can take a cold-turkey plunge and cut carbs in half (or further) to make fat loss happen quickly, while others might have to adopt a more gradual approach to avoid some of the stumbling blocks in the transition to fat-adaptation. Bear in mind that extracting yourself from decades of sugar dependency can initially challenge your energy, appetite, and hormonal functions—often in measure with just how severe that sugar dependency was.

First ditch sweetened drinks, sugars, and grains. Then get a good handle on your average daily carb intake with journaling and online calculators, and see how things work for you.

Your health and likely your life span will be determined by the proportion of fat versus sugar you burn over a lifetime.

—Dr. Ron Rosedale
author of The Rosedale Diet

Fat

Consuming healthy fats from animal and plant sources supports optimal function of all the systems in your body. Ingesting fat helps you feel full and satisfied in a way that ingesting carbohydrates, generally speaking, cannot. Because fat has little or no impact on blood glucose levels or insulin production, and takes far longer to leave your stomach and metabolize than carbohydrates, you will feel a deep and long-lasting satisfaction from consuming high-quality fat in your diet.

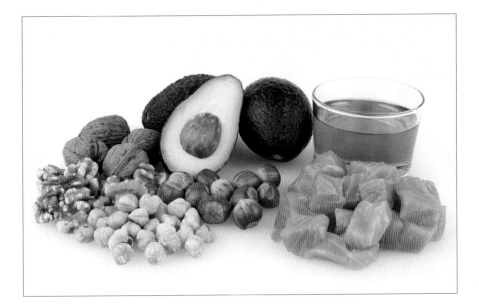

After decades of fat being maligned and misunderstood, mainstream health and medical science is finally embracing the reality that fat is not a direct catalyst for heart disease or weight gain. For instance, take the highly respected Nurses' Health Study, which tracked the dietary habits of 90,000 nurses over two decades. It is the largest epidemiological study of women in history, leading to the publication of 265 scientific papers in leading journals. The study showed no statistically significant association between total fat intake (or cholesterol intake) and heart disease. Many other studies have attempted to establish a firm connection, yet none have demonstrated that a high-fat diet by itself causes heart disease.

> *The Nurses' Health Study (involving 90,000 nurses over two decades) showed no statistically significant association between total fat intake (or cholesterol intake) and heart disease.*

So how can it be that low-fat eating became conventional wisdom? I believe that the otherwise well-meaning, well-educated folks in the low-fat camp are influenced by a few factors that lead them to the party-line conclusion that a high-fat diet is unhealthy.

Failure to distinguish between good fats and bad fats: The skyrocketing rates of obesity, heart disease, and cancer from eating a diet high in both processed carbs and highly refined polyunsaturated or chemically altered fats have unfairly led to all fats being villainized indiscriminately. Indeed, consuming certain dangerous fats is, from a health perspective, one of the most objectionable behaviors in modern life; but other fats are extremely healthy and nutritious. Processed junk foods are laden with partially hydrogenated trans fats, "Franken-fats" created by adding hydrogen to liquid oils to make them more solid. Solidifying fats in this manner effectively extends shelf life—a boon, for sure, for the food industry's pocketbook. Yet from a health standpoint, trans fats can be devastating. A report in *The New England Journal of Medicine* reviewed numerous studies and found a strong link between consumption of trans fats and heart disease. Trans fats prevent the synthesis of prostacyclin (a cardio-protective lipid molecule that helps blood vessels dilate) and can make cells more rigid and less fluid when incorporated into cell membranes. Because your brain, nervous system, and vascular system are highly dependent upon healthy cell membranes, any dysfunction in these critical areas can be devastating. Research also shows that consumption of trans fatty acids from partially hydrogenated oils may promote inflammation, aging, and cancer.

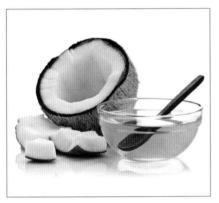

Coconut oil: very, very good. High in health-promoting medium-chain triglyceride (MCT).

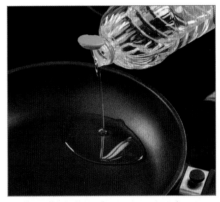

Refined high polyunsaturated vegetable oil: very, very bad. Full of free radicals!

Any consumer with a basic concern for health has undoubtedly heard about the dangers of partially hydrogenated trans fats. Less appreciated are the dangers of refined polyunsaturated vegetable and seed oils (canola, corn, soybean, safflower, sunflower, grapeseed, peanut, etc.), buttery spreads made with polyunsaturated vegetable oils, and assorted packaged or frozen processed foods manufactured with these oils. Scan labels in just about any aisle of the grocery store and you will see how these toxic agents are ubiquitous in our food supply. Because they've been stripped of any saving nutritional grace that could compensate for their fragile chemical structure (such as vitamin C, polyphenols, and other antioxidant phytochemicals), refined polyunsaturated fats—unlike the whole foods they were extracted from—are easily oxidized by light, heat, or oxygen. Ingestion of these free radicals in a bottle, tub, or package will disrupt healthy hormone and immune function upon consumption, and over time lead to more cellular damage throughout your body.

It's especially risky to cook with these unstable oils, as the heat causes significant oxidative damage to the molecules. As Dr. Cate Shanahan explains, studies reveal that the ingestion of a simple order of French fries causes an immediate disruption in the normal dilation of arteries (such as that which occurs in response to exercise), and that this disruption in healthy cardiovascular function can last for up to 24 hours.

Carbs making fat look bad: Fat is calorically dense at nine calories per gram. If you consume excessive carbs (150 to 300 grams or more per day), produce a high level of insulin, and eat any appreciable amount of fat along with your high-carb diet, your fat intake will contribute directly to making you fat. Excess carbs raise insulin levels, which steers both carbs and fat (and even excess protein via gluconeogenesis, as we learned) into your fat cells, making high amounts of carbs and fat together more problematic than either macronutrient on its own.

Propaganda and flawed science manipulated into conventional wisdom: The machinations of public policy bureaucracy often leave rational thinking in the dust in favor of protecting and promoting corporate interests and the reputations of politicians. While I am all in favor of capitalism, it's unsettling how much decision-making power is controlled by corporations that spend billions of marketing dollars molding and shaping conventional dietary wisdom in the direction of profits, with little regard for health.

In the story of how saturated fat came to be vilified, American scientist Ancel Keys is a central character. Keys was an eloquent and dynamic early promoter of the link between saturated fat intake, cholesterol levels, and heart disease. Keys achieved notoriety in the 1960s for his efforts to transition the public away from saturated fats to replacements such as polyunsaturated oils or low-fat eating in general—as well as his remarkably successful use of the American Heart Association to cement his theories into public policy. It has taken decades, at a dawdling pace, to recognize the folly of his health suggestions. For example, Keys was unable to explain the existence of healthy high-fat populations like the Inuit and Masai. While some of his earlier observational work (comparing fat intake and heart disease rates among different cultures) seemed to show a link between saturated fat and heart disease, his data were taken to show causation, a dreadful misinterpretation. (Just because two things co-occur, that does not mean one causes the other.)

The Framingham Study, Nurses' Health Study, and recent meta-analyses (reviews that aggregate data from numerous related research studies) have strongly refuted the oversimplified direct association between fat and disease that unfortunately became entrenched in conventional wisdom. (In fairness, Keys also did some great work helping to popularize the Mediterranean diet—highlighted by the liberal intake of healthy fats—even spending his last few decades living in a small town in Italy and studying the residents' dietary habits.)

On a bureaucratic level, the U.S. government has time and again shown a penchant for doggedly defending the status quo, while vigorously squashing voices opposing conventional wisdom. A prime example of the influence of power and money on the development of public policy is found in the FDA's so-called "imitation policy," passed in 1973 (without congressional approval, thanks to some clever legal maneuvering). The legislation relieved food manufacturers from having to use that pesky "imitation" designation on labels of foods created with artificial ingredients (coffee creamers, egg substitutes, processed cheeses, whipped cream, and hundreds more), as long as manufacturers added synthetic vitamins to their concoctions to approximate the benefits of similar whole foods.

Mary Enig, Ph.D., a renowned nutritionist, lipid biochemistry expert, and author of *Know Your Fats,* from the University of Maryland, spent her career battling conventional wisdom's take on fat intake and heart disease. In the 1970s she was a central figure in challenging the corruption and misinformation dispensed by the USDA and the U.S. Senate's McGovern Committee (headed by former presidential candidate George McGovern). Influenced by highly questionable and lobby-influenced testimony, the committee published its report directing Americans to replace saturated fat with polyunsaturated fatty acids and to limit fat intake in general, which was then disastrously replaced with excessive processed carbohydrates.

On the heels of these cultural turning points, government-funded research over the following decades tended to fall in line with the committee recommendations. The notion that all fats are bad gained momentum and was adopted as conventional wisdom. Today leading health authorities are now presenting a more responsible big-picture perspective about the role of fats in a healthy diet and the dangers of eating chemically altered fats in particular. But it will take the general public—and especially low-fat enthusiasts—many more years to embrace and implement what is now validated by scientific research.

The Wonderful World of Ketones

While most cells in our body can easily burn both fats and glucose, there are a few select cells that function only on glucose (some brain cells, red blood cells, and kidney cells, for example). Without glucose, those cells would cease to function, and we would not last very long. The minimum daily glucose requirement to keep those systems running has been estimated at between 150 and 200 grams per day, but recent research shows that after a little adaptation, some of these cells can operate effectively on a fuel your body manufactures itself known as ketones, dramatically reducing your overall glucose requirement.

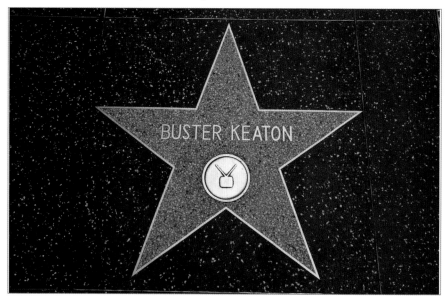

Bust out some ketones by restricting carb intake once you are fat-adapted.

Ketones are produced in the liver as a byproduct of fat metabolism when blood glucose and insulin levels are very low. Brain cells and cardiac and skeletal muscles utilize ketones in the same manner they use glucose, making ketones a highly effective, clean-burning substitute for the energy provided by ingested carbohydrates. As you might imagine, ketones were crucial to human evolution, since our ancestors rarely had steady access to carbohydrates like we do today. In fact, they may have gone weeks or months without appreciable carbs, so they had to evolve systems to manufacture glucose (gluconeogenesis) or glucose substitutes like ketones.

Your body evolved to utilize ketones in the same manner as glucose; a key survival component throughout human evolution.

Ketone burning helped keep Grok alive during short periods of starvation or longer periods when meat (protein and fats) was plentiful but plants (carbs) were not. Ketones are safe, desirable, energy-efficient forms of fuel. They are quite literally the fourth macronutrient fuel source, but they come from inside your body instead of from your plate. After just a few weeks of reducing carb intake, and therefore insulin production, and increasing the relative amounts of healthy fats in your diet, you will send signals to your genes that result in an increased production (an "upregulation") of the metabolic "machinery" used to effectively burn both fats and ketones throughout your body. When your body becomes efficient at using fat and ketones for energy, you are said to be fat- and keto-adapted.

> *Ketones are an internally manufactured energy source that the body burns in the same manner as glucose—except more cleanly!*

•••••••••• **GROK TALK** ••••••••••

Why Glucose Is Dirty and Ketones Are Clean

The benefits of being keto- and fat-adapted extend far beyond weight loss. Quite frankly, glucose burns "dirty" in your body, creating considerable metabolic waste products, inflammation, and oxidative damage; while fat and ketones burn "clean." Glucose is metabolized for energy quickly and easily, but mitochondria and oxygen are not required for glucose burning. Hence, you can lose out on the free-radical protection that mitochondria provide during calorie burning. When you are locked in a carbohydrate-dependency diet, your mitochondria can actually atrophy. This atrophy increases your susceptibility to all forms of oxidative stress, not just from diet but from chronic exercise, pollution, and the stress of hectic modern life. Note: glucose can also be burned with oxygen and mitochondria, but even then more free radicals are generated in comparison to burning fat and ketones.

The best way to optimize mitochondrial function and protect yourself against general free radical damage is to become fat- and keto-adapted. Utilizing lots of oxygen and mitochondria to metabolize calories, requiring fewer calories to survive (because insulin and hunger hormones are moderated when you are fat-adapted), engaging in Intermittent Fasting, and dipping into that rarified state of ketone burning—even if it's just occasionally—all support mitochondrial biogenesis. Mitochondrial biogenesis is the manufacture of additional mitochondria (and optimizing the functioning of existing mitochondria) to better diffuse the oxidative stress of burning calories and simply being a living, breathing human.

Ketone burning has been shown by science to facilitate rapid fat reduction, improve the function and development of mito-chondria (the energy centers of our cells), exert a potent anti-inflammatory effect, improve immune function, boost cellular repair, con-trol epilepsy, deliver assorted benefits to cognitive function (especially for those with dementia, autism, and ADHD), and even fight can-cer (by starving cancer cells of their main fuel, glucose.) Check out *The Art and Science of Low Carbohydrate Living* by Dr. Steven Phinney and Dr. Jeff Volek for a com-prehensive education with scientific detail about the wonders of ketones for the aforementioned conditions, and watch Dr. Dom D'Agostino's TEDx Talk "Starv-ing Cancer" for details on that subject. Interestingly, the therapeutic benefits of ketone burning have prompted the manufacture of consumable sources of ketones, allowing one to override the delicate macronutrient restrictions and achieve elevated blood ketone levels.

PROTEIN 20%
CARB 10%
FAT 70%

KETOGENIC DIET
● PROTEIN
● FAT
● CARBS
(approximates)

After reaching sufficient fat-adaptation through a sustained period of primal-style eating, people who take the next step and commit to a ketogenic eating pattern (requiring even further carb restriction) report accelerated fat reduction, improved mental clarity, and better endurance performance. (See Chapter 7 in *Primal Endurance* for some amazing accounts of elite athletes performing world-class endurance feats fueled by fat and ketones.) Interestingly, many cells actually prefer to burn ketones over glucose, given the choice between the two. Cardiac muscle, skeletal muscle, and even certain brain cells thrive on the four-and-a-half calories per gram delivered by ketones. After a little keto-adaptation, the brain can do very well getting 75 percent of its energy from ketones.

Ketones can't be stored conveniently the way fats (and excess glucose) can be stored in fat cells or the way glucose can be stored as glycogen.

Ketones simply circulate in the bloodstream where they are available to be picked up by any cells that want and need the energy they provide. *Ketosis* is the scientific name for a relative condition in the body where ketones start to accumulate in the bloodstream to a point beyond which they can be utilized for energy. Despite the flawed assertions from some mainstream dietary authorities, there is nothing dangerous or undesirable about being in ketosis, per se. It is a natural, normal part of human energy production and metabolism. In fact, most everyone wakes up in a state of mild ketosis from fasting overnight (unless you are a midnight snacker!), or any other time you don't ingest carbs for a prolonged period of time.

That said, ketosis is a very delicate metabolic state. Once you consume even a moderate amount of carbs (or enough protein to get converted into carbs), you'll be spit right out of ketosis and back into a glucose-burning state. It's most likely a state early humans encountered frequently, but not permanently. And while existing studies on ketosis have been promising, very long-term sustained ketosis—say, years and beyond—remains something of an experiment, with potential negative repercussions for gut health and hormone function if occasional carb refeeds don't occur. (Contrary to popular belief, there aren't any known examples of human populations who live entirely in ketosis. Even the traditional Inuit diet isn't ketogenic because of it's too-high-for-ketosis protein intake; plus, a widespread genetic mutation causes Inuit to burn long-chain fatty acids for heat instead of producing ketones.) Bottom line: intermittent macronutrient changes are more in line with our evolutionary past than any permanent dietary state, and most people—excepting those with specific athletic goals or health conditions that benefit from ketosis—should think of ketosis as a cyclical tool, rather than a state to strive for indefinitely.

If you are not presently keto-adapted—and most people who eat a moderate-to-high-carb diet are not—and then you abruptly decide to fast in the name of cleansing or weight loss, the ketones you manufacture in the absence of dietary carb intake aren't yet able to be burned efficiently. Instead, you excrete the ketones you make via breathing and elimination. Some describe the smell of ketone breath as that of overly ripe apples or nail polish remover. If you are new to primal eating, you will require a few weeks to reprogram your genes to become more efficient at burning ketones. As your body adapts to a genetically optimal low-carbohydrate eating pattern, you will *burn* ketones effectively and *excrete* fewer, thereby further reducing your glucose requirements.

Some people—including some misinformed doctors and dietitians—maintain a distorted, negative view of ketones and ketosis. I believe these criticisms arise because the diets in question allow for only 20 grams or less of carbs per day, a level that does not allow for the plentiful intake of nutrient-rich vegetables. While we are not meant to run predominantly on carbohydrate energy, we do depend heavily on the nutrients offered by vegetables and most fruits. Other people may be mistaking ketosis for *ketoacidosis*, a potentially deadly condition that affects insulin-dependent diabetics and alcoholics and which is completely different from nutritional ketosis.

Under normal Primal Blueprint maintenance eating patterns, you rarely enter a state of ketosis because of the dietary emphasis on high-nutrient-value carbs like vegetables. The Carbohydrate Curve maintenance zone of 100 to 150 grams of carbohydrates daily is still quite low by comparison to the Standard American Diet, but it's too high to launch you into serious ketone burning. This is just fine, of course, but learning about ketosis and trying it now and then to accelerate weight loss (and enjoy other metabolic benefits) or to experiment with endurance performance gains is something to consider, especially as you get further into primal living and become highly fat-adapted.

On the Primal Blueprint accelerated fat-loss program (detailed in Chapter 9), you will eat in what I call the sweet spot—a level of mild ketosis—by consuming 50 to 100 grams of carbs per day. Here, your carbs are low enough to enable quick fat reduction, your protein is optimized to preserve lean muscle mass, and you have plenty of fat to keep you completely satisfied at meals and throughout the day.

Understanding how you metabolize protein, fat, carbohydrates, and ketones, and controlling the rates at which each one burns by improving your diet and exercise habits, you needn't agonize over day-to-day calorie counting. As long as you are eating primal-aligned foods, you will be able to naturally maintain your ideal body composition and mitigate your risk of diet-related health conditions and diseases.

My doctor told me to stop having intimate dinners
for four. Unless there are three other people.

—Orson Welles

CHAPTER SUMMARY

1. The dated "calories in, calories out" equation for weight management fails to recognize context, particularly the hormonal disregulation caused by wildly excessive insulin production. If you are locked into a fat-storage pattern due to high-carb eating patterns, this will override attempts to lose weight through caloric deficits.

2. Daily macronutrient need calculations start with protein, since protein is essential for building and repairing healthy tissues and organs. The updated Primal Blueprint recommendation for average daily intake is 0.7 grams per pound (1.5 grams per kilo) of lean body mass. Consuming higher amounts of protein is stressful to liver and kidneys, and (when carb dependent) often converted into glucose via gluconeogenesis. Furthermore, a pattern of excess protein consumption stimulates growth factors and accelerates cell division, leading to increased cancer risk and reduced life span.

3. Wildly excessive carbohydrate intake is the foremost health-undermining behavior of the Standard American Diet. Carbohydrate intake prompts insulin production, which prompts fat storage. Dial back carbs and you will drop excess body fat. The primal approach recommends ditching grains, sugars, and sweetened beverages and obtaining whatever level of carbs are desired from high-nutrient-value sources like vegetables, fruits, sweet potatoes, and wild rice. The various intake ranges on the Primal Blueprint Carbohydrate Curve reflect how one can achieve weight-loss goals, optimize general health, and minimize disease risk. Primal Blueprint-style eating affords abundant intake of vegetables, sensible intake of fruits, and high-nutrient-value carbs as desired by fitness/activity goals and personal preference—usually landing in the neighborhood of 150 grams per day.

4. When protein intake is optimized according to lean mass, and carb intake is moderated per primal guidelines, fat becomes the primary source of caloric energy and dietary satisfaction. Fat has been maligned by conventional wisdom for a few reasons: failure to distinguish between good and bad fats, high carb intake making fat problematic, and propaganda and flawed science. Saturated fat is healthy and optimal to cook with. Monounsaturated fats and omega-3 fats offer excellent health benefits. Refined high polyunsaturated vegetable oils and chemically altered vegetable oils inflict oxidative damage on the body and should be eliminated.

5. Ketones are an *internally* manufactured energy source, a byproduct of fat metabolism in the liver when blood glucose levels are low due to disciplined restriction of dietary carbs. The brain, heart, and skeletal muscles use ketones in a similar manner to glucose, but it burns with much less oxidative stress than glucose and actually delivers a potent anti-inflammatory effect. Ketones were a critical component of evolution, enabling humans to survive during periods of insufficient dietary calories. Today, breaking science shows ketones to have incredible promise for fat loss, improving cognitive conditions and seizures, boosting endurance performance, and fighting cancer. Becoming keto- and fat-adapted means that you are efficient at burning internal sources of energy and no longer dependent upon regular meals to sustain energy or concentration.

CHAPTER FIVE

PRIMAL BLUEPRINT LAW #1: EAT PLANTS AND ANIMALS

(Insects Optional)

IN THIS CHAPTER

I detail the health benefits of eating Primal Blueprint style and explain how to choose the best products in the categories of animal foods (meat, fish, fowl, eggs, and even insects) and plant foods (vegetables, fruits, nuts, seeds, and their butters, and herbs and spices), as well as moderation foods (coffee, high-fat dairy, high-nutrient-value carbs, dark chocolate), and certain high-quality nutritional supplements.

While you likely have a basic understanding of what carbohydrate, protein, and fat do in the body, it's important to examine the role of each nutrient further from a Primal Blueprint perspective. This is particularly true in light of the massive misinformation, distortion, and confusion presented by opposing camps on the issue of the optimal macronutrient balance in the diet.

Locally grown, pesticide-free, or certified organic vegetables and fruits are the safest and richest in micronutrients. They are packed with phytochemicals, antioxidants, vitamins, and minerals that support health and help prevent disease. Emphasize locally grown, in-season, high-antioxidant fruits, such as berries, but avoid excessive year-round consumption. Local, pasture-raised, or certified organic animal foods are healthy and nutritious and will help you reduce excess body fat and build lean muscle. They are free from the offensive ingredients (hormones, pesticides, and antibiotics) and processing methods commonly found with mass-produced foods. Eggs are healthy and rich in fat-soluble vitamins. They have been mistakenly maligned due to the flawed assertion that their high cholesterol content is a heart disease risk factor. The higher cost of buying local or organic plant and animal products pales in comparison to the health care costs of long-term conditions like type 2 diabetes that are strongly influenced by poor dietary habits.

Nuts, seeds, and their derivative butters are nutritious, satisfying foods that make a popular primal-approved snack replacement for typical grain-based snacks. Coconut products are great sources of the hard-to-obtain medium-chain fatty acids, and they're great substitutes for conventional cooking oils and baking ingredients. While fruits are teeming with good nutrition, some moderation is warranted due to our propensity for frequent year-round consumption versus only eating these dietary carbs when in season. In fairness, our excessive levels of total dietary carb intake are due to the inclusion of processed foods and beverages containing the objectionable high fructose corn syrup.

Herbs and spices deliver excellent antioxidant and anti-inflammatory benefits, and they enhance food's flavor. Foods to enjoy in moderation include coffee (don't use as an energy crutch), high-fat dairy products, and high-nutrient-value carbs (sweet potatoes, squash, wild rice, quinoa).

Prebiotics and probiotics have gained recognition as an important component of healthy eating and optimal immune and digestive function. Prebiotics, aka resistant starches, feed probiotics. Best sources are raw potato starch and green bananas, and, interestingly, cooked and cooled white rice and russet potatoes. Probiotics are found in fermented foods such as yogurt, kefir, sauerkraut, kombucha, and pickles. Dark chocolate is the Primal Blueprint-approved treat (75-percent cacao or higher is ideal). It's rich and satisfying, high in antioxidants, phytonutrients, brain-stimulating compounds, and even resistant starch.

Hydration is a complex issue, particularly for athletes. While minimally active people can use thirst as a guide, and not worry about the outdated "eight glasses per day" dogma, more active types must pay more attention to hydration and electrolyte balance issues and take a preemptive approach to maintaining adequate hydration.

Certain supplements, such as a comprehensive multivitamin, omega-3 fish oil, prebiotics, probiotics, protein powder/meal replacement, and vitamin D for the sun-challenged, can be useful to shore up deficiencies in our hectic modern life.

If we're not supposed to eat animals,
how come they're made out of meat?

—Tom Snyder

PRIMAL BLUEPRINT FOOD PYRAMID

for effortless weight loss, vibrant health, and maximum longevity

- Nutritious, satisfying, high-nutrient-value, low-insulin-stimulating foods.
- Low carbohydrate, moderate protein, ample nutritious fats.
- Flexible choices and meal habits by personal preference.
- Free of grains, sugars, and refined vegetable oils.

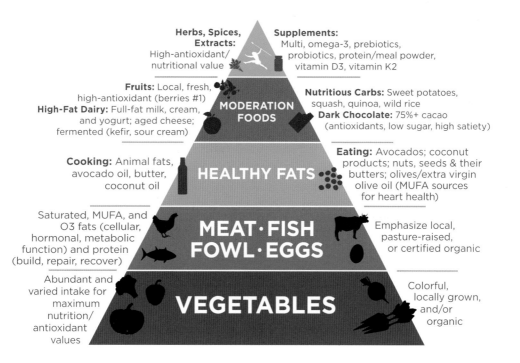

Herbs, Spices, Extracts: High-antioxidant/nutritional value

Supplements: Multi, omega-3, prebiotics, probiotics, protein/meal powder, vitamin D3, vitamin K2

Fruits: Local, fresh, high-antioxidant (berries #1)
High-Fat Dairy: Full-fat milk, cream, and yogurt; aged cheese; fermented (kefir, sour cream)

MODERATION FOODS

Nutritious Carbs: Sweet potatoes, squash, quinoa, wild rice
Dark Chocolate: 75%+ cacao (antioxidants, low sugar, high satiety)

Cooking: Animal fats, avocado oil, butter, coconut oil

HEALTHY FATS

Eating: Avocados; coconut products; nuts, seeds & their butters; olives/extra virgin olive oil (MUFA sources for heart health)

Saturated, MUFA, and O3 fats (cellular, hormonal, metabolic function) and protein (build, repair, recover)

MEAT·FISH FOWL·EGGS

Emphasize local, pasture-raised, or certified organic

Abundant and varied intake for maximum nutrition/antioxidant values

VEGETABLES

Colorful, locally grown, and/or organic

Perhaps the most fundamental element of the evolutionary health movement is the simple assertion that humans have evolved into omnivorous creatures adapted to consume a variety of plants (vegetables, fruits, nuts, seeds, and their butters, and herbs and spices) and animals (meat, fish, fowl, eggs, and even insects), and are wholly unequipped to consume the refined sugars, grains, and industrial oils that comprise a huge proportion of our modern diet. Plant foods are the main sources of vitamins, minerals, antioxidants, anti-inflammatory agents, and thousands of other healthful phytonutrients in the human diet. Animal foods are calorically dense and satiating, offering the best forms of healthy protein and fat. They should represent the bulk of your caloric intake, while vegetables will represent the bulk of the space on your plate.

> *Humans have evolved into omnivorous creatures adapted to consume a variety of plants (vegetables, fruits, nuts, seeds, and their butters, and herbs and spices) and animals (meat, fish, fowl, eggs, and even insects), and are wholly unequipped to consume the refined sugars, grains, and industrial oils that comprise a huge proportion of our modern diet.*

In hunter-gatherer times, a significant portion of calories in the human diet (estimates range from 45 to 85 percent, depending on geography) came from eating a variety of animal life, including insects, grubs, amphibians, birds, eggs, fish and shellfish, small mammals, and some larger mammals. In general, those living closer to the equator consumed more plants and less animal food, while those at colder latitudes with fewer plant options consumed more meat.

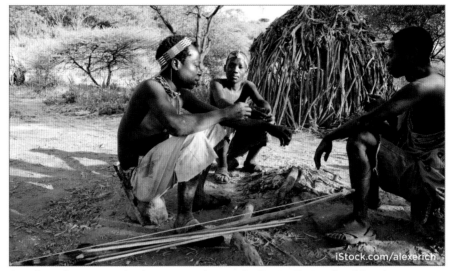

Studies of present-day hunter-gatherers indicate that animal foods are a centerpiece.

These estimates are based in part on studies of contemporary hunter-gatherers who still live traditionally (that is, whose lifestyles have not been radically changed by the incursion of outside cultures and dietary practices like the SAD). Among those still living traditionally, the Hiwi in Venezuela have a diet that is 75 percent animal foods. The Aché in Paraguay eat 78 percent game meat. The traditional-living Inuit in arctic Canada and Alaska famously eat 96 percent animal foods. On the other end of the spectrum, the remaining hunter-gatherer Hadza of Tanzania eat 48 percent animals, 52 percent plants. The !Kung Bushmen of the Kalahari eat 31 percent animals, 28 percent nuts, and 41 percent other plants. No 7-11 Slurpees to be found!

These meat sources provided generous amounts of protein and all types of essential fatty acids and vitamins. Grok often ate as much as 300 or 400 grams of protein and up to 200 or more grams of fat in a day during times of plenty—and yet maintained a svelte physique. Of course, he also ate zero refined carbohydrates, produced moderate levels of insulin, and excelled at using stored fat as fuel. These macronutrient profiles allowed him to build or preserve muscle and provided ample fuel for both long treks and short bursts of speed.

Animal foods are healthy and nutritious and will help you reduce excess body fat, build lean muscle, and generally obtain peak performance. I highly respect those who have philosophical objections to consuming animal products. However, I must maintain that the widely held modern belief that saturated fat and cholesterol in animal foods are directly correlated with obesity and heart disease, or that vegetarianism is somehow healthier, has been proven by science to be grossly inaccurate. Like it or not, our bodies have evolved for 2.5 million years on animal foods, ever since meat eating facilitated survival and became a catalyst for population expansion. (Our ability to migrate to the higher latitudes depended on us developing "meat-adaptive" genes.)

No culture or society has ever survived for an extended period of time on a meatless diet. While it would seem to be much easier to live and evolve without having to run around and kill animals, the truth is that we need the concentrated, nutrient-rich energy source of meat, fish, fowl, and eggs to support accelerated brain development—our distinguishing feature that brought humans to the top of the food chain.

Remarkably, about 500 calories a day are required just to fuel the human brain (both primitive and modern brains). Anthropological evidence strongly suggests that it was saturated fats, protein, and omega-3 fatty acids from animal foods that provided both the raw materials and the energy necessary for the human brain to grow larger and more sophisticated through evolution. Our ability to catch and cook meat (cooking makes meat easier to chew, swallow, and digest) was critical in our branching up and away from our mostly vegetarian ape cousins.

The vegan/vegetarian eating strategy has numerous health benefits, but adherents often default to eating a fair amout of nutrient-deficient

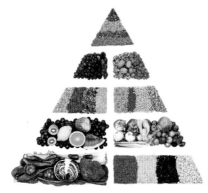

There are many positives about the vegan pyramid, particularly the colorful, high-antioxidant vegetables and fruits. However, this eating pattern results in excess carbs, excess insulin, and insufficient nutritious fats due to restriction of high-nutrient-value animal foods like meat, fish, fowl, and eggs.

high-carbohydrate foods simply to obtain sufficient calories. If you first ditch sugars, grains, bad oils, *and* also decide to avoid animal products, you are going to have a very difficult time getting enough high-quality protein, fat, and overall calories (while avoiding toxic modern foods) to remain healthy and vibrant.

> *Animals (meat, fish, fowl, and eggs)*
> *and plants (vegetables, fruits, nuts, seeds,*
> *and herbs and spices) should represent nearly*
> *the entire composition of your diet.*

Unfortunately, over the last few generations, conventional wisdom has disparaged not only red meat but all forms of saturated fat. Starting back in the 1960s and 1970s, we were aggressively steered away from traditional cooking with animal fats (butter, poultry fat, lard, tallow) in favor of cooking with refined high polyunsaturated vegetable/seed oils. This saturated-fat-phobic "margarine movement" has now been widely exposed as a disaster. Saturated fats are temperature stable at high heat, making them the most appropriate choice for cooking. As we learned in Chapter 3, refined high polyunsaturated oils are easily oxidized during processing and further oxidized when heated, making the ingestion of these oils among the most dangerous elements of the modern diet. The "Primal-Approved Fats and Oils" section later in this chapter lists my favorite fats and oils, as well as which ones to avoid.

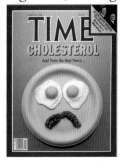

Fortunately, everyone is in agreement that brightly colored vegetables and fruits are healthy, supplying high levels of antioxidants, flavonoids, carotenoids, and myriad other important phytonutrients that serve as a powerful first line of defense against oxidative damage from aging, stress, and inflammation. Moreover, antioxidants and other phytonutrients appear to contain cancer-fighting properties, support immune function, aid in digestion, and help preserve muscle mass, a critical component of longevity for those of advanced age.

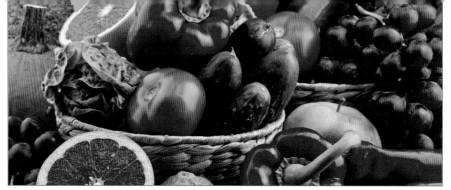

Color is good in the diet! Veggies and fruits deliver assorted antioxidant, anti-inflammatory, anti-aging, anti-cancer, and antimicrobial properties.

While leading a healthy, balanced lifestyle will activate the genes that make our built-in antioxidant systems (catalase, superoxide dismutase, and glutathione) fight hard against cellular and DNA breakdown, research suggests that we may require additional antioxidant support from foods and supplements. Of course, most processed foods, meats, and refined carbohydrates are devoid of antioxidants, while vegetables, fruits, and nuts are the best sources of these natural antioxidants.

Remember the discussion of oxidation as a central heart disease component? Well, antioxidants protect against oxidative damage in the body. It follows that if you want to be healthy and prevent disease, vegetables (and fruits, with a bit of moderation and selectivity) must play a prominent role in your diet. For a quick primer, red plants (beets, red bell peppers, radishes, dark cabbage, pomegranates, cherries, watermelon) have been shown to help reduce the risk of prostate cancer as well as some tumors. Green fruits and vegetables (avocados, limes, bell peppers, zucchini) are high in antioxidants and phytonutrients, deliver a powerful anti-aging effect, and are especially helpful for vision. Yellow and orange fruits and vegetables (bananas, papayas, carrots, butternut squash, pineapple) offer beta-carotene for immune support as well as bromelain, which has been shown to aid in digestion, joint health, and the reduction of inflammatory conditions. Cruciferous ("cross"-shaped, with a branch and leaves) vegetables, including broccoli, Brussels sprouts, kale, arugula, turnips, bok choy, horseradish, and cauliflower, have demonstrated specific anti-cancer, anti-aging, and antimicrobial properties. Nuts and seeds provide high levels of beneficial unsaturated fatty acids, fiber, phytonutrients, antioxidants (e.g., vitamin E and selenium), and a host of essential nutrients (e.g., manganese, magnesium, zinc, iron, chromium, phosphorous, and folate).

PALEO VERSUS PRIMAL: SPLITTIN' HAIRS

I often get questions about the distinctions between paleo and primal. Paleo is an abbreviation for Paleolithic—the historical time period predating civilization. Primal is a more generic term conveying the basic, fundamental, essential, and original elements of being human. In the context of the Primal Blueprint, it's about applying evolutionary science to create a blueprint for healthy living today.

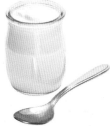

With regard to diet, the precise use of the term "paleo" requires the application of a strict litmus test: did the food/ingredient exist in Paleolithic times? *Yes* means you can eat it (meat, fish, fowl, eggs, vegetables, fruits, nuts, seeds); *No* means it's not paleo (grains, sugars, vegetable oils, and also dark chocolate and cheese). Hence, primal is less strict than paleo. If dark chocolate or high-fat dairy products offer nutritional benefits and are not oppositional to our genetic expectations for health, they are primal approved—even if they were not part of the human diet 10,000 years ago.

Anyone asking about the distinction between paleo and primal is likely well-informed about, and committed to, an alternative and enlightened approach to optimum health. It's important to not waste time or energy splitting hairs about the nuances of one person's message or interpretation when the different approaches are extremely similar, especially in contrast to the Standard American Diet. While healthy debate and constructive feedback help to advance the evolutionary health movement in general, we must all respect the importance of remaining amicable and staying focused on the big picture: rejecting disastrously flawed conventional wisdom in favor of a simple, back-to-basics, evolutionary-based approach to healthy living.

Grok never ate dark chocolate... but he certainly would have if it were offered to him.

The rest of this chapter will detail the health benefits of each of the entries on the Primal Blueprint Food Pyramid and how to make the best consumption choices.

MEAT AND FOWL

Many of the conventional wisdom health objections to eating animal foods can easily be countered by eating local, pasture-raised, 100 percent grass-fed, or USDA certified organic sources of meat. This suggestion is highly recommended due to the generally poor quality of much of today's mass-produced feedlot animal products, which typically contain hormones (to grow the animals bigger quickly and therefore increase profits), pesticides (ingested from their own inferior food sources; vegetarian advocates claim that 80 to 90 percent of your total dietary pesticide exposure comes from eating meat, although that's disputed by the EPA), and antibiotics (to prevent widespread illness resulting from consuming immune-suppressing feed and living in filthy, cramped feedlots and coops).

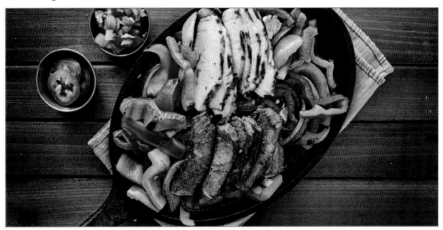

Furthermore, today's feedlot cattle, chickens, and other animals are usually fed a diet of fortified grains, which have a similar effect on their bodies as on a human's! If you purchase meat at an ordinary supermarket chain, there's a good chance you'll end up eating a malnourished, insulin-resistant, and quite possibly diseased animal whose meat is higher in omega-6 fats (thanks to grain feeding) —a far cry nutritionally from Grok's fresh, lean, wild kills. Finally, humane reasons compel many to avoid meat. The animals we typically dine on consume half of our crop harvest; their waste pollutes air, rivers, and streams; and they are subjected to horrifying treatment at unsanitary production facilities (as detailed in such books as *Fast Food Nation, The Omnivore's Dilemma, Diet for a New America*, and even *Skinny Bitch*).

My favorite animal is steak.

—Fran Lebowitz

For these reasons, I strongly urge you to look for local sources of pasture-raised meat whenever possible, which are typically found at farmers' markets. If local, pasture-raised meats are not available, the next best alternative is USDA certified organic. Clearly, there is a continuum here where you can find options that are various degrees away from ideal. While the ultimate dining experience in this category would be to consume as much of the entire body as possible of a wild animal who consumed a nutritious, high-omega-3 diet (including a delicious bone broth made from the carcass), there aren't many of them running around the continent these days. Beyond local, pasture-raised animals from small farms or USDA certified organic animals, there is minimal regulation in this industry, and assorted other descriptors such as "free-range" and "all-natural" have limited significance. (More on this topic later in this chapter.)

Fortunately, the popularity of eating locally and/or organic is skyrocketing, so you should have good luck finding healthier animal products in your area. If not, you can utilize some of the excellent resources on the Internet, such as americangrassfedbeef.com and eatwild.com. I order wagyu-style ground beef and other cuts from grass-fed cattle in Montana, packed in ice and shipped directly to my home from thompsonriverranch.com.

Besides being free of hormones, pesticides, and antibiotics, pasture-raised animals offer two to six times more omega-3 and monounsaturated fats than feedlot animals do. If, for reasons of budget or availability, you find yourself eating a less-than-ideal source of meat, always choose the leanest possible cuts and simply trim the excess fat. This will significantly limit your potential exposure to these toxins, because environmental pollutants and toxins build up in adipose tissue—fat. Of course, you can add back some delicious fat by cooking the now leaner meat in grass-fed butter!

It's important to acknowledge that over the past decade, some studies about red meat consumption have prompted alarming headlines that "excessive" consumption of red meat may be associated with a slightly increased risk for cancer and heart disease. In reality, many of these studies are a matter of mistaking correlation for causation. That is, they assume that because someone who eats more red meat is also at higher risk for a certain disease, that means the red meat is *causing* that disease—when in fact, the risk factor could instead be the hamburger buns the red meat is sandwiched between, the fries or soda that accompany it, the less healthy lifestyle that typical meat-eaters in the West often embrace… you get the picture.

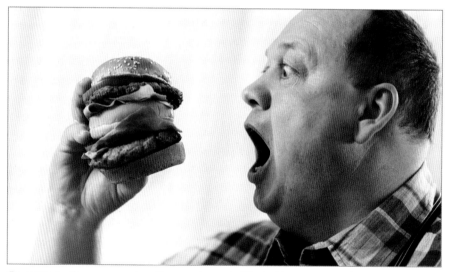

Recent studies suggest eating red meat (it's in there somewhere…) is unhealthy… Ya think? In other news, throwing the baby out with the bathwater can harm your child.

Likewise, although excessive carbohydrate intake—like that inherent in the Standard American Diet—negatively affects how we metabolize meat, none of these studies take that into account. (Remember that carbs and fats consumed together increase triglyceride production in the liver, and emerging evidence suggests that certain bacteria found in the guts of heavy grain-eaters may convert substances in red meat to harmful compounds.) Furthermore, most of these studies (in which participants self-report their dietary intake) include in the general "red meat" category all manner of popular processed meats (chemically-treated hot dogs, breakfast sausage, jerky, bacon, bologna, salami, etc.), which generally contain nitrosamines and other potential carcinogens. These agents have been shown to accelerate the formation and growth of cancer cells throughout the body.

Authors of these studies also offer another possible explanation for the increased risks: overcooking of meat. You may have heard that some forms of seared, burned, or overcooked meat may contain heat-altered chemical byproducts called heterocyclic amines (or HCAs) and polycyclic aromatic hydrocarbons (or PAHs) that may be carcinogenic if consumed frequently over long periods of time. Since mankind has been cooking with fire for hundreds of thousands of years, it's apparent that we have developed a host of natural genetic adaptations to allow us to eat most properly cooked foods without problems.

Furthermore, some studies indicate that consuming antioxidant-rich foods (such as vegetables, fruits, herbs and spices, and even red wine and dark chocolate) along with cooked meats can essentially neutralize any potentially harmful byproducts of overcooking. Of course, the Primal Blueprint would argue that eating only "clean" meats (pastured or organic whenever possible), avoiding nitrosamine-laden processed meats, using appropriate cooking techniques (like slow-roasting, stewing, or using crock pots or sous-vide cookers), lightly cooking red meat, enjoying a variety of different forms of animal foods, eschewing deep-fried or high-heat barbecued meats, eating certain forms of meat raw (sushi, tartare, etc.), and including high-antioxidant fruits and vegetables with your meat consumption will likely eliminate any possible risk altogether.

Making the best purchasing decisions about meat requires a good understanding of the labeling/categorizing terminology. It's easy to be fooled by meaningless accolades that might be slapped on inferior quality products, because regulations in this area are minimal. Following is a description of common labels on meat products to assist you in making the most discretionary purchases:

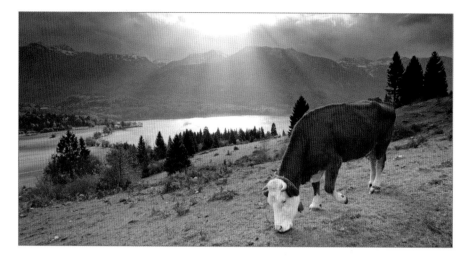

Local, Pasture-Raised: The premier choice for meat; the ultimate in sustainability and minimal carbon footprint. A locally raised chicken, cow, or lamb grazing in the open pasture consumes a variety of grass, grubs, worms, and bugs that are rich in nutrients such as omega-3 fatty acids and assorted vitamins and minerals that are deficient in CAFO (concentrated animal feeding operation) animals. Note that the onus is on the consumer to research farms and find a trustworthy source. Being pasture-raised does not guarantee, for example, that the animals are not given hormones. Ideally, you can establish a relationship with a local farmer or rancher (perhaps through a farmers' market or food co-op) and inquire about their methods, and even visit the farm if you are so inclined.

Certified Organic: Raised on grass or grain feed without antibiotics, hormones, genetic engineering, irradiation, sewage sludge, or artificial ingredients. Afforded "conditions which allow for exercise, freedom of movement, and reduction of stress appropriate to the species." Suppliers are subject to regular inspection by USDA-approved third parties. Animals may not be locally raised (and in fact may have traveled a great distance to your market) and have possibly received grain-based feed to supplement calories obtained on the free range. This results in a slightly-to-significantly less optimal nutritional profile than a 100-percent pasture-raised/grass-fed animal.

Certified: USDA evaluated the meat for class, grade, or other quality characteristics (e.g., Certified Angus Beef).

Chemical-Free: This vague term is not defined or recognized by the USDA and has virtually no significant meaning on a package.

Country of Origin Labeled (COOL): Specifies where the animal was raised, slaughtered, and processed—sometimes including multiple locations (USDA regulated). As with purchasing produce, buying meat from local sources when possible is preferred.

Free Range: Indicates an animal was given "access" to outdoors. Has no legal definition or third-party verification and is often abused by growers. "Access" can refer to a large indoor facility (where animals have been conditioned to remain) with a door to a small outdoor area. No guarantee that meat is free from hormones and antibiotics.

Fresh: Implies that the meat has not been frozen (internal temperature dropping below 26 degrees Fahrenheit) prior to sale; no relevance to how animal was raised, fed, or slaughtered, and not third-party verified.

Grass-Fed, Grass-Finished, Pasture-Raised: Animals afforded access to grass, but no guarantee of grain-free diet unless a "100 percent" qualifier appears on label. Even then, no guarantee that meat is free from hormones or antibiotics. Terms are not regulated or third-party verified and are thus inferior to USDA certified organic.

Hormone/Antibiotic Free: No legal definition or third-party verification. Suggests an improvement from conventional products, but inferior to USDA certified organic.

Humane Designations: Animal Welfare Approved, American Humane Certified, Certified Humane Raised & Handled, or Free Farmed are common terms. The first designation, from the Animal Welfare Institute, certifies that animals were treated humanely throughout all life stages. Their designation (and the others) has strict standards for outdoor access; diets free of hormones, pesticides, or antibiotics; and freedom from overcrowded conditions. Furthermore, the terms are third-party verified. Humane-certified animals are probably a suitable choice in the absence of local or USDA certified organic meat.

Kosher: Meats prepared under rabbinical supervision and guidelines. The designation relates more to slaughtering methods, segregation of implements and production facilities (i.e., meat cannot be mixed with dairy products, etc.), and other factors that may or may not be related to health quality.

Natural: Meat free of artificial flavors, colorings, and preservatives. No relevance to how animal was raised, fed, or slaughtered, and not third-party verified.

Vegetarian Diet: This pertains to the animal's diet only and does not guarantee that the animal had access to pastures or humane treatment. Absent any special label designations, you are likely buying a mass-produced animal raised on feedlot grains with pesticide residues, growth hormones, and antibiotics. Such animals are often treated inhumanely.

FISH

Fish offer a rich source of omega-3 fatty acids (particularly the important omega-3 fractions known as DHA and EPA that are not present in most other foods), complete protein, B complex vitamins, selenium, vitamin D, vitamin E, zinc, iron, magnesium, phosphorous, antioxidants, and other nutrients. A 2006 study by the Harvard School of Public Health concluded that regular consumption of fish helps dramatically reduce the risk of heart disease and that the benefits (particularly the omega-3 content) outweigh the potential risks of ingesting toxins from polluted waters.

Regular consumption of fish has been shown to exert a strong anti-inflammatory effect, reduce risk for heart disease, help protect against asthma in children, moderate chronic lung disease, reduce the risk of breast and other cancers by stunting tumor growth, and ease the symptoms of rheumatoid arthritis and certain bone and joint diseases. Nursing and pregnant women enjoy a host of benefits from fish consumption, including support for fetal and early childhood brain and retinal development and a lowered risk of premature birth.

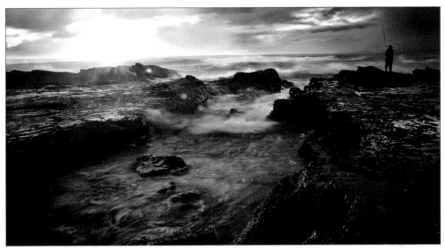

Humans typically followed the seashore in their migration to every corner of the globe. Archeological evidence of Paleolithic fishing sites proves the central role fish played in our ancestors' ability to survive and thrive.

While the benefits of eating fish are substantial, you should learn to choose wisely to avoid fish possibly tainted with environmental toxins and to try and avoid or minimize certain objectionable farmed species (although some other farmed species are fine; we'll cover the particulars shortly). The risk of ingesting fish tainted by environmental contaminants (heavy metals such as mercury, polychlorinated biphenyls [PCBs], dioxins, and other toxins) can be countered by emphasizing fish caught by domestic operations in remote, pollution-free ocean waters. The healthiest sources of fish are small, oily cold-water fish, such as, sardines, mackerel, anchovies, wild-caught salmon, and herring (SMASH hits in your diet!)

Certain fish at the top of the marine food chain, such as swordfish and shark, should be limited or avoided due to their tendency to accumulate concentrated contaminants. However, the threat of mercury poisoning from fish consumption generally has been exaggerated. The Western Pacific Regional Fishery Management Council, based in Hawaii, asserts that most every Pacific Ocean fish except swordfish and shark contain substantially high enough levels of selenium (a potent antioxidant) to negate concerns about mercury toxicity. "Our favorite fish are more likely to protect against mercury toxicity than cause it," according to the Council.

The reason to avoid some species of farmed fish is that they are often raised under unsanitary conditions similar to those of ranch animals and are exposed to high levels of dangerous chemicals such as dioxins, dieldrin, toxaphene, and other pesticides or toxic residue. These chemicals (from contaminated sediments in their fish meal) are easily absorbed into fat cells. Farmed fish may be routinely exposed to their own waste. Salmon are often fed artificial dyes to help their flesh match the deep pink color of wild varieties of salmon (derived from the molecules of carotenoids containing the pigment astaxanthin). The benefits of carotenoids that salmon get from their wild diet of crustaceans like tiny shrimp are then passed on to us when we eat them. Antibiotics are also used in farmed salmon to fight infections and disease typically caused by living in cramped quarters. The waste from a large salmon farm is estimated to equal the sewage from a city of 10,000 people and is believed to deliver assorted negative effects on the surrounding marine ecosystem. A 2004 report in the journal *Science* warned that farmed salmon contained 10 times the amount of toxins of wild salmon and should

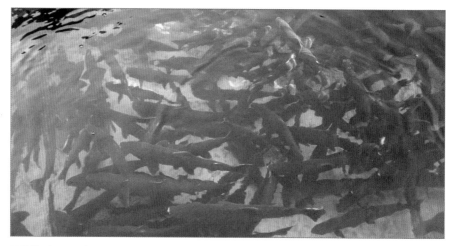

While farmed Atlantic salmon still offer decent nutritional benefits, they are an inferior choice to wild-caught salmon.

be eaten rarely—once every five months—due to their high cancer risk. Furthermore, the watchdog organization Food and Water Watch states that it takes around 42 pounds of wild fish to create the feed product necessary to produce 10 pounds of farmed fish, so there are sustainability concerns here too.

While wild salmon offers 19 to 27 percent of its total fat in omega-3s, farmed Atlantic salmon (by far the most common salmon offered at markets and restaurants) generally contain lower amounts of omega-3s, less protein, and higher levels of omega-6 fats (obtained from their commercial feed, unlike the omega-3-rich algae that nourishes wild fish). Of additional concern are the estimated three million salmon that escape from their pens into the ocean each year, contaminating and genetically diluting nearby wild salmon.

Use discretion and look for the various species of wild-caught Pacific salmon (Chinook, Sockeye, Coho, Pink, Chum), even if your budget requires that you choose less expensive frozen or canned products at times. You can also look for farmed Coho salmon as a healthy, budget-friendly alternative, especially from freshwater tanks. Farmed Atlantic salmon comes with concerns about industrial and environmental contamination and inferior nutritional value. If you're dining out, even at a nice place, it's probably farmed Atlantic; Atlantic is the species, not the location where it was caught.

Now that you've been warned of the risks of some types of farmed fish, know that there are certain other categories of farmed fish with minimal toxin levels and superior nutritional profiles that make them acceptable to consume. You just have to do a little homework. If you do choose to eat farmed fish, insist on domestic sources to alleviate the risk posed by polluted waters and lax chemical regulations in high-producing countries like China and other Asian neighbors. It might be best to also avoid wild-caught fish from Asia if you live on distant continents, due to these quality control uncertainties, as well as the lengthy transit time. Yep, look more closely at the perfect looking, incredibly low-priced stuff on display at the big box store—it's most likely from Asia. These industrialized products are quite a bit different from sitting down to a quality sushi experience in Tokyo.

Barramundi, catfish, crayfish, and tilapia from domestic farms have impressive nutritional profiles and minimal toxin risks. Farmed trout from the United States or Canada is nutritionally comparable with wild trout, with minimal contaminant concerns, making it another sensible choice. Farmed shellfish are okay because they don't eat artificial foods and have similar living circumstances as wild shellfish, i.e., they are attached to a fixed object. However, make a strong effort to eat fresh over frozen shellfish.

If you are wild about salmon and willing to endure the trade-off of a big carbon footprint and substantial expense to get a quality product, you can find better and better options at specialty fish markets, quality supermarkets, big box stores, and online resources like wildpacificsalmon.com, seabeef.com, jdockseafood.com, or vitalchoice.com. The first site, wildpacificsalmon.com, offers a choice of a half-dozen different species, all caught in Alaska and shipped across the United States via FedEx next-day in vacuum-packed, cold-insulated containers. This site also features extensive details about the benefits of eating wild salmon and the dangers of eating farmed salmon.

For smart shopping, cultivate a relationship with a local dedicated fish market or farmers' market vendor who are far more likely to carry fresh, local fish than a supermarket or big box store. When shopping, take aggressive, close-up sniffs of the offerings. Odor should be nonexistent for freshwater fish and perhaps a faint ocean smell for saltwater fish. Bad fish will have the unmistakable smell of, well, bad fish. There are also a growing number of reputable online sources for high-quality fish (if you don't mind the carbon footprint of shipping fish from far away). If you're lucky—and not landlocked—you might have access to a community-supported fishery (CSF) program in which you can purchase a share of local, sustainable seafood (modeled after traditional CSAs that deliver local produce on a regular schedule).

Finally, be advised that the safety, quality, and sustainability of fish are in constant flux. Check resources such as the Marine Stewardship Council (msc.org), Monterey Bay Aquarium Seafood Watch (montereybayaquarium.org), and the Environmental Defense Fund (edf.com) for up-to-date information.

Many farmed fish, especially the prevalent Atlantic salmon, should be avoided because they are raised in unsanitary, waste-infested waters and have dangerous chemical additives in their diets.

EGGS

Eggs can be freely enjoyed as an excellent source of healthy protein, fat, B complex vitamins, choline, and folate. Be sure to obtain local, pasture-raised, or organic chicken eggs. Chickens afforded their natural omnivorous diet of bugs, lizards, worms, and grass can produce eggs with up to 10 times more omega-3s than conventionally raised eggs. Anyone who has tried a farm-fresh egg from a pasture-raised chicken can attest to the incredible flavor intensity—and distinctive orange-tinted yolk (from beta-carotene)—compared to a conventional egg. The conventional wisdom "heart-healthy" concept of discarding the yolk to avoid cholesterol is misguided, as the yolk is one of the most nutrient-rich foods on the planet, particularly when it comes from a pasture-raised hen. In contrast, egg whites, besides being a good source of complete protein, have otherwise a rather low nutrient content.

If the outdated dire warnings about eating eggs are still echoing in your ears, know that recent scientific research has found that those concerns about eggs are completely unfounded. A Harvard Medical School study that followed 115,000 individuals over a span of 8 to 14 years found no correlation between egg consumption and heart disease or stroke. A 2008 study published in the *International Journal of Obesity* suggests that eating two eggs for breakfast is

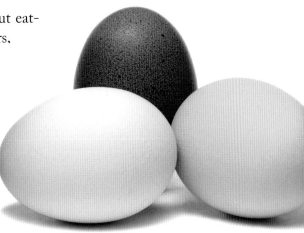

healthier than eating a bagel. Your local farmers' market should be teeming with pasture-raised eggs. Otherwise, most quality grocers, health food stores, co-ops, and national chains (e.g., Trader Joe's and Whole Foods Market) stock abundant sources of organic eggs. If you have trouble finding organic eggs near you, visit localharvest.org and perform a zip code search. Look for some unique suppliers and try other types of eggs. Duck eggs have delicious, intense flavor. You may also enjoy emu, goose, ostrich, pheasant, or quail eggs. Since these eggs aren't mass-produced, they are certain to be unaffected by problems associated with mass-produced chicken eggs.

Eliminating processed or packaged foods and sweetened beverages and growing your own fruits and vegetables can reduce your budget and improve your dietary quality.

GOING PRIMAL ON A DIME

I understand that buying organic animal products can be cost-prohibitive. I acknowledge the criticism of primal/paleo as an "elitist" diet and elaborate on this philosophical issue in Chapter 10. For now, I'll stand as a strong advocate for healthy living and getting your priorities straight, including budgeting for the best foods you can afford—even if this means your diet may potentially become more expensive and cumbersome (though it might not, if you do a little legwork).

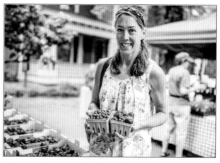

Shop frequently for fresh, primal-approved foods—prioritize health and enjoyment of every bite of food that you eat!

If you sharply cut back or eliminate processed carbohydrates from your diet, you avoid the vast majority of the high-cost (and high-profit), low-nutritional-value products in the store. Shifting from bottled waters, juices, designer coffees, and all other sweetened beverages to emphasize water, tea, or even making your own probiotic-rich kombucha at home will save a substantial amount of money. Switching from designer snacks such as synthetic energy bars and meal replacements (Kelly Korg spends about 70 bucks a month on her twice-daily SlimFast shakes) to such basics as nuts, seeds, nut butters, homemade trail mixes or jerky, sardines, or hard-boiled eggs can reduce your budget while also improving dietary quality.

Consider growing your own fruits and vegetables in your backyard garden, in containers on your balcony or patio, or in a patch rented from an urban community garden. Perhaps there is even a co-op or farmers' market in your area where you can trade time volunteering for food. "Cowpooling" (divvying up a butchered, local animal amongst friends) can also be economical. Ultimately, clever primal purchasing strategies can actually get you close to breaking even with your pre-Primal-Blueprint grocery expenses. Visit MarksDailyApple.com and enter "primal budget eating" in the search bar for numerous articles on the subject.

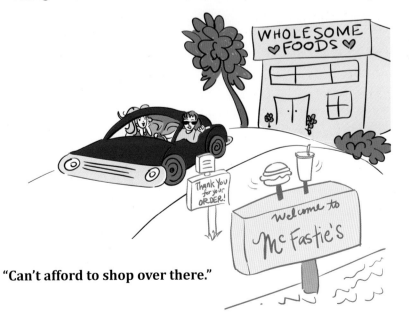

"Can't afford to shop over there."

As a health advocate, I am sensitive to sounding judgmental or critical when I present the Primal Blueprint principles. Rather than moralize endlessly about right or wrong, I prefer to present you with information and empower you to make your own decisions, understand the consequences of those decisions, and walk the path that you have chosen. Then, if you depart from the healthiest path now and then, rather than beat yourself up, simply acknowledge, accept, and recalibrate back to choices that bring happiness and satisfaction the next time you decide what to eat, whether to work out, or what time to go to bed.

Few things demand more freedom from moralization or outside control than deciding how to spend your hard-earned money. Yet, as we are all susceptible to the relentless consumerist messages to consume processed, conveniently packaged food, it might be helpful to reexamine the budget, particularly when considering your diet and health. Deciding to eat higher-quality food, may require more of your time, energy, and expense compared to simply grabbing what you can on the go or on the cheap. However, because food, as your fuel source, is such a critical component of health, it can be argued that your return on investment is far greater than any other lifestyle change you can make. Not to sound trite, but such an investment in your health today, can pay dividends far more impactful and longer lasting than you might ever see in your 401(k).

Granted, real-world concerns may result in you sometimes falling short of the ideal spelled out in these pages. It's important to remember the big-picture view that the Primal Blueprint is a way of life, not a boot camp. If you are purposefully choosing fruit that stimulates a lower glycemic response, or you find yourself eating conventional hamburger at the company picnic but are diligent enough to toss the buns in the garbage before you dig in, congratulations are in order for the momentum and awareness you have already created. Every step you take toward living primally puts you that much closer to your health and fitness goals—and makes you that much more adept at righting the course when the inevitable deviations happen.

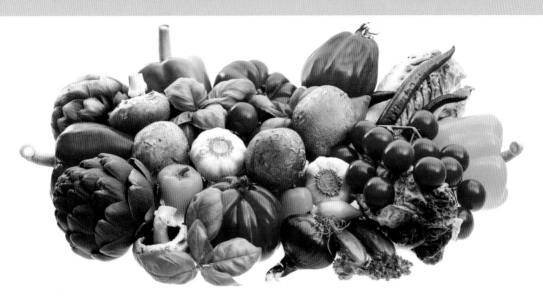

VEGETABLES

It's hard to criticize vegetables, but the shiny, buffed-up conventionally grown vegetables on display in our local supermarkets are often nutritionally inferior to locally grown produce. Conventional produce is sprayed with pesticides, picked too early and then artificially ripened by exposure to ethylene gas, and shipped far from its distant origins (thumbs-down from a carbon footprint perspective). Genetically modified produce does grow bigger and more colorful, but at what cost to our health? All these mechanized processing methods compromise the nutritional content of our food.

It is preferable to select locally grown, in-season vegetables whenever possible, and to opt for pesticide-free or organic if they are available. Pesticide-free is the best way to completely avoid pesticide exposure because while the organic certification limits use of synthetic chemicals, it still allows for the use of some harmful natural pesticides. The best way to ensure that your produce is grown using your preferred methods is by contacting the local farmers supplying your produce and inquiring directly about their growing practices. In the absence of freshly picked, locally grown veggies, certified organic supermarket vegetables are the next best option. These will have less exposure to chemicals and a higher nutritional value accordingly. It's also important to acknowledge that organic veggies might also suffer from the aforementioned lengthy journeys from farm to your shopping basket. (I will address these issues again in the "Fruit" section later in this chapter).

Local Is the Way to Go

Your best bet with fruits and vegetables is to stay local, and yep, that means your produce intake will vary wildly according to the season. Even in temperate Southern California, the farmers' market offerings in the summer (berries and pitted fruits abound) are nothing like the winter (squash and other root vegetables abound, no berries in sight). Go with the flow and eat what's available in your area. Obvious allowances must be made for those living in produce-challenged climates or during the winter months to ensure that you get enough colorful, high-antioxidant vegetables into your daily routine. Bonus points should be awarded if some of your fruits and vegetables come from home-preserved supplies of canned, frozen, dried, or fermented supplies that you were resourceful enough to stock during the plentiful growing season.

If, for reasons of budget or availability, you decide to eat conventionally grown produce, understand that certain veggies have lesser pesticide concerns while others have higher levels of residue exposure and warrant more discretion. Choosing pesticide-free or organic is critical when it comes to vegetables that have a large, edible surface area (leafy greens, including spinach and lettuce, are treated with some of the most potent pesticides) or a skin that is consumed (bell peppers are perhaps the most pesticide-tainted vegetable; also avoid conventional celery, cucumbers, and carrots). On the other hand, for vegetables with tough, inedible outer covers like avocados and squash, the edible portion is well protected, so there is less risk of ingesting objectionable chemicals. However, the risk is not zero, and there are still serious environmental concerns associated with conventional agricultural methods, so you might choose to purchase pesticide-free or organic produce across the board if you are able. If you do find yourself purchasing high-exposure-risk conventional produce, be sure to wash them with soap, soak them in a solution of two parts water to one part white vinegar (then rinse with plain water), or use a fruit/vegetable wash solution, which you can find in any health food store.

It may take some acclimation to center your diet around vegetables because we are so accustomed to centering our meals around heaping servings of grain foods. Don't follow the example of restaurants that serve skimpy vegetable portions seemingly just for decoration; prepare heaping servings that almost crowd out everything else on your plate! Enjoy vegetables raw, steamed, baked, or grilled—even slathered in butter if you like. Cook or slice up extra portions for easy preparation or snacking the following day. Reject your attachment to cultural meal traditions centered on grains and get wild and colorful with your meals. Have some steamed carrots and beets with your eggs for breakfast or kale, squash, and chicken for lunch. Try some of the many delicious vegetable-focused recipes at MarksDailyApple.com, *The Primal Blueprint Cookbook*, or the *Primal Blueprint Quick & Easy Meals*. Grab some stuff you've never tried before and ask your grocer about the best preparation methods.

If you aren't much of a cook and find yourself falling short of abundant vegetable consumption despite good intentions, how about preparing a morning vegetable smoothie to hit your quota? You can obtain abundant servings more easily this way and generally boost the overall nutrient content of your diet. Since it's easier to consume extra calories and feel less satiated when drinking liquids, strive to balance the macronutrient content of your smoothies so you don't get a blood sugar spike. Throw in a few ice cubes, some big piles of leafy greens, beets, carrots, and whatever other veggies you've got around, and add just a small palmful of frozen fruit (frozen, peeled bananas provide good bulk for a smoothie) for sweetness. Then, include a scoop or two of protein/meal replacement powder (microfiltered whey is the highest quality powdered protein supplement) and fats in the form of coconut milk, avocado, and even a tablespoon of olive, avocado, or coconut oil. Delicious!

While virtually all vegetables offer excellent nutritional value, some offer particularly high levels of antioxidants. One of the best objective resources to determine the antioxidant power of any vegetable, fruit, herb, or other food is the USDA's ORAC (Oxygen Radical Absorbance Capacity) report. I like to aim for at least 10,000 ORAC units a day, which is easily obtained from a few servings of the top fruits and vegetables (the USDA recommends a much lower number, between 3,000 and 5,000 per day). Here (in alphabetical order, not rank order; don't worry, they're all gold medal winners) is a list of some of the highest antioxidant vegetables. Make a special effort to include these regularly in your meals:

1. Avocado
2. Beets
3. Broccoli
4. Brussels sprouts
5. Carrots
6. Cauliflower
7. Eggplant
8. Garlic
9. Kale
10. Onions
11. Red bell pepper
12. Spinach
13. Yellow squash

NUTS, SEEDS, AND THEIR DERIVATIVE BUTTERS

Nuts and seeds are concentrated foods that represent an energy source (some might call it a "life force") for future generations of their plant—packed with protein, fatty acids, enzymes, antioxidants, and abundant vitamins and minerals. You can conveniently carry and eat nuts and seeds anytime, anywhere, making them a favored primal snack.

At the time of the original publication of *The Primal Blueprint*, the evolutionary health world was buzzing with concerns about the dangers of an imbalanced omega-6:omega-3 dietary ratio. While our hunter-gatherer ancestors probably had a nearly 1:1 ratio, modern diets are believed to be grossly out of balance, as in 20:1 in favor of omega-6, or even much worse for a SAD junk food eater. Even disciplined primal enthusiasts would end up with imbalanced omega-6:omega-3 ratios, which was purported to promote systemic inflammation. Consequently, I and other thought leaders in the primal/paleo scene suggested moderating intake of all nuts, due to their uniformly higher ratio of omega-6 to omega-3 (except macadamia, which is mostly monounsaturated, and hence inconsequentially low in both omega-6 and omega-3). Plus, nuts were getting pushback due to some juicy gossip that primal enthusiasts tended to overdo it snacking on "approved" foods like nuts, a habit that could easily derail their efforts to reduce excess body fat.

While omega-6 fats are indeed inflammatory in isolation, nuts and seeds tend to be rich in antioxidants (such as vitamin E) that counteract the oxidation-prone nature of the delicate polyunsaturated fats they also contain. To sweeten the deal, nuts and seeds also provide a wide spectrum of phytochemicals and hard-to-find-elsewhere minerals (like selenium and copper), in turn boosting the overall nutritional quality of your diet. And some nuts, especially almonds and pistachios, contain prebiotic compounds that improve intestinal health and immunity through gut-mediated pathways.

Numerous respected studies (Iowa Women's Health Study of 40,000 women, Harvard School of Public Health's Nurses' Health Study of 127,000 women, and Physicians' Health Study of 22,000 men are among the most prominent) suggest that regular consumption of nuts significantly reduces the risk of heart disease, diabetes, and other health problems.

Although overdosing on omega-6 still isn't a great idea, the reality is that when we look at the overall omega-6:omega-3 ratio of the diet, it's pretty hard to reach an unhealthy level of omega-6 when eating primally. Once you take away vegetable oils and grains and eat more seafood and pasture-raised meats, your omega-6:omega-3 ratio will generally be favorable even if you have a hefty nut and seed intake. As mentioned in Chapter 3, it's likely that the "omega-6 inflammation" effect is mainly from consuming highly oxidized refined vegetable oils (high in omega-6) that have been stripped of the antioxidants present in the foods they were expelled from and that are further oxidized when they are heated to high temperatures during cooking. That leaves nuts and seeds, which are not subjected to such harsh processing methods, in the clear.

The buzz about the modern dietary omega-6:omega-3 imbalance has misled primal enthusiasts to minimize or avoid healthy sources of omega-6 like nuts. The real inflammatory damage comes from consumption of high polyunsaturated, high-omega-6 oxidized vegetable oils.

While all nuts, seeds, and nut butters are thumbs-up primal approved, realize that the ever-popular peanuts should be avoided. Peanuts are technically categorized as a legume, not a nut. (See the discussion of legumes in Chapter 6.) They are highly allergenic for sensitive people and also can contain dangerous molds that produce aflatoxin, a potent carcinogen. Obviously, it's wise to also avoid nuts that have been processed with sugary or oily coatings or other offensive ingredients. Read the labels of many nut products (even simple, clean-looking, nuts-only products), and you will frequently notice these sinister vegetable/seed oils used in the preparation.

Use a mini food processor to grind nuts and then sprinkle on salads, over baked vegetables, or even into omelets. Whole nuts (in the shell) will last up to a year without spoiling. Shelled nuts have shorter shelf lives, and sliced or blended nuts less again. Store nuts in the refrigerator (or freezer, if longer than six months) to prolong freshness. If your nuts have a rancid, oily smell or any discoloration, fleckings, or signs of mold, discard them. Concern about pesticide exposure from nuts is minimal due to protection offered by their shells. Don't worry about looking for organic nuts, as shells protect the end product from any potential pesticide exposure during growing (less than one percent of U.S. tree nut farmland is certified organic anyway.)

Nut and seed butters offer a versatile and great-tasting way to spread your intake of nuts and seeds over different meals and snacks. Take care to choose cold-processed butters that are simply ground up (at low temperatures and free of added ingredients except salt, which is fine), and refrigerate them at all times. Many health proponents claim raw nuts, seeds, and butters have superior nutritional value to those that have been roasted, so choose raw products if you can find them. You don't have to stick exclusively with raw nuts, but make sure the nuts you choose have been minimally processed (e.g., dry roasted) and do not have any added oil or sugar ingredients on the label.

While rare and expensive, coconut butter and macadamia nut butter are absolutely delicious treats, especially when you spread on dark chocolate. Among the more common products, almond butter is recommended due to its high protein content (20 percent of total calories) and impressive levels of antioxidants, phytonutrients, vitamins, minerals, and plant sterols that support health and lower disease risk.

As we get nuts over nuts, we must admit that the "dangers" of overdoing it have some validity. If you are used to frequent, perhaps even absent-minded, snacking to get through the day, and you are trying to fill the void of energy bars, potato chips, sweetened Starbucks creations, and other popular mid-afternoon snack fare, it's entirely possible that you could overdo nut intake to the extent that you compromise fat-loss efforts. You could certainly have worse problems as a primal convert than eating too many nuts, but as you become more and more fat-adapted through sustained primal-style eating, you will want to start paying more attention to your natural appetite and satiety levels both during and between meals. When you enjoy a snack of nuts or nut butter with full attention and appreciation, you realize that a little goes a long way toward sustaining your energy for hours afterward.

As you fine-tune all of your food consumption in this manner, you will break free from the metabolic problems and emotional anxiety that come from missing meals whilst immersed in carbohydrate dependency. Over time, you will naturally trend in the direction of requiring fewer calories to maintain healthy metabolic function and a high satisfaction level with your diet. This means effortless long-term weight management and enhanced longevity, primal style!

COCONUT PRODUCTS

Integrating coconut products (oil, milk, butter, flakes, and flour) into your diet provides a variety of health benefits and can conveniently replace SAD foods such as milk, wheat flour, and polyunsaturated cooking oils. Coconut is an excellent source of a special type of fat—medium-chain fatty acids—

that are difficult to find even in a healthy diet. While all vegetable oils comprise some ratio of monounsaturated, polyunsaturated, or saturated fatty acids, there is another classification based on molecular size or length of the carbon chain within each fatty acid. Nearly all oils we consume are classified as long-chain fatty acids. Coconut's distinctive medium-chain composition has been shown to offer protection from heart disease, cancer, diabetes, and many other degenerative illnesses; to improve fat metabolism; to protect against liver damage from alcohol and other toxins; and to deliver anti-inflammatory and immune-supporting properties.

Nearly one-third of the global population has had coconut as a dietary centerpiece of their traditional diets for centuries. Of particular note are Polynesian cultures that are remarkably free of heart disease with diets heavy in coconut and saturated fat intake. Asian Pacific cultures love the healing properties of coconut and use coconut extensively in their traditional medicine, particularly for skin and digestive conditions, since it offers potent antimicrobial properties.

Due to its high saturated fat content, coconut oil is resistant to oxidation and free radical formation, even when heated to high temperatures during cooking. Unfortunately, coconut has been maligned along with other saturated fats for several decades, beginning with the Standard American Diet's migration to polyunsaturated oils in the 1960s. Coconut is indeed the most saturated of all vegetable oils; at 92 percent saturated, it's solid at room temperature but will liquefy in temperate weather (76°F/24°C). While it may seem like a minor issue, cooking and preparing recipes with coconut oil or other saturated fats like butter instead of polyunsaturated oils can be one of the healthiest dietary changes you can make. *The Primal Blueprint Cookbook* and *Primal Blueprint Quick & Easy Meals* have extensive recipes featuring coconut or substituting familiar ingredients (flour, milk, refined high polyunsaturated oils) with coconut products.

To get on the coconut bandwagon, grab a jar of coconut oil at a health food store or finer market and use it for pan-frying. Get some coconut milk and use it as a liquid base for smoothies and for replacing dairy milk. With cans, choose the full fat variety, not "light." With cartons, check the label to avoid those with added sweeteners.

Get some coconut flakes and enjoy them in smoothies, sprinkled on salads, or with nuts as a trail mix. On those special occasions when you need a carbohydrate beverage during or after exercise, coconut water is a good choice for its natural electrolytes, vitamins, minerals, trace elements, amino acids, antioxidants, phytonutrients and cytokinins (plant hormones with anti-aging properties); just watch out for brands with added sugar (again, read the label). Try some coconut butter (hard to find, try a health food store or the Internet, or try making your own by pureeing coconut flakes) as a delicious spread on vegetables or dabbed onto some squares of dark chocolate. Visit MarksDailyApple.com and review the many posts on coconut (including some amazing desserts) as you explore this wonderful new dietary centerpiece.

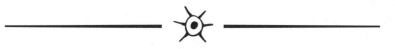

MARK'S FAVORITE PRIMAL SNACKS

Beef Jerky: How primal can you get? Branch out and try buffalo, turkey, and venison. Choose natural products or make your own; avoid the greasy gas station fare with sugar, vegetable oils, preservatives, and other unhealthy additives.

Celery: Enjoy with big gobs of cream cheese or nut butter.

Cottage Cheese: Enjoy the full-fat variety with nuts, berries, balsamic vinegar, or other creative toppings.

Dark Chocolate: Any lingering sweet tooth issues relating to your transition to primal eating can be assuaged with a couple/few/several squares of dark chocolate. Look for 75-percent or greater cacao content.

Fish: Canned tuna or sardines (packed in olive oil or water—avoid soybean oil, cottonseed oil, or other vegetable-oil-packed brands) can easily replace a full meal for nutrient intake and satiety.

Fresh Berries: Raspberries, blueberries, blackberries, strawberries, and the rest are the top-rated fruits for their high-antioxidant, low-glycemic properties. Serve them with homemade whipped cream for a great dessert option.

Green Bananas: Smother in almond butter for a nice dose of resistant starch as well as a filling snack.

Hard-Boiled Eggs: Sprinkle some salt, spices, and a little olive oil in a baggie, and then roll the peeled egg around in the bag for a tasty snack.

Nuts and Seeds: Almonds, macadamias, pecans, walnuts; pumpkin, sunflower, sesame seeds, and the rest, as well as all nut butters except peanut butter.

Olives: Great source of monounsaturated fatty acids and a big reason for the compliments lavished on the Mediterranean diet.

Trail Mix: Make your own with assorted nuts, seeds, coconut flakes or chunks, small bits of dried fruit, and even dark chocolate (if your creation can be stored in cool temperatures). Avoid the high-sugar store offerings filled with too much dried fruit, yogurt-covered raisins, M&M's, milk chocolate, peanuts, or other sugary or heavily processed items.

Website: MarksDailyApple.com has hundreds of postings for snack and recipe ideas, including some creative make-your-own primal snacks. We also have dozens of our ever-popular "top 10 lists" for everything you can think of relating to meat, vegetables, fruits, seasonal favorites, recipes, foods to avoid, and healthy dietary habits.

FRUITS

While fruits are outstanding sources of fiber, vitamins, minerals, phenols, antioxidants, and other micronutrients, some moderation and selectivity with your consumption is warranted. While our ancestors had to forage for fruit that might have only ripened for a few months of the year, we now have all manner of fruits available year-round. Furthermore, modern cultivation and chemical treatments have resulted in fruits that are often larger and sweeter than their wild counterparts. If you're in

Oregon picking wild blackberries in the summer, knock yourself out and enjoy abundant servings of one of the most nutritious foods on the planet. On the other hand, when you see those golf ball-sized blackberries on display at the big box store in January, imported from Chile, pause to reflect how this might not be as primal-aligned as the stuff you plucked off the top rung of the ladder back in summertime.

The main problem I have with fruit consumption is the fruit calories contributing to excessive total carbohydrate intake in the modern diet. If you are able to ditch grains, sugars, and especially the many hidden sources of processed fructose in today's processed food offerings, your fruit consumption becomes far less problematic. However, if you are diligently trying to reduce excess body fat and consuming heaps of fruit (perhaps inspired by Weight Watchers giving fruit a zero "PointsPlus" score for calorie counting purposes), it's important to recognize that fruit can contribute to fat storage more easily than other forms of carbohydrate because of the way it is processed in the body.

Fructose is the predominant carbohydrate contained in fruit. (Fruits also have smaller amounts of sucrose and glucose in ratios that vary by fruit.) When consumed, fructose is not burned in the bloodstream right away like other carb forms; it must be processed in the liver first. The liver converts fructose into usable carbohydrate in the form of glucose, but if you already have sufficient glucose in the bloodstream, and your muscle and liver glycogen stores are full, the liver will convert fructose into triglycerides (fat). High levels of triglycerides in the

Fruit calories get processed in the liver, the same place carbs get converted into fat. Zero points for people who don't acknowledge this!

bloodstream is one of the most prominent risk factors for cardiovascular disease. High blood triglycerides also interfere with the function of the important appetite and satiety hormone leptin. Poor leptin signaling causes you to eat more and, hormonally speaking, be more likely to store your calories as fat than burn them.

Studies that link fructose to metabolic and cardiovascular risk usually employ diets with excessive fructose consumption, more than one might normally eat in terms of percentage of daily calories. Particularly if you are eating primal-style, it's hard to eat enough fructose in whole-food form to cause serious damage. Nevertheless, eating excessive levels of fruit can counteract some of the health benefits provided by a more moderate intake. It's not my desire to scare you away from eating fruit, but simply to help you recognize that fruit is a lipogenic (fat-forming) carbohydrate source, so it should be consumed sensibly with that fact in mind. The best approach is to try and emulate Grok by eating fruits grown locally during their natural local ripening seasons (I'll grant you some latitude—literally—if you live in a fruit-challenged climate), especially if you are trying to shed excess body fat.

Individuals who are sensitive to fructose should show even more discretion with their fruit consumption. Scientists now believe that possibly one-third of the population is fructose intolerant (technically they suffer from "fructose malabsorption"). With fructose malabsorption, a significant portion of fructose consumed remains unprocessed in the small intestine. This causes excess water to be drawn into the small intestine, and the poorly digested matter to ferment in the large intestine. Symptoms of fructose malabsorption resemble those of irritable bowel syndrome (IBS) and include digestive disturbances such as flatulence, cramps, bloating, and diarrhea. Research suggests that significant numbers of people diagnosed with IBS might suffer from fructose malabsorption and could benefit from a diet low in fructose and fructans (fructose polymers—found in foods like agave, artichokes, asparagus, leeks, garlic, and onions).

To determine if you have fructose malabsorption, your doctor can give you a simple, non-invasive hydrogen breath test that measures your ability to process fructose in the hours after ingestion. Another suggestion for those with fructose sensitivities is to exercise immediately after consumption. This speeds transit time out the small intestine, lessening the chance for bloating in the small intestine and fermentation in the large intestine.

Interestingly, studies have linked fructose malabsorption to depression, especially among women. Scientists attribute this finding to the fact that fructose can interfere with tryptophan, which is a chemical precursor to serotonin, a main "feel good" neurotransmitter. If you suffer from digestive disorders or depression, it might be a good idea to try cutting fructose out of your diet for 21 days or longer to see if your symptoms improve.

Choosing the Best Fruits

Three major categories that affect fruit quality are growing methods, nutritional value (antioxidant levels as well as how much the sugar content affects your metabolism), and risk of pesticide exposure. The "Fruit Power Rankings" sidebar in this section details which types of fruits to enjoy in abundance, which to eat in moderation, and which to strictly avoid. Regarding growing methods, fruit grown locally without the use of synthetic pesticides is the best choice, followed by certified organic. As with vegetables, these growing methods offer superior nutritional value and eliminate the health risks associated with conventionally grown fruits. Some experts estimate that organic fruits are 10 times richer in key micronutrients than their conventional counterparts. Organic fruits must manufacture higher levels of antioxidants to defend themselves against pests—something conventional fruits don't have to worry about thanks to their treatment with synthetic chemicals. But remember, organic farming can still employ natural pesticides, so depending on the farm and the crop, organic produce can still contain residue from potentially toxic substances.

Likewise, organic fruits from distant lands can be less tasty and nutritious because of their premature picking and long transit time to market. Even if local fruit is not certified organic, your local farmer likely uses less offensive growing methods than do large commercial operations (not to mention the fact that you can directly ask

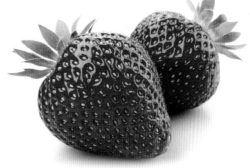

them). Also local farmers allow the fruit to mature before picking so it is bursting with great nutrition and taste. Those living in areas with thriving farmers' markets and food co-ops might even encounter fruits designated as wild. As the term conveys, these fruits are as good as it gets… if you can find them. If you are so inclined, you may want to visit seedsavers.org or seedsofchange.com to purchase seeds and plant your own wild-variety of fruit trees, berry bushes, and vegetable plants.

Be strict (particularly with children, due to their substantially higher risk of harm from pesticides) about avoiding conventionally grown fruits with soft, edible skins that are difficult to wash, such as berries. You can be less strict about fruits with tough, inedible skins that peel because they offer a protective barrier against chemical ingestion. If you must eat conventional fruits, wash your fruit thoroughly with soap or a special solution. Avoid genetically modified fruit, a concept that elicits serious health and philosophical concerns and is about as far away from Grok as you can get. Genetically modified organisms (GMOs) have not been subject to sufficient research to guarantee their health and safety.

All fruits offer a host of nutritional benefits, but some (detailed in the sidebar) are relatively low in antioxidant values while having a high impact on your blood glucose and insulin production. *Paleo Diet* author Loren Cordain, Ph.D., ranks common fruits according to their "Total Metabolic Fructose" (TMF) to take this factor into consideration. Fruits with high TMF scores (sometimes referred to as "high-sugar" or "high-glycemic" fruits) warrant moderation, particularly if you are trying to reduce excess body fat.

In light of the popularity of juicing, it's important to note that whole fruits are vastly superior to juice—even the most nutritious, freshly squeezed glass. Juice is generally higher in sugar and lower in many other micronutrients than its produce sources because juicing eliminates the nutrient-rich skin and fiber and provides a more-concentrated, less-filling source of carbohydrates than whole foods do. Recall that Kelly Korg's 24-ounce Strawberry Surf Rider smoothie contained 71 grams of sugar. That's like eating 51 large strawberries! (Can you say *Cool Hand Luke*?) I strongly suggest passing on juice in favor of whole foods.

If your eyes are bouncing up and down the page sorting out which fruits are good and bad, relax! If you've scrapped sugars, grains, and refined vegetable/seed oils to become preoccupied with prioritizing your fruit choices, you're progressing nicely. I'm certainly not advocating sitting forlornly off to the side at the Fourth of July picnic, watching others eat the hot dogs, corn on the cob, and watermelon. By all means enjoy the watermelon guilt-free (just forget the former two and smuggle in your own smoked wild salmon for a main course!). Simply use a bit of restraint for certain fruits, particularly if you are pursuing ambitious fat-reduction goals.

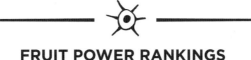

FRUIT POWER RANKINGS

You can be more selective by considering a fruit's growing methods, pesticide risk, and glycemic/antioxidant values (high-antioxidant, low-glycemic fruits being the best), and TMF scores. Each list is ranked in order of best to worst.

Growing Methods

1. **Wild:** Hard to find—plant your own, forage, or hit the farmers' market!
2. **Local pesticide-free:** Superior choice for nutritional value, taste, and safety.
3. **Local organic**: Similar to the above, but organic can still contain pesticides (just not synthetic ones).
4. **Local conventional:** Superior to remote organic due to freshness and ideal picking time. Wash thoroughly with soap or vegetable solution.
5. **Remote pesticide-free or organic:** Ranks below local conventional due to negative effects of transportation and premature picking.
6. **Remote conventional:** Avoid due to diminished nutritional value and pesticide risk. (Hint: if it's out of season in your area, don't eat it!)

7. **GMO fruit:** Putting aside the debate on the validity of the dangers of eating genetically modified foods, it's seems reasonable to avoid GMO fruits if for no reason other than principle. Like ya can't find something in the other six categories?!

Nutritional Value

This list comes from my unscientific blending of antioxidant values, glycemic index values, and total metabolic fructose values. You may find it useful, but please default to the big picture—enjoy local, seasonal fruit and ditch grains, sugars, and bad oils!

1. **Outstanding:** High-antioxidant, low-glycemic, low-TMF fruits, including all berries, most stone (pitted) fruits (cherries, peaches, apricots), avocado, casaba melon, lemon, lime, tomato, and guava.
2. **Good:** Lower-antioxidant, higher-glycemic, medium-TMF fruits, including apples, bananas, cantaloupe, cherries, grapefruit, kiwi, and pomegranates.
3. **Moderate or restrict:** Low-antioxidant, high-glycemic, higher-TMF fruits, including dates, dried fruits (all), grapes, mangoes, melons, nectarines, oranges, papayas, pineapples, plums, and tangerines.

Pesticide Risk

1. **Low risk:** Fruit with tough, inedible skin, including bananas, avocados, melons, oranges, tangerines, mandarins, pineapples, kiwis, mangoes, and papayas.
2. **High risk:** Fruit with soft, edible skin, including apples, apricots, cherries, concentrated juices, grapes, nectarines, peaches, pears, raisins, raspberries, strawberries, and tomatoes.

Mark's Top 10 Favorite Fruits

Naturally, everything on this list assumes a locally grown, pesticide-free, or organic variety. Consult the three previous sections to ensure your pesticide risk is minimized and you otherwise choose the most nutritious fruit possible—and avoid problematic fruits. These are in my personal rank order, but again, anything on this list is great.

1. Blueberries, strawberries, raspberries, blackberries, cranberries, and nearly all other berries
2. Avocados
3. Cherries
4. Apples
5. Peaches
6. Pears
7. Figs
8. Grapefruit
9. Kiwis
10. Apricots

HERBS AND SPICES

No discussion of healthy eating would be complete without the inclusion of herbs and spices. Although these tasty additions provide minimal calories, they are packed with significant amounts of important micronutrients. Extensive evidence suggests that herbs and spices support cardiovascular and metabolic health, may help prevent cancer and other diseases, and improve mental health and cognition. Some of the highest antioxidant values (from ORAC scores) among all foods can be found in herbs and spices. Certain marinades and herbal preparations are so powerful in their antioxidant capacity that they have been shown to mitigate or eliminate potential issues that may arise from overcooking meat.

Herbs are generally green plants or plant parts used to add flavor to foods. Herbal extracts have been used for thousands of years in Eastern medicine and continue to enjoy widespread popularity today for their powerful immune- and health-supporting properties. Spices, on the other hand, are typically dried seeds, fruits, and plant parts. Spices are used to enhance flavor, add color, or help prevent bacterial growth on food.

You can bet that Grok partook of the many varieties of plants he encountered. Throughout history, herbs and spices have played a large role in the human diet and even in culture as a whole. During the Middle Ages, spices were a currency with substantial economic value. Their popularity to enhance flavor and preserve food was the catalyst for the fervent exploration of the globe by such explorers as Marco Polo, Columbus, and Magellan.

The specific health properties of individual herbs and spices could fill an entire book. A couple of headliners that are easy to integrate into everyday meals include turmeric (offers potent anti-inflammatory effects and high antioxidant value) and cinnamon (regulates blood sugar and demonstrates high antibacterial, anti-inflammatory, and antioxidant values). Visit MarksDailyApple.com for extensive coverage of numerous herb and spice benefits.

MODERATION FOODS

While they may not be exactly what our ancestors ate, moderate consumption of the following foods and beverages can add some nutritional benefit to your diet without negative consequences, provided they are not overemphasized. Furthermore, I want to make the Primal Blueprint as accessible and enjoyable to as many people as possible. If you are pursuing ambitious fat-reduction goals, you will probably want to eliminate some of these from the picture.

Coffee

Coffee is often called the most popular drug in the world because its effects on the central nervous system are significant enough to qualify as drug-like. Opinion and research varies on the subject of caffeine's effects on the body and whether or not it's a healthy habit. Personally, I enjoy a morning cup of coffee—especially after adding heavy cream and a pinch

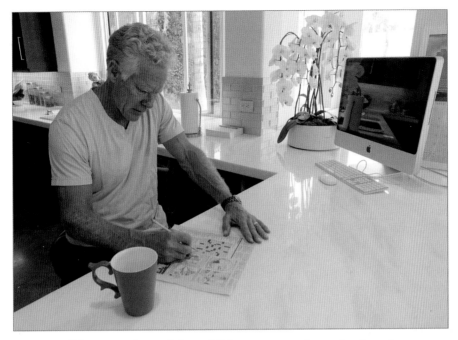

of sugar. (Yes, a pinch won't hurt.) It's a warm and comforting element to my morning routine, especially on those freezing cold winter mornings in Malibu. (Don't scoff, I'm allowed a little hyperbole here. After all, I grew up in Maine!) I never abuse the potential stimulant effects of caffeine and feel comfortable that my coffee "habit"—when viewed in the context of my deliberate morning ritual—benefits my mental, physical, and emotional health. Furthermore, if I miss my morning cup, I'm not a basket case; I think this is a good litmus test to make sure you are not abusing caffeine.

I'd say that coffee is fine to enjoy in moderation, but I do have some concerns with the widespread use of caffeine—in coffee or elsewhere, especially the high-sugar "energy drinks" and single-dose booster products—as a crutch to boost unsatisfactory energy levels. This concern is especially relevant for devoted fitness enthusiasts or high-stress Type-A personalities who really love their coffee. Hot-wired folks who trigger the fight or flight response frequently in their jam-packed, high-performing daily lives can mask symptoms of fatigue and dig a deeper hole for themselves due to the influence of caffeine on the central nervous system—keeping them awake pounding the keyboard or pedaling more miles when they might be naturally inclined to, and better served by, sleeping in or napping. Proper diet, exercise, sleep, and other lifestyle habits *should* enable you to wake up feeling refreshed and energized each morning and to avoid afternoon blues caused primarily by high-carbohydrate eating habits, along with sleep deficiencies and other lifestyle shortcomings.

Some studies suggest that caffeine can actually reduce risk of heart disease and cancer and enhance fat metabolism, particularly during exercise. Other studies are inconclusive, while still others suggest that caffeine is harmful to the cardiovascular system and does not enhance fat metabolism. I'm particularly concerned about how caffeine stimulates the sympathetic (fight or flight) nervous system. Athletes, high-stimulation business executives, multitasking moms, and other high-energy types should strive to balance potential overstimulation of the sympathetic nervous system with a nurturing of the parasympathetic (rest and digest) nervous system. Many habitual caffeine users might be better off spending six minutes doing some deliberate deep breathing exercises in the park instead of spending six minutes in line at Starbucks ordering up their daily venti designer creation for $5.14. (Multiply that expense by 365 and you have a romantic Hawaiian getaway for two.)

Obviously, your tolerance for caffeine is personal and, in fact, is believed to have a strong genetic influence. Recent research suggests that variants of a gene called CYP1A2 determine whether your liver metabolizes caffeine quickly or slowly. If you are a fast metabolizer, those studies saying caffeine reduces risk of heart disease and cognitive decline might apply to you. If you are a slow metabolizer, caffeine might make you might feel more jittery, have a longer-duration effect, and significantly raise your risk of heart disease, cognitive diseases like Parkinson's and Alzheimer's, high blood pressure, aggravated PMS symptoms, and sleep disturbances. While you can do Internet-based DNA testing to reveal your genetic caffeine sensitivity, and the particulars of many other diet, fitness, and lifestyle genetic traits, you can discern whether you are slow or fast metabolizer pretty easily on your own. Just note how long and how significantly caffeine ingestion affects you. If you have one cup of coffee at 2 P.M. and have trouble sleeping that night, you are surely a slow metabolizer!

High-Fat Dairy Products

Some purists in the paleo diet world avoid all dairy products on the grounds that dairy products didn't exist in hunter-gatherer times. On the other hand, our hunter-gatherer ancestors very likely consumed the milk in mammary glands and in the young animals' stomachs they ate on occasion (along with kidney, liver, heart, lung, intestines, bone marrow, and brain). Hence, the talking point from strict paleo enthusiasts that our ancestors completely avoided dairy is not entirely accurate. The Primal Blueprint stance is that certain forms of dairy can provide excellent nutrition and enjoyment for those who can tolerate dairy consumption without digestive distress.

The best dairy choices are raw, fermented, unpasteurized, unsweetened, and high-fat options such as ghee, butter, full cream, aged cheese, cottage cheese, cream cheese, Greek-style full-fat yogurt, half and half, kefir, and raw whole milk. Stick to pasture-raised/grass-fed or organic dairy products to avoid the hormones, pesticides, and antibiotics common in mainstream dairy products. Eliminate fruit-sweetened yogurt, frozen desserts, and other high-carb dairy offerings. Stay completely away from regular pasteurized, homogenized two-percent and skim milk. These are just more carbohydrate bombs to disturb your progress toward becoming fat-adapted.

Fermented dairy products may help you avoid the immune system issues and allergenic reactions that many have toward the lactose and casein (an objectionable protein I'll discuss further shortly) in cow's milk. They also offer a good source of probiotics (healthy bacteria for your intestines—more on these later in the chapter). Raw dairy products undergo the least processing, increasing their nutritional value. High-fat dairy products have low levels of carbohydrates and little to no casein. And how can you not love an eating style that supports your enjoyment of butter and heavy cream (both of which are almost entirely comprised of healthy saturated animal fat)?

Cheese does have broad appeal and can play a minor role in a healthy diet. Play it snooty and go for the high-quality, aged stuff—not the industrialized ooze found in mini-mart nacho machines. Aged cheese is a fermented food, so it contains little to no lactose. Cheese offers high-quality fats and proteins, as well as many other essential nutrients. Raw cheese (hard to find, but worth the effort) offers the most nutritional value since it's minimally processed.

Having offered possible options of what might constitute acceptable dairy, let's now look at why milk doesn't necessarily "do a body good." Lactose is a carbohydrate in milk that is difficult to digest for many who stop producing lactase (the enzyme that helps digest lactose) after age three or four. This is in alignment with our genetically programmed transition away from breastfeeding in early childhood (breast milk contains significant lactose).

Casein is a protein that can have autoimmune-stimulating properties and can initiate very serious allergic reactions in some people, particularly those who have experienced "leaky gut" syndrome as a result of a concurrent intolerance to grains. Casein is believed to contribute to or exacerbate conditions such as celiac disease, Crohn's disease, irritable bowel syndrome, asthma, and possibly autism in some people. *Paleo Diet*

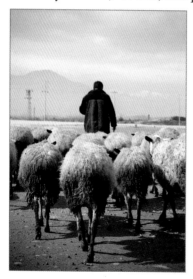

author Loren Cordain notes that a substance known as epidermal growth factor (EGF) in milk and other dairy products can increase cancer risk and tumor progression and also suggests that milk and other dairy products worsen acne. Success has been reported treating these conditions holistically with a wheat- and dairy-free diet.

Those of distinct herding ancestry have a very high rate of lactose tolerance, a fascinating example of a rapid genetic adaptation to selection pressure.

Milk doesn't necessarily "do a body good,"
at least not the usual store-bought kind.
The calcium benefits are overstated,
and it often contains agents such as lactose,
casein, hormones, pesticides, and antibiotics.

Interestingly, almost all people of distinct herder ancestry (and hence ancestrally high dairy consumption)—such as Northern Europeans and Scandinavians—possess the genes that allow them to tolerate lactose throughout their lives. This lactose persistence among ancestral herders is believed to be a rare example of recent genetic change through selection pressure in the manner of evolution. (I discuss this topic at length in the Primal Blueprint Q&A Appendix at MarksDailyApple.com/the-book/references.) On the other hand, the bulk of Asians, Africans, Native Americans, South Americans, and generally the vast majority of the global adult population become lactose intolerant by the time they reach adulthood.

While the severely lactose intolerant are quite aware of their immediate adverse reactions to consuming high-lactose milk products, you may be slightly intolerant without even realizing it. If you take a closer look at your consumption of milk products, you may connect incidences of bloating, gas, or cramping (especially when you do high-impact exercise in proximity with milk consumption). You may even notice a slight worsening of inflammatory or autoimmune conditions like allergies, asthma, acne, sinus trouble, or arthritis around milk consumption. As we discussed with gluten, most of us have no good reason to consume the low-fat and nonfat milk products that deliver a significant dose of lactose sugar, and we have plenty of reasons to avoid these foods.

The downsides of lactose intolerance and casein allergy do not even address the consequences of consuming the hormones, pesticides, and antibiotics contained in commercial milk and dairy products. Fortunately, the dangers and objections of the commonly used recombinant bovine growth hormone (rBGH—an agent given to cows to increase their milk production) are well publicized, leading some forward-thinking nations to ban its use and inspiring sophisticated consumers to steer clear of milk made with rBGH.

Milk's modern processing methods also present health objections. Milk that is homogenized and pasteurized is certainly free of dangerous bacteria, but it is also devoid of beneficial bacteria, vitamins, and enzymes due to the heating process. Furthermore, the homogenization process compromises the otherwise healthy milk fats by reducing the size of the fat globules, interfering with their digestibility.

For those who recoil at the suggestion to limit intake of milk, let's examine further some of the flawed conventional wisdom about dairy. Yes, most dairy is an excellent source of calcium, but we don't need nearly as much calcium as we have been led to believe. The United States and other Western nations with high dairy intake nevertheless have high rates of osteoporosis, suggesting that calcium is not the be-all and end-all for bone health. Experts agree that magnesium, vitamin D, vitamin K, potassium, and other agents are also extremely important to maintain bone density. It's also evident that aggressive efforts to boost calcium intake in the name of bone health can result in imbalances such as magnesium deficiency, because these two agents compete for the same absorption pathways.

For your calcium needs, you are better off consuming easily assimilated, high-calcium foods that don't have the nutritional objections of dairy. These include leafy greens, nuts, seeds, oranges, broccoli, and sweet potatoes, and calcium-rich fish, including wild salmon and sardines (especially "bones in"). These foods also happen to be excellent sources of magnesium, helping you naturally achieve an optimal balance of these nutrients.

What's more, many experts believe that vitamin D synthesis (predominantly from sun exposure, and only minimally from diet, as I will detail in Chapter 8) might be more critical than calcium to bone health. It is also believed that chronic stress may play a huge role in osteoporosis, since the stress hormone cortisol inhibits calcium uptake by bones, rendering ingested calcium less effective. How about that? Taking a break from your busy day to de-stress and bagging some rays in your lounge chair might be better for your bones than drinking a glass of milk or swallowing a bunch of calcium horse pills!

Approved Oils and Cooking Fats

For cooking, animal fats (butter, ghee, lard, recycled bacon grease, poultry fat, and tallow), avocado oil, and coconut oil are great choices because they are temperature-stable even under high heat. The best oil to consume with meals is domestically grown, extra virgin, first-cold-press olive oil. (I'll explain the importance of these distinctions shortly.) Olive oil, the most monounsaturated oil, offers proven cardiovascular benefits (raises HDL and lowers LDL cholesterol) and has powerful anti-inflammatory and antioxidant properties. It's okay for cooking at low heat, but be careful because monounsaturated oils are less temperature stable than the saturated fats that are more ideal for cooking.

As you probably know, various processing methods dramatically affect the health quality of olive oil, with extra virgin designated as the purest form. Unfortunately, the use of the "extra virgin" moniker is loosely regulated, and there is a tremendous disparity in quality between fresher domestic products and inferior imports from Greece, Italy, or Spain (which comprise the vast majority of products on the market). As with fruit, you should strive for oil produced locally or at least domestically for maximum freshness. The additional distinction "first cold press only" suggests that the olives have been pressed only once and bottled immediately instead of being repeatedly pressed for maximum crop yield. (This is the most common method, particularly with the large bottle/low price imports.) You may have to contact the manufacturer to determine whether your bottle is indeed first cold press only.

You'll notice the difference with a single taste of a domestic, first-cold-press extra virgin olive oil in comparison with a much blander, duller-tasting extra virgin import. The aroma and taste are incredibly powerful—the high level of tocopherols (a potent antioxidant) may actually sting the back of your throat! In my estimation, nothing beats a primal Big Ass Salad (made famous by a YouTube video I posted years ago called "2 Minute Salad") with a generous drizzling of olive oil.

High-omega-3 oils are a good way to bump up your omega-3 intake if you don't eat a lot of oily, cold-water fish. Omega-3 fish oil capsules are a convenient daily supplement, or you can get bottled omega-3 oils at a health food store, fine supermarket, or Internet source. These oils are extremely delicate and easily suffer damage from exposure to heat, light, oxygen, and time. Thus, you'll often find them refrigerated and in small containers.

If you are considering an omega-3 supplement, look for something other than flax oil. While flax is the most common offering and is high in omega-3, recent research suggests that the predominant type of omega-3 found in flax oil, alpha-linoleic acid (ALA), is difficult to assimilate in the body. When you ingest ALA, it must undergo a difficult enzymatic conversion into the more useful omega-3 fractions—docosahexanoic acid (DHA) and eicosapentanoic acid (EPA)—not a good bang for your buck when you look at the price tags on the boutique omega-3 oils.

Some alternative high-omega-3 offerings you might find are borage, cod liver, krill, salmon, and hemp seed. Always compare the expiration dates on a few bottles within the same brand and buy the one with the most amount of time left on it. It's best to store all oils (all kinds, but especially high-omega-3s) in the refrigerator and to use them quickly—usually within six weeks of opening. Remember, while omega-3 oils are healthy, they are still subject to rancidity and, when exposed to air, will oxidize a bit. If you detect a slightly rancid smell in any oil or if it's been on the shelf for more than six months, discard the product immediately.

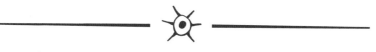

PRIMAL-APPROVED FATS AND OILS

The list of approved oils (in alphabetical order) contains a variety of saturated and unsaturated types with different ideal uses. Review the list carefully, stockpile your fridge, and be sure to stick to the best intended use for each.

1. Animal Fats: Chicken, duck, or goose fat; lard (pork fat); beef or lamb tallow; recycled bacon grease; and other animal fats are excellent for cooking because their saturated composition makes them temperature stable—they won't oxidize under high heat.

2. Avocado Oil: A recent riser in popularity due to its subtle flavor, nutritional similarity to olive oil (mostly monounsaturated fat), and high smoke point of 400 degrees F (204 degrees C). Buy dark bottles and store in a cool, dark location to prevent oxidation.

3. Butter: An excellent choice for cooking or enhancing the taste of steamed vegetables, butter is a good source of vitamins A and E as well as selenium.

4. Coconut Oil: Temperature stability and numerous health and immune-supporting benefits make it an excellent choice for cooking. Find an organic brand and try it in the Primal Energy Bar or Primal Chocolate Mousse recipes at MarksDailyApple.com!

5. Dark Roasted Sesame Oil: This oil's intense flavor makes it a great choice for wok vegetables, meat, or salads. Some alternative healers promote its antibacterial properties to heal wounds and prevent infection.

6. High-Omega-3 Oils: These delicate oils are a great addition to salads or protein shakes for an omega-3 boost. Choose borage, cod liver, krill, salmon, or hemp seed as alternatives to flax.

7. Macadamia Nut Oil: Along with lending a smooth, buttery taste to cold dishes, this high-monounsaturated-fat oil can tolerate heat (smoke point 413 degrees F, or 210 degrees C), making it an excellent—albeit pricey—option for cooking and sautéing.

8. Marine Oils: Typically delivered in capsule or soft-gel supplement form, these fish or krill oils are an excellent source of omega-3s.

9. Olive Oil: Choose locally or domestically grown, first cold press only, extra virgin, and savor the flavor! Best not to cook at high temps with olive oil due to temperature fragility, but low temperature (e.g., sautéing of veggies) is okay.

10. Palm Oil: The unprocessed variety (not to be confused with widely used partially hydrogenated palm oil) is great for cooking.

High-Nutrient-Value Carbs

High-nutrient-value carbs don't have the objectionable properties of the nutritionally devoid, pro-inflammatory, insulin-spiking sweetened beverages and sugary treats, nor the drawbacks of the minimal nutrition and anti-nutrients present in grains. While vegetables and fruits are obviously high-nutrient-value carbs, we've covered them in their own categories, so this section is technically "other" or "supplemental" high-nutrient-value carbs. Sweet potatoes and yams are the most popular supplemental carbs for primal enthusiasts. Assorted other starchy root vegetables (beet, carrot, cassava, lotus root, rutabaga, taro) could potentially be placed in this category, but we generally just drop these and other starchy plants (pumpkin, squash, zucchini) into the regular vegetables category.

Quinoa and wild rice are also favorable high-nutrient-value carb choices, providing a grain-like texture to meals without the anti-nutrient objections of cereal grains. Quinoa is technically not a grain, but a chenopod—closely related to beets, spinach, and tumbleweeds. It's a complete protein (containing all nine essential amino acids, with 12 to 18 percent of total calories as protein), and it's gluten-free. Wild rice is also not a true grain but rather an aquatic grass. It offers a better nutritional profile than grains, a nearly complete array of essential amino acids (14 percent of calories as protein), and is gluten-free.

Since fruit was listed as a moderation food, consuming fruit more liberally could also be considered as a supplemental carb choice. Also, if you don't have leaky gut issues or autoimmune sensitivities, you may find legumes to be another favorable option, especially when you soak them to minimize anti-nutrient concerns. As you will soon learn in the discussion about prebiotics and probiotics, eating white rice and white potatoes, cooked and then served cool, provide a source of resistant starch. Resistant starch promotes healthy intestinal flora but does not count as a carbohydrate source, since the "cooked and cooled" condition renders the carbohydrate calories indigestible. So while warmed white rice and white potatoes are not advised (sweet potatoes and yams are much more nutritious and less glycemic), the cold versions have unique health-boosting properties. Sushi rolls anyone? Yes, a little confusing—more shortly!

Note that while the Primal Blueprint is accurately described as a low-carbohydrate diet when compared with the Standard American Diet baseline of excessive refined carbohydrates, we must be careful with using blanket statements that could give a distorted impression of what primal eating is all about. The main goal of the primal lifestyle is not low-carb eating, per se. Most importantly, the Primal Blueprint honors flexibility and personal preference, while also respecting the evolutionary health premise that we should eat foods promoting optimal gene expression and avoid foods we have not evolved to consume. It's here that we differ a bit from a strict paleo philosophy, which suggests that we only eat foods that existed prior to 10,000 years ago in hunter-gatherer times. I thought about going there, but realized society would be doomed without dark chocolate....

Determining your optimal level of dietary carb intake, particularly the level at which you partake in high-nutrient-value/supplemental carbs, starts with an evaluation of your body composition. If you carry excess body fat and want to get rid of it, the most direct and reliable route to is to dial back your average daily carb intake per the Carbohydrate Curve guidelines. This goal tends to be an immediate priority for a large percentage of primal enthusiasts and healthy living enthusiasts in general. When you ditch sugars and grains, you are well on your way to down-regulating sugar-burning genes and upregulating fat-burning genes to achieve long-term satisfaction with your body composition—without having to stress about calorie counting or obsessive exercise. However, if the pace of your results, or heaven forbid a lack of results, in dropping fat is troubling you, consider making a more ambitious short-term restriction of not only refined carbs but also the high-nutrient-value carbs mentioned in this section, as well as fruits and dark chocolate, until you are pleased with your body composition. Notice I didn't mention restricting vegetables. Even if you are aggressively pursuing fat loss, there is no need to restrict these nutritional powerhouses. Furthermore, experts assert that so much glucose energy is required to digest vegetables that you are pretty much looking at a wash when it comes to counting carbs per the Primal Blueprint Carbohydrate Curve.

Personal experimentation will determine where high-nutrient-value carbs fit into your eating pattern. High-calorie-burning athletes, and other high-energy/fast-metabolizer folks, might find these carbs occupying a more prominent role in their diets than other primal enthusiasts. These unique individuals (assumed to have optimal body composition) require a requisite amount of dietary carbs to replenish their depleted muscle glycogen after workouts and/or fuel their generally high-calorie-burning lifestyles. Also, some women struggling with metabolic or hormonal issues when eating primally might also feel better when sweet potatoes, quinoa, and wild rice make regular appearances on their dinner plate, or when they make certain to get regular doses of dark chocolate. Jeanne Calment, the human longevity record holder at 122 years (1875–1997—search YouTube for her sharp-witted interview delivered at age 119!), reportedly consumed a kilogram (2.2 pounds) of dark chocolate per week!

Interestingly, for endurance athletes who have long reigned supreme in the massive carbohydrate intake category, the paradigm is changing quickly. Breaking science and anecdotal evidence from many world-class performers are revealing remarkable benefits from fat-adapted endurance training employing a lower-carb/higher-fat diet. That's right, they are going long without the obsessive ingestion of carbohydrates that has long defined the training and dietary patterns of endurance performers. But that's a topic for a whole 'nuther book… and it's called *Primal Endurance*!

DEALING WITH PRIMAL STRUGGLES

While the Primal Blueprint approach to dropping excess body fat is pretty straightforward (cut grains and sugars, moderate insulin, burn fat) there are some practical nuances that can make the application of these principles a bit more complex. The rate and rigorousness at which you transition from your SAD patterns—or whatever pre-primal patterns you were engaged in—to primal-style eating is personal, and the smoothness of the transition is sensitive to many variables. Some primal enthusiasts, particularly females who transition to primal after decades of high-carb eating and yo-yo dieting, report experiencing fatigue, sleep disturbances (either insomnia or excessive sleeping), thyroid disturbances (particularly lower-than-normal body temperature), gut health disturbances (because many carbohydrate foods contain healthful resistant starches), and difficulty losing excess body fat. These problems can occur immediately after going primal and also after a sustained period of minimized carb intake.

The weight-loss stalls are possibly due in part to muscles becoming a bit insulin resistant in order to prioritize glucose delivery to the brain when carb intake is minimized. After initial weight-loss success, your body might recalibrate to store what carbs you do eat as fat. Females more frequently report this phenomenon because they are hardwired to store enough fat to ensure reproductive success, not cut down to a six-pack. The practice of occasional carb "refeeding" (brief periods of higher carb consumption inside a general low-carb eating pattern) is believed to rekindle insulin sensitivity in a low-carb eater. Refeeds may be effective especially when your fat-reduction efforts stall.

If you experience malaise or any other disturbances in overall wellbeing after going primal, it's best to tap the brakes a bit and more gradually reduce average daily carb intake. You can add in more high-nutrient-value carbs (but there is a never a reason to chow on grains or sugars!), and discover a strategy that allows you to enjoy effortless weight management, adequate recovery from exercise, healthy hormone function, and stable energy, mood, and appetite throughout the day.

Forget love—I'd rather fall in chocolate!
—Sandra J. Dykes

Dark Chocolate

Dark chocolate is the Primal Blueprint preferred treat because along with being delicious and satisfying (even for a sweet tooth—after a little bit of acclimation), it's actually a highly nutritious food. The antioxidant values (measured on the ORAC scale) of raw, unprocessed cacao beans are among the highest-scoring foods ever tested—higher than blueberries! Dark chocolate is rich in various other health-promoting agents, including phenolic phytochemicals, or flavonoids, that have been shown to improve cognitive function. Flavonoids also improve blood flow to the skin and offer protection from sunburn. Dark chocolate also contains phenylethylamine, a powerful opioid peptide that increases alertness and produces a feeling of wellbeing and contentment similar to the feeling of falling in love. Phenylethylamine, often called the "love drug," is a likely reason why chocolate is considered the most craved food in the world. One prominent flavonoid in dark chocolate called epicatechin stimulates the production of nitric oxide (NO), helping your arteries become more relaxed and supple.

The higher percentage cacao the better. Less sugar = more nutrition. Strive to get used to bars that are 75-percent cacao or higher.

Other antioxidant compounds in dark chocolate have been found to decrease oxidized LDL cholesterol and increase HDL cholesterol.

Dark chocolate products are made from the cacao bean, which can be processed into chocolate liquor, cocoa butter, or cocoa powder. The liquor (also called unsweetened chocolate, bittersweet chocolate, or cocoa mass) is produced by grinding the center of the bean (aka the "nib") into liquid. The butter is the fat component of the cacao bean that gives chocolate it's unique taste and texture. The powder is made by pressing the cocoa butter out of the bean and grinding it into powder. The percentage listed on the label (e.g., "85-percent dark chocolate") refers to the percentage of ingredients by weight that are derived from the bean. The higher the cacao percentage, the more intense the chocolate flavor, the less sweet flavor, and the more health benefits you enjoy. In contrast, milk chocolate has a higher sugar content and a lower percentage of cacao.

If you are a "more is better" type and want to get maximum health benefits, 100-percent cacao is available (it's often used for cooking) but it has no sweetness whatsoever (it contains simply cocoa solids and cocoa butter) and tastes extremely bitter. Most primal enthusiasts take their chocolate up to 85-percent cacao content to enjoy a pleasant bittersweet

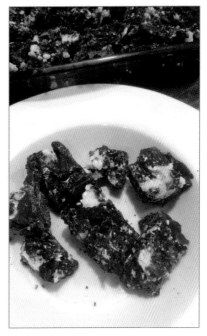

taste. Note that "cacao" (pronounced "kuh-kay-oh") is the correct term for the plant that yields the cocoa butter, powder, and chocolate liquor. When examining labels or reading about chocolate, you can consider the terms cacao and cocoa to be interchangeable for practical purposes.

Once you get used to the rich taste of high-cacao-content dark chocolate, you'll likely lose your affinity for milk chocolate, which will consequently

Brad Kearns's full-on primal-approved dark chocolate-macadamia nut-coconut butter-almond butter bark was a huge hit at PrimalCon. This delicious treat is around 80-percent fat, so it delivers high satiety without spiking insulin.

seem too sweet. Read labels when choosing your brand, looking for more fat and fewer carbs. One of my favorites, Trader Joe's Dark Chocolate Lover's Chocolate Bar (85-percent cacao) contains 50 grams of fat, 34 grams of carbs, and 10 grams of protein in a 3.5-ounce bar.

Organic chocolate offers you the comfort of greater oversight of the growing, harvesting, and processing procedures—important due to the fact that conventional cacao beans have a high pesticide content and commonly arrive from countries with questionable growing regulations and safety standards. Many dark chocolate bars—even the organic ones—are made with soy lecithin, a common emulsifier that stabilizes food ingredients. Like the vast majority of soy products in the U.S.A., soy lecithin is typically derived from genetically modified crops. If you are sensitive to soy or want to avoid the minimal amount of GMO soy in a chocolate bar, you can find soy-free brands with a little investigation. The Primal Chocolate line at EatingEvolved.com, SantaBarbaraChocolate.com, and RaakaChocolate.com offer soy-free products.

PREBIOTICS AND PROBIOTICS FOR GUT HEALTH

Gut health has become a hot topic in progressive health circles lately. The gut is home to around 40 trillion (in a typical average-sized healthy adult; we have a similar total number of human cells when you count small red blood cells) microorganisms in the form of bacteria and yeast, also called flora. Gut bacteria set up shop during our evolutionary development, as *Homo sapiens* were constantly exposed to microbes in the course of routine daily life. Grok walked barefoot in the dirt, worked and played in the dirt, and ate dirt at pretty much every meal. Hey, when you never wash your hands or your food (or anything else, for that matter), you pretty much can't avoid it. With all that soil came billions of soil-based organisms (mostly bacteria and yeast) that entered his system daily and populated his gut. Most were friendly bacteria that actually helped him better digest food and ward off infections. In fact, much of Grok's (and our) immune system evolved to depend on healthy flora living in us symbiotically. Grok also ate the occasional unfriendly organism that had the potential to cause illness, but as long as the healthy flora well outnumbered the bad guys, all was well.

A mounting body of research links the state of the bacteria in your intestinal tract to various diseases, and many doctors now consider microbial diversity (how many different types of gut microbes you have—more is better) to be an important health marker. The immune system in particular depends upon a healthy balance of bacteria in the gastrointestinal tract, a state characterized by a predominance of "friendly" bacteria over the "bad" bacteria that can cause illness. Contrary to the oversimplified layman's view of germs and bacteria as universally bad and dangerous, our bodies are constantly covered and populated by all manner of germs and bacteria, both good and bad, no matter how hard we try to scrub and cleanse everything we eat and touch.

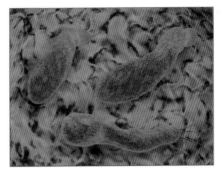

Emerging science suggests our gut health has a strong influence on immune function, hormonal function, weight management, and even athletic performance.

Beneficial bacteria are the most important line of defense for your immune system. They help quell inflammation, neutralize toxic substances, turn fiber into special health-promoting fatty acids, and even produce important nutrients like B vitamins and vitamin K. Interestingly, 90 percent of the production of your body's critical "feel good" neurotransmitter serotonin happens in the gut, regulated by intestinal enterochromaffin (EC) cells and other forms of intestinal bacteria. Gut microbes also produce other adaptive hormones like dopamine and noradrenaline.

What's more, recent research draws a connection between healthy gut flora and improved athletic performance. Exercise has been shown to promote increased microbial diversity, and a study out of University College Cork in Ireland revealed that a group of elite athletes had twice the diversity of gut flora as average folks. (It is worth noting, too, that these researchers found that protein consumption was positively correlated with microbial diversity—good news for primal omnivores!) High microbial diversity is believed to help increase antioxidant production, increase exercise time to exhaustion, regulate inflammation, improve resistance to illness (especially during heavy training), and improve tolerance to exercising in the heat.

The problem today is that not only do we avoid dirt, but we also pursue cleanliness and sterility to the extent that we dramatically minimize our exposure to all forms of bacteria. Our genes developed a reliance on a regular and consistent supply of soil-based organisms to optimize immune and digestive function and to become adept at fighting off pathogens. Unfortunately, our modern propensity for excessive sanitation of meals and living environments has weakened our defenses by providing insufficient exposure to routine environmental germs. This, combined with excess exposure to non-primal stuff like sugar, grains (especially the leaky-gut-promoting lectins), oxidized vegetable oils, alcohol, tobacco, antibiotics and other pharmaceuticals, insufficient vitamin D, and chronic stress, can destroy healthy bacteria and allow harmful bacteria to proliferate.

Healthy bacteria usually render harmful bacteria benign, but if harmful bacteria are able to gain a foothold in your bloodstream and digestive tract, they can cause assorted health disruptions and diseases. Conditions associated with poor gut health include constipation, irritable bowel syndrome, diarrhea, and acid reflux; conditions outside the intestinal tract such as allergies, asthma, acne, migraines, psoriasis, autoimmune disorders, and systemic inflammation; and an increased risk of obesity, diabetes, and heart disease. Research has even linked disturbed gut flora to an increased likelihood of autism and mental health disorders, including depression, obsessive-compulsive disorder, and anxiety and panic attacks.

It is unfortunately a common occurrence for harmful bacteria to compromise gut health and promote digestive, immune system, and mood and cognitive dysfunction. This can be caused by poor dietary habits, environmental stressors, adverse lifestyle practices (too much stress, not enough sleep, excessive exercise, etc.), and especially the use of antibiotics. Antibiotics wipe out both healthy and harmful bacteria in the name of treating illness. Unfortunately, without an aggressive effort to repopulate your gut with healthy bacteria, coming off antibiotics leaves you vulnerable and defenseless against harmful microorganisms in the intestinal tract, right when you are hoping to get better from the original illness.

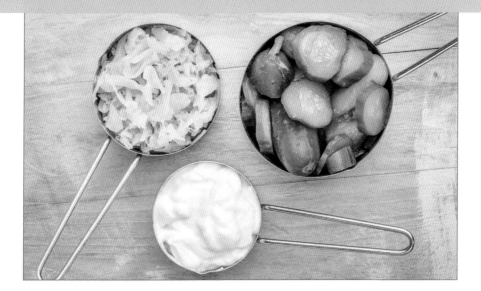

Food Sources of Probiotics and Prebiotics

Besides embracing healthy lifestyle habits (adequate sleep and sunlight, good stress management, nutrient-dense diet, etc.), healthy intestinal flora is promoted by the consumption of *probiotics*. These are healthful living organisms present in certain foods that, when consumed, take up residence in your digestive tract. Fermented foods such as yogurt, kefir, sauerkraut, pickles, kimchi, fermented soy products (miso, tempeh), kombucha drinks, and even dark chocolate are rich in health-promoting probiotics. Probiotics are also popular in liquid or capsule supplement form. Polyphenols, abundant in blueberries, red wine, green tea, and high-cacao-percentage dark chocolate, can also benefit your gut microbiome. Probiotics (and polyphenols) can be considered agents in certain foods that help populate your digestive tract with healthy bacteria. Probiotics, however, need their own type of food to survive in the form of *prebiotics*.

Prebiotics are indigestible agents present in certain foods (or supplements) that nourish the healthy bacteria already living in your digestive tract. Resistant starch is the best dietary source of prebiotics. Unlike regular starch in complex carbohydrate form, resistant starch is indigestible (it "resists" digestion) when consumed. Instead of being processed like regular food calories, resistant starch travels through the small intestine unscathed and into the colon. There, friendly bacteria called *bifidobacteria* metabolize these special starches into a short chain fatty acid called butyrate that is the prime energy source for your colonic cells. Butyrate communicates with your immune system, helping to regulate inflammatory processes. Resistant starch consumption has also been shown to boost insulin sensitivity, improve the integrity of your gut lining (combating the aforementioned leaky gut), reduce fasting blood sugar levels, and lessen the glucose and insulin responses to high-carb meals.

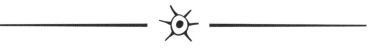

TYPES OF RESISTANCE STARCHES

Technically speaking, there are four different categories of resistant starch as follows:

RS1: found in indigestible plant cell walls (coating) around beans, grains, and seeds.

RS2: found in raw potatoes, bananas, and plantains. These foods, high in amylose, become digestible when they are cooked (potatoes) or ripen (bananas and plantains).

RS3: aka retrograded starch, formed when certain starches are cooked and then cooled—potatoes, grains, and legumes.

RS4: a chemically modified starch that does not exist in nature, known as "hi-maize resistant starch."

Resistant starch boosts the integrity and function of your gut, flushes away harmful microbes by binding to them and escorting them out in feces, and even contributes to satiety. Recent research from the University of Toronto showed that supplementation with resistant starch decreased hunger and reduced subsequent food intake. Numerous other studies tell a similar tale: resistant starch helps promote lowered body fat and increased lean mass, as well as improved thyroid function, better sleep, and more mental calmness.

Prebiotics are present in an assortment of foods such as asparagus, Jerusalem artichokes, bananas, plantains, onions, garlic, leeks, red wine, honey, and even whole grains and legumes. However, to pursue maximum health benefits, a strategic approach of taking concentrated sources of resistant starch such as potato starch, tapioca starch, or plantain flour, or emphasizing foods that are very high in resistant starch such as green bananas, is recommended.

Many experts agree that raw, unmodified potato starch is the fastest and most reliable way to up your resistant starch intake. However, some people—especially those with compromised gut health—may want to proceed with caution (try adding only a teaspoon a day at first and increase gradually), as it is possible to experience gastrointestinal distress (gas, bloating, constipation) from the sudden alteration in typical dietary habits. If you notice any digestive trouble as you attempt to add potato starch or other resistant starches to your diet, reduce intake for a while. Also, consider emphasizing whole-food sources over powdered forms. Some of the best whole-food sources of resistant starch include:

Green Bananas and Plantains: That's right, going green is key. Ripe bananas and plantains provide mostly carbohydrates and minimal resistant starch, but the nutrient composition is quite different when you consume these tropical fruits unripe. A typical green banana contains only 6 grams of carbs, while a ripe banana contains around 25 grams. Bananas and plantains in unripe form provide an abundance of resistant starch and fewer carbohydrate calories, making them particularly appealing to carb-conscious primal eaters.

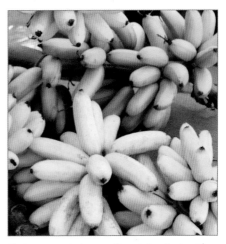

Get a good dose of resistant starch from green bananas—they're delicious! Okay, not really—they're pretty chalky... but a few smears of almond butter make them tolerable.

Cooked and Cooled Potatoes, Rice, or Legumes: Yes, the "cooked and cooled" qualifier is critical here because cooking followed by cooling alters the structure of the carbohydrates in these foods to render them resistant to normal digestion. If you eat a warm baked potato or a steaming bowl

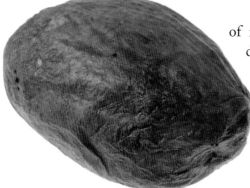

of rice, these carbohydrates will be in digestible form with little to no resistant starch. Instead, consume them cold after they have been cooked to get a good dose of resistant starch.

Ahh, an ice cold bowl of rice and a potato really hit the spot... in your gut!

Flours: You can also obtain resistant starch by supplementing smoothies or soups with isolated starch sources such as raw potato starch, plantain flour, green banana flour, and cassava/tapioca starch. There are around eight grams of resistant starch in a single tablespoon of raw potato starch, which is believed to be the most reliable form of supplementary starch.

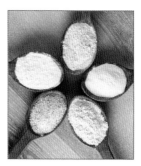

HYDRATION: OBEY YOUR THIRST, AND USE YOUR BRAIN TOO!

The original *Primal Blueprint* book delivered a pretty simple and primal take on the issue of hydration. The message was essentially "obey your thirst." The updated Primal Blueprint message on hydration is now significantly more nuanced. Your thirst mechanism and your kidneys indeed do an excellent job keeping you hydrated and electrolyte-balanced, and most people—especially minimally active people—needn't concern themselves with anything beyond a sensible daily intake of all kinds of fluids, eating plenty of high-water-content fruits and vegetables, and of course heeding general sensations of thirst.

However, in recent years, some leading scientists and peak performance experts seem to be paying attention to the hydration issue more than ever before. Dr. Kelly Starrett, one of the world's leading mobility/rehabilitation experts and author of *Becoming a Supple Leopard*, is constantly harping on his athletes and students to hydrate conscientiously.

Dr. Phil Maffetone, a pioneer in the world of aerobic training and balancing health with fitness pursuits, coach of legendary triathletes Mark Allen, Tim DeBoom, and Mike Pigg, and author of *The Big Book of Endurance Training and Racing*, mentions hydration often and considers suboptimal hydration a stumbling block to peak performance and quick recovery for athletes of all levels. Dr. Stacy Sims, an Environmental Exercise Physiologist and Nutrition Scientist and cofounder of Osmo Nutrition, has produced detailed research and commentary about how hydration affects hormones, blood volume, and overall performance and recovery for athletes.

Interestingly, there are some significant differences of opinion among experts when you dig into the details of hydration, especially when it comes to recommendations for athletes. My desire here is to give you an easy-to-understand overview that can guide you to best practices and winning decisions about hydration. First off, let's marvel at the amazing ability of our kidneys and endocrine system to promote optimum fluid levels in your bloodstream. Leading scientists like Dr. Heinz Valtin, former chair of physiology at Dartmouth Medical School and one of the world's foremost experts on kidney function, explains that your internal mechanisms enable hydration homeostasis even when your water intake fluctuates significantly. If you get a bit low on fluids, an agent known as vasopressin (an antidiuretic hormone, aka AVP) goes to work increasing the absorption of water from the kidneys and returning it to the bloodstream. If your blood becomes concentrated by about two percent (meaning you are on your way to becoming dehydrated), your thirst mechanism will kick in big time, telling you to consume additional fluids. It is only when your blood becomes concentrated by five percent—way past the point of experiencing significant thirst—that the medical concerns regarding dehydration present themselves. On the flip side, if your blood concentration (osmolality) decreases, indicating that you are overhydrated, your body will act to increase urine production and draw on its sodium reserves to restore balance.

These systems evolved to run very efficiently, so for otherwise-healthy adults, simply drinking to thirst is the best recommendation. Remember, too, that we do get some of our hydration needs (up to 20 percent, according to the Mayo Clinic) met through solid foods, especially primal people who consume ample amounts of high-water-content fruits and vegetables. To make sure your body is actually absorbing the water you ingest, Dr. Sims also recommends salting your food (especially in light of the fact that primal adherents tend to eat a relatively low-sodium diet). Sodium plays a key role in absorption, so unless you have, for example, a heart or kidney disorder for which you have been prescribed a low-sodium diet, don't be afraid to reach for the salt shaker—sea salt or pink salt being more nutritious than regular old iodized salt.

So why all the fuss about hydration for athletes? Because athletes' bodies are under higher-than-average physical and metabolic stress. Their hydration needs are greater and also harder to satisfy. Perhaps counterintuitively, the harder and longer they work, the less appropriate the "drink to thirst" recommendation might be. The reason is twofold. First, when athletes are under stress from strenuous exercise, in high temperature and/or humid climates, or just totally immersed in their effort, they simply might not be accurately attuned to their bodies' thirst mechanism. Plus, when AVP is released in response to signs the body is becoming dehydrated—as inevitably happens during intense physical exertion—one of the effects is that thirst sensation is muted. The kidneys are doing as asked by dumping more water into the bloodstream; exercise continues, but the athlete is potentially digging into a dehydration hole—maybe not at that particular workout, but they could be initiating a downward spiral that takes some time to unfurl. For example, you might come into a workout with slightly concentrated blood volume for whatever reason and perform a session that is intense, prolonged, in hot weather, or any combination of these, further depleting you of fluids and perhaps electrolytes. Because your body is so adept at adapting on the fly, you might not experience compromised performance during this workout. You might drink to your thirst over the ensuing 12 hours or whatever, feel fine, deliver clear urine, and soon perform another challenging workout. If you repeat this scenario a few times, things could get dicey. Over time, you will probably notice a decrease in performance, an increase in recovery time, and increased propensity for injury.

One important addition to these guidelines, and one which is especially important for athletes: do not force yourself to drink more than you need. There *is* such a thing as too much water. Hyponatremia is a serious and occasionally fatal condition in which sodium levels become too diluted in the blood. Among athletes, hyponatremia usually results from overconsumption of water. If you are minimally active and can't remember the last time you moistened a t-shirt with sweat, you are at low risk unless you force yourself to drink well beyond what is appealing or comfortable. For anyone engaging in sports, especially endurance sports such as running and triathlon, exercise-associated hyponatremia (EAH) is a real concern. Dr. Timothy Noakes, one of the world's leading endurance exercise physiologists, founding member of the IOC's Olympic Science Academy, and author of many books including the epic *Lore of Running* (widely regarded as the most informative book ever written on the physiology of endurance performance), was among the first to sound the alarm about EAH. In his book *Waterlogged*, he chronicles the alarming frequency of hyponatremia among marathon runners. According to Dr. Noakes, flawed research published in the 1960s, concurrent with the rise of the sports energy industry (Gatorade, and then many others), made us afraid to become even a little dehydrated during exercise. Athletes were increasingly encouraged to push water and sports drinks early and often, regardless of actual thirst. As a result, athletes starting falling sick during races. There have been a significant number of fatalities in endurance events (and radio station water drinking contests) from hyponatremia in recent years.

For endurance athletes especially, there is a delicate balance that must be achieved between too much and too little water. Athletes who are out training and racing hour after hour must work extra hard to listen to their bodies and to consider factors such as environment, temperature, perspiration, diet, and so on, when deciding how and when to drink. For training sessions and races lasting more than three or four hours, it is probably wiser to implement a hydration plan rather than relying only on thirst to guide fluid intake. Dr. Sims also advises athletes to drink a solution that includes sodium, glucose, and sucrose—but not maltodextrin and fructose!—because the salt and sugars will help the intestines absorb water efficiently. (Note that the sugars here are not for fueling, but rather for facilitating fluid uptake.) This can be done using an engineered sports drink, but carefully read the label. (Hint: many popular sports drinks contain ingredients you do not want to consume during

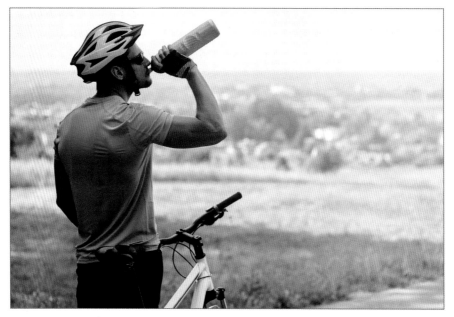

sports, or ever!) You can also just add a pinch of salt (or, if you are prone to leaky gut issues, use sodium citrate or carbonate instead of salt) and a splash of maple syrup to your water bottle on the way out the door.

This is one reason training is so important; it provides the opportunity for learning about and experimenting with individual hydration needs. The time to start thinking about hydration is not when you are over-stressed, overheated, and exhausted. This could land you in serious trou-ble. I remember one occasion decades ago where I came home from a long, hot training run so tired that I just collapsed on the couch. I was too tired to shower, refuel, or rehydrate. When I woke up around 90 minutes later, I didn't feel so good—headache, dizzy, nauseous—telltale signs that I was significantly dehydrated, yet I hadn't even noticed feeling thirsty on the run. Just like with your diet, hydrating optimally might take some experimenting and tinkering to get right, and common sense will be a reliable guide to make sure you don't under- or overdo it. In general, the best advice for most fitness enthusiasts is still to drink to thirst. If during exercise water sounds and tastes good, drink; if it sounds horrible, wait a while. Add a little sodium and glucose plus sucrose to maximize absorption. After a workout, focus on rehydrating slowly over a few hours instead of gulping a ton of water that the body will just dump back out. For athletes engaged in long endurance training and events, or extreme challenges like CrossFit Games (or doing too many CrossFit workouts in the course of a week!), implement a methodical hydration plan.

A final caveat: as Dr. Sims reminds us, "women are not small men!" She and others have begun to shed light on the fact that women need to take extra care to adapt their hydration strategies to their menstrual cycles. During the high-hormone phase (the one to two weeks before their periods), when estrogen and progesterone are elevated, women have lower plasma volume and decreased sodium, which essentially means they are predisposed to hyponatremia. Because they are already physiologically on the road to hyponatremia, it is important that they not overhydrate. Women in this phase especially need to take care to ingest sodium in their diets and in their water, and they need to carefully monitor their hydration. Dr. Sims recommends drinking to thirst during the high-hormone phase to be safe, unless they are ingesting fluids with the proper balance of sodium and glucose/fructose.

FINALLY, A WORD ABOUT SUPPLEMENTS

I must start this section with a disclaimer: I own and operate a supplement company called Primal Nutrition, and I've spent several decades researching, formulating, and selling nutritional supplements such as vitamins and meal-replacement formulas. I'm not an impartial party on this issue, and I've taken a fair amount of heat from haters who claim that my involvement with supplements taints the purity of my primal message. If you are not enthusiastic about the topic of supplements, I remind you that you are free to skip this section and jump to the next chapter!

That said, here's the reality of where I'm coming from: modern life presents many, many challenges to living in a strict primal fashion and closely adhering to the dietary and lifestyle habits of our ancestors. I'll admit that a devoted health enthusiast—a hard-core primal follower—can orchestrate a dietary pattern and an exceptional stress-management strategy that optimizes nutritional intake and renders a supplement strategy unnecessary. Despite claims from the olestra folks, we have yet to invent a manufactured product that outdoes a steak salad for nutritional benefit.

My angle has always been personal: I recommend diet, exercise, and lifestyle patterns that I have personally tried and found to be successful. I design and market supplements that I use and benefit from in my own life, simple as that. And while you can bet I'm a pretty hard-core primal guy, I also travel on airplanes, stress over business challenges, overdo exercise now and then, and experience assorted other pressures that challenge my immune function, digestive tract, and ability to manage stress. I use supplements when my primal-but-also-modern lifestyle requires additional support to optimize my health and wellbeing. Supplements should be considered just that: "supplements" to a foundation of healthy dietary choices and lifestyle habits.

If you are interested, following is some brief commentary about certain supplement categories that might help you shore up any shortcomings and also make it more convenient and realistic to stay primal-aligned in your hectic modern life.

Multivitamin/Mineral/Antioxidant Formula

Eating, exercising, and living according to the Primal Blueprint will help mitigate much of the oxidative damage modern humans sustain as a result of eating the Standard American Diet, performing chronic or insufficient exercise, getting inadequate sleep and sunlight, and coping with generally excessive stress levels. Your internal antioxidant systems work quite well when you're healthy and stress-balanced. However, pushing the limits with subpar nutrition, jet travel, emotional stress, or chronic exercise, for example, can quickly compromise your digestive, immune, and endocrine systems, along with other aspects of general health.

We need a broad mix of antioxidants on a daily basis, because they work in different ways and in different parts of the cell. Too much of any single antioxidant (in the absence of others) has been shown to have potentially negative effects, as a few recent studies about taking vitamin E only and experiencing negative results have demonstrated. Unfortunately, many of our ancestors' best sources of dietary vitamins, minerals, and antioxidants have all but disappeared, or have been rendered impotent, by today's aggressive factory farming techniques. In the fruit industry, for example, obtaining the highest possible sugar content and visual appeal has replaced nutritional value as the priority. Even if you are diligent about selecting locally grown produce farmed with the least objectionable methods possible, you are probably still not getting the nutrient density our ancestors would have enjoyed. Your best efforts will come up short, nutritionally speaking, thanks to widespread depletion of minerals in the soil and to manipulation of the crops that have made them in some cases unrecognizable from the ones our ancestors would have foraged in the wild. (For example, modern wheat is very different from the ancient varietals of the grain, which is one reason—among many—that it poses such a serious health concern.)

When you take a quality broad-spectrum antioxidant formula (containing hard-to-get nutrients such as full-spectrum vitamin E—not just alpha-tocopherol; mixed carotenoids—not just beta-carotene; tocotrienols, n-acetyl-cysteine, alpha-lipoic acid, curcumin, resveratrol, milk thistle, CoQ10, and quercetin, to name a few), the agents work synergistically to mitigate oxidative damage and recycle back to their potent antioxidant form. For that reason, I choose to take a high-potency multivitamin loaded with extra antioxidants every day.

Omega-3 Fish Oil

In Grok's day, virtually every animal he consumed was a decent source of vital omega-3 fatty acids. The fish he caught ate algae to produce omega-3 fatty acids rich in EPA and DHA (which helped build the larger human brain over a couple hundred thousand years). The animals he hunted grazed on plants that generated high levels of omega-3. Even the vegetation Grok consumed provided higher levels of omega-3s than the levels found in today's plants.

The richest source of dietary omega-3s, by far, is oily, cold-water fish. If you are not a big seafood fan, a fish or krill oil supplement is a convenient way to boost your omega-3 intake. The research on fish oils is extraordinarily positive, showing such benefits as decreased risk for heart disease and cancer, lowering of triglycerides, improvement in joint mobility, decreased insulin resistance, and improved brain function and mood. The drug companies are even starting to recognize the power of this "natural medicine" and have begun promoting prescription fish oil (at four times the price of a comparable supplement, of course!).

As healthy as my own diet is, I rarely go a day without taking a few grams of omega-3 fish oil. The key is to supplement wisely, adding fish oil to round out a nutritious primal diet—rather than going overboard to reach a sky-high omega-3 level that even Grok wouldn't be capable of achieving.

Probiotics

You don't necessarily need to take probiotics every day, because once these "seeds" have been planted in a healthy gut, they tend to multiply and flourish easily on their own. Rather, consider taking extra probiotics under times of significant stress, when you have been sick, when you are traveling (particularly to foreign countries where unfamiliar bacteria—even good stuff from good foods—can overwhelm your digestive system), when you detect any sign of compromised immune function (remember, the gut is the first line of defense for your immune system), and especially in the aftermath of taking a course of antibiotics.

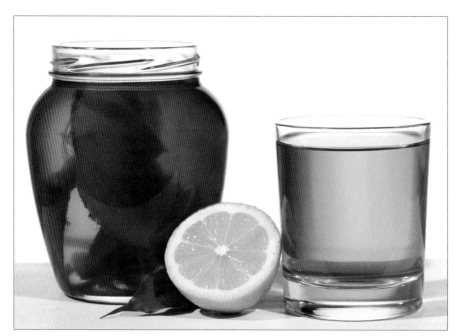

Kombucha is a fermented, lightly effervescent sweetened tea beverage harvested from a symbiotic bacteria colony—a great source of probiotics.

Prebiotics

The right array of prebiotics in your diet makes for a very happy, diverse gut microbiome, which in turn benefits nearly every other aspect of your health. By eating a variety of primal plant foods, you'll naturally be getting some prebiotics in your diet. But to seriously revamp a compromised gut—from a history of antibiotic use, certain medications, too much stress, chronic infections, or otherwise suboptimal lifestyle and diet—you might benefit from more prebiotics than diet alone can deliver, and supplementation may be in order. Although a variety of different prebiotics are currently on the market, the "resistant starch" we discussed earlier in this chapter, which is found abundantly in raw potato starch or green bananas, is remarkably effective and relatively affordable. Resistant starch can directly feed your most beneficial microbes and, especially in conjunction with probiotics, help repopulate your gut with powerful health-promoting bacteria.

Protein Powder/Meal Replacement

Restricting your intake of processed carbs often means being at a loss for quick, convenient snacks or small meals. We are so conditioned to reach for a bagel, an energy bar, chips, crackers, and other grain-based products or sweets for snacks, we often run short on convenient, transportable, nonperishable options for an afternoon pickup snack or mini meal. While not exactly primal, protein powders/meal replacements do combine the best of 21st-century technology with a true primal intent: get me a fast, good-tasting source of nutrients without too many carbs or unhealthy fats.

I prefer micro-filtered whey protein to obtain an impressive profile of all the essential and nonessential amino acids, and coconut milk solids to provide healthy fats that can be delivered in a powdered formula. I recommend finding a product that tastes great when mixed only with water so you don't have to add sugary juices or milk just to choke it down. You can always throw in a piece of fruit for added calories or flavor, if you choose. If I am in a hurry and want a quick, high-protein start to my day, my morning smoothie shake takes less than a minute to make and covers the bases I need covered. Adding some omega-3 oil covers you on two critical primal areas. Micro-filtered whey, while derived from dairy, has insignificant amounts of lactose, so it's fine for most all lactose-intolerant folks.

Another popular practice in the primal community is to start the day with a macronutrient balanced "green" smoothie, full of nutritious leafy greens and other veggies, protein powder, and healthy fats like coconut milk, avocado, or even coconut oil. Here, you get a concentrated dose of antioxidants and other nutrients, even when you are not hungry for a proper meal, but you don't get the sugar bomb of most commercial "green" smoothies that are commonly prepared in a base of fruit juice or contain high volumes of berries for taste, but are devoid of sufficient fat or protein. A primal-style green smoothie with ample protein, fat, and carbs from fruits and veggies can especially benefit the athletic/high-calorie-burning primal folks who practice Intermittent Fasting and consume high-fat meals. Being extremely calorically efficient and not needing regular meals is great to optimize cell repair and promote insulin sensitivity and longevity, but it's also possible to fall behind nutritionally because you don't require regular meals or massive calories to function. A green smoothie is like an insurance policy against the potential drawbacks of fasting or primal-style meals that are rich in other nutritional attributes (e.g., steak, eggs, fish, etc.), but a little light on the colorful vegetables that are meant to be consumed in abundance.

Vitamin D

There's no question that the best way to obtain vitamin D is how nature intended: directly from the sun. Even an excellent diet provides for only a fraction of your needs in comparison to regularly exposing large skin surface areas of your body to direct sunlight at the times of day and year of peak solar intensity. While obtaining enough sun exposure to manufacture adequate levels of vitamin D would have been no problem for Grok, many modern citizens are vitamin D deficient, mainly because of our predominantly indoor lifestyles and aversion to deliberate sun exposure due to misguided fears about skin cancer.

This is such an important topic—and such a pervasive problem in modern society—that an entire primal law is dedicated to it, which I'll cover in detail in Chapter 8. There I provide a basic strategy to get adequate sun exposure so that you can maintain a sufficient blood level of vitamin D year-round (since vitamin D can be stored in your fat cells for winter use). That said, if you look at the extreme disparity between our sun exposure in modern life versus our ancestors' experience, it follows that most of us can benefit from vitamin D supplementation, especially in wintertime and if you fall into one or more of the high-risk categories: those living at latitudes extremely distant from the equator, with dark skin living outside tropical latitudes, with indoor-dominant lifestyles, or those who are elderly, obese, or with Metabolic Syndrome.

Again, this is an area where conventional wisdom is behind the curve. Vitamin D deficiency is not recognized as the extreme public health problem that it is. What qualifies as "normal" on traditional blood tests is actually deficient in the opinion of many vitamin D advocates. Dermatologists constantly admonish us to avoid the sun, and we are misled into thinking that eating vitamin D-fortified foods (like those great high-sugar breakfast cereals) will keep us covered in this area.

More on all this in the "Primal Blueprint Law #8: Get Plenty of Sunlight" section of Chapter 8. For now, know that expert vitamin D advocates recommend obtaining an average of 4,000 International Units (I.U.) per day of vitamin D. For reference, you can easily bag 5,000-10,000 I.U. during a single half-hour sunbathing session in the summer-time. On the diet front, eating nutritious, primal-aligned meals (especially emphasizing oily, cold-water fish) will deliver maybe 1,000 I.U. on a good day, while experts estimate a SAD eating pattern delivers around 300 I.U. per day. Consequently, I recommend supplementing with at least 2,000 I.U. of vitamin D per day when you are not getting frequent sun exposure. That said, getting your blood tested is essential to supplementing optimally, instead of indiscriminately. I am fair-skinned, live at 34 degrees latitude in Los Angeles, and get a ton of sun exposure during the summer, but I still supplement during the winter to be extra sure that my blood levels are adequate.

The aforementioned supplement categories represent what I believe to be the most useful products to consider for supplementation, but there are numerous other product categories and individual supplements that address more specialized needs. Among them are phosphatidylserine (PS), which improves cognitive function and moderates cortisol spikes in the bloodstream, and buffering joint compounds (glucosamine, chondroitin, MSM, and enzyme cofactors), which support connective tissue and alleviate pain. A knowledgeable healthcare practitioner may recommend other products to address your particular needs.

Supplement Quality

Regardless of what brand of products you choose, you should be extremely vigilant in an industry that is minimally regulated by the FDA. Good manufacturers have a tightly controlled production environment where every single raw material that goes into the finished product is easily sourced and certified by the supplier. Contact your supplement manufacturers and ask if they obtain "Certificates of Assay" attesting to the source, potency, and purity of each ingredient. Ask if their products are produced in a pharmaceutical-grade manufacturing environment. Ask whether they adhere to the "Good Manufacturing Practices" (GMP) that is overseen by the Food and Drug Administration. Notice how well products are sealed when presented for retail sale.

You will be able to quickly discern from email replies (or lack thereof) or phone conversations whether the manufacturer of the supplements you consume, or are considering consuming, has its act together. Examine labels and choose supplements that are free of common fillers and additives such as colorings, waxes, preservatives, and other chemicals. They'll be listed under "inactive" or "other" ingredients. You'll be surprised to discover just how prevalent these agents are in many of the leading vitamin brands and discount products available through big-box retailers and in supermarkets and drugstores. Understand that premium quality supplements are considerably more expensive than the giant bottles found on the shelves of warehouse stores. Many, but not all, products in the latter category offer minimal potency and bioavailability (ease of digestion and utilization by the body) and bring literal accuracy to the expression "pissing away your money."

CHAPTER SUMMARY

1. Meat and Fowl: Choose local, pasture-raised animal products (or, next best, USDA certified organic animal products) to avoid today's poor quality mass-produced feedlot animals that are fattened up with grains and laden with hormones, pesticides, and antibiotics. Regarding the headlines about red meat consumption causing cancer, it's important to avoid heavily processed meats (bologna, hot dogs, cheap bacon, jerkies and sausage) and, to be safe, avoid overcooking meat (which produces carcinogens).

2. Fish: Fish are a rich source of omega-3 fats and many other vitamins, minerals, and nutrients, and they have strong anti-inflammatory, antioxidant effects. Emphasize wild-caught fish from remote, pollution-free waters. Oily, cold-water fish (anchovies, herring, mackerel, salmon, sardines) have the highest level of omega-3 fatty acids. Choose only acceptable farmed fish (Coho salmon, shellfish, domestic trout, and certain other domestic species), and avoid other farmed fish (including the popular Atlantic salmon), fish at the top of the food chain (shark, swordfish), fish caught by environmentally objectionable commercial methods, or imports from Asia (both wild-caught and farmed).

3. Eggs: Eggs are one of the most nutritious foods on the planet—especially the yolks! Local, pasture-raised chickens deliver more omega-3s and other nutrients than commercially raised chickens. Think outside the chicken coop and try other types of eggs like duck, quail, and goose.

4. Vegetables: Vegetables should play a central role in your diet and comprise the largest section of your daily "plate." Brightly colored foods have high levels of antioxidants, phenols, fiber, vitamins, minerals, and other micronutrients. Consuming vegetables (and fruits) helps boost immune function and reduces disease risk. Dark leafy greens are an excellent choice to consume regularly as a base for any main course. Eating vegetables liberally (and seasonal fruits with some moderation and selectivity) will result in satisfactory macronutrient ratios.

It's essential to select locally grown, organic, pesticide-free vegetables for maximum nutritional value and health safety whenever possible. Be strict about going organic and/or pesticide-free with vegetables (and fruits) that have a large surface area (leafy greens) or a soft open skin (bell peppers, carrots, winter squash, berries, peaches). You can be less strict with plants that have a tough, inedible skin (bananas, avocados, melons, oranges).

5. Nuts and seeds, and their derivative butters: Nuts and seeds are rich sources of micronutrients, and phytochemicals. While nuts and seeds are invariably higher in omega-6 than omega-3, their nutritional benefits outweigh any concerns about inflammatory balance. Choose raw or minimally processed products, and avoid nuts processed with vegetable oils or with sugary coatings. Store all nuts, seeds, and butters in the fridge or freezer to prevent rancidity and extend shelf life.

6. Coconut Products: Coconut's medium-chain fatty acids offer exceptional health benefits and are difficult to obtain, even in a healthy diet. Coconut oil, milk, flakes, and other derivatives can be great substitutes for offensive SAD ingredients. Coconut oil is excellent for cooking due to its high saturated fat composition.

7. Fruits: Fruits offer an outstanding source of fiber, vitamins, minerals, antioxidants, and other phytochemicals. Choose wisely by sticking to locally grown, in-season, pesticide-free fruits that are high in antioxidants. Fresh berries offer excellent antioxidant and nutrient levels. Some moderation is warranted with fruit due to year-round availability of sweet fruits and the high prevalence of processed fructose in the modern diet. This is particularly true for those wanting to reduce body fat, since a major carbohydrate in fruit (fructose) is easily converted into fat in the liver.

8. Herbs and Spices: Herbs and spices offer tremendous macronutrient and antioxidant values and can enhance your enjoyment of meals. Strive for organic/pesticide-free sources of herbs to avoid pesticide risk.

9. Moderation Foods: The moderation foods category suggests that certain foods offer health benefits and are not objectionable like sugars, grains, and bad oils, but they don't need to be a dietary centerpiece. These foods include coffee (don't use as an energy crutch); high-fat dairy (preference for raw, fermented products); approved fats and oils (saturated for cooking, extra virgin olive oil and avocado oil for eating); high-nutrient-value carbs (sweet potatoes, quinoa, wild rice, extra fruit—moderate consumption based on body composition, fitness goals, and hormonal concerns); and dark chocolate (75-percent cacao or greater—a satisfying, high-antioxidant, low-sugar treat).

10. Prebiotics and Probiotics for Gut Health: The burgeoning scientific interest in gut health suggests that a healthy and diverse gut microbiome is essential for optimal immune and digestive function and overall health. Consuming ample sources of *probiotics* (friendly intestinal bacteria) and *prebiotics* (the resistant starches that feed probiotics) helps ensure that friendly intestinal bacteria predominate over harmful bacterial. Stressful lifestyle circumstances, unhealthy diets, and especially antibiotic consumption can compromise healthy intestinal flora. To help friendly bacteria flourish, consume prebiotics in the form of raw potato starch, green bananas, or cooked and cooled white rice and/or russet potatoes. Probiotics are found in high levels in fermented foods (yogurt, kefir, sauerkraut, pickles, kimchi, kombucha, and fermented soy products like miso and tempeh) or in supplement form (liquids or capsules). Probiotics are also found in other healthy foods like vegetables and dark chocolate.

11. Hydration: The updated primal position on hydration extends beyond the simple "obey your thirst" admonition to consider females' and hard training athletes' unique needs. While the thirst mechanism and kidneys generally do an excellent job at regulating hydration, it's possible that high-stress exercise can mute the thirst mechanism. This is especially true over time if training hard in warm temperatures. Hence, a methodical strategy is recommended to ensure optimal hydration both before and after workouts. Females also should be mindful of how hydration needs vary according to the menstrual cycle. Beware of overhydration to the extent of triggering the dangerous condition of hyponatremia (diluted sodium due to excessive fluid intake). Never force fluid consumption unnaturally. To optimize rehydration, consume fluids steadily over time instead of in a single dump that might overwhelm the body and just be excreted. Also, a bit of sodium, glucose, and sucrose can assist with more efficient fluid absorption in the intestines.

12. Supplements: Supplements can play a useful role in adapting primal recommendations to the realities of hectic modern life. Supplements offer a convenient source of concentrated nutrition that helps account for nutrient deficiencies in today's food supply (due to depleted soil or objectionable conventional growing and production methods, for example). The following categories offer comprehensive protection and added support for even the healthiest of diets: multivitamin/mineral/antioxidant formula, omega-3 fish oil, probiotic capsules or liquid, raw potato starch prebiotics, protein powder/meal replacement, and vitamin D capsules.

CHAPTER SIX

PRIMAL BLUEPRINT LAW #2: AVOID POISONOUS THINGS

"Drop Your Fork and Step Away from the Plate!"

IN THIS CHAPTER

I detail the health risks of eating "poisonous things." In Grok's day, poisonous plants could drop him on the spot. Today our poisons are factory-produced items in bright packages that poison you more insidiously over decades. We explore the cultural factors that default us to eating an unhealthy diet and consider strategies for resisting these manipulative influences.

Topping the list of foods to avoid are sugar and sweetened beverages, grains (yes, even whole grains), and refined vegetable oils. Unfortunately, these comprise a huge percentage of calories in the Standard American Diet. I detail why the low-fat, grain-based diet recommended by conventional wisdom for decades is unhealthy

Grains—even whole grains—have minimal nutritional value in comparison to primal plant and animal foods, stimulate excess insulin production, and contain anti-nutrients (lectins, gluten, and phytates) that compromise gut health, hamper immune function, and promote systemic inflammation. Ironically, the whole grains we've been taught to emphasize contain higher levels of these harmful anti-nutrients.

Sugar drives excess insulin production and fat storage; disturbs your appetite, satiety, and fat-storage hormones (locking you into a carbohydrate-dependency/fat-storage pattern); suppresses immune function; is pro-inflammatory; causes oxidative damage to important cells and organs throughout the body; and overstimulates the HPA axis (the fight or flight response). Sweetened beverages are especially problematic because they are less filling than whole foods, often leading to extreme overconsumption.

While healthful fats play a central role in the primal eating style, bad fats are possibly the most destructive of anything else you can eat. The dangers of consuming chemically altered partially hydrogenated trans fats are well publicized, but consuming refined, high polyunsaturated vegetable and seed oils (and the many processed and frozen foods made with vegetable oils) also generates an immediate and severe toxic effect. Ingesting these oils wreaks havoc at the cellular level, promoting inflammation, aging, and cancer. As trans fats become increasingly taboo in the public eye, they are being replaced by a new agent called interesterified fats, a different type of artificial "franken-fat" that might be even more deleterious to health.

While legumes have more nutrition and lower anti-nutrient levels than grains, they still deliver big insulin hits. Furthermore, those with sensitive digestive tracts can experience inflammatory, autoimmune, and leaky gut issues. Hence, legumes are considered unnecessary in the Primal Blueprint.

Alcohol was originally categorized as a "sensible indulgence" by the Primal Blueprint, but after years of research and rethinking, it's presented here with a more sobering message. After all, it is a poison, and many primal-aligned eaters might struggle to reduce excess body fat due to even a moderate amount of regular alcohol consumption.

When you see the golden arches, you are probably
on your way to the pearly gates.

—William Castelli, M.D.
Director of the Framingham Heart Study

'd like you to reflect for a moment on your priorities and your vision of a long, happy, healthy, fit life. Often, today's culture of rampant consumerism and instant gratification compromises our admirable long-term life goals. Emphasizing a diet of fresh, nutritious food, or meeting even a modest quota for daily movement and physical activity can be challenging, especially when you are starting from scratch and trying to build momentum for healthy new habits. It's easy to feel discouraged when we stumble from our goals, especially if we compare ourselves to others. It's hard for our confidence not to crack from such comparisons or to formulate excuses and rationalizations about our failure to meet diet and exercise goals.

Even when we wake up with noble intentions to do the right thing, it's easy to miss the mark and make bad choices. Health-conscious athletes are habituated to pound nutritionally devoid, insulin-spiking "energy foods." Purification/detox diets based on dubious science, such as eating nothing but brown rice for a week (talk about a long, hot insulin bath!) are equally damaging. Many of our eating habits are influenced more by cultural or social trends rather than sound science. In addition, many of our eating habits are informed more by emotion or stress, than by hunger.

Savoring the occasional rich treat on a special occasion is one thing. It is an entirely different story to habitually or mindlessly ingest hot dogs at the ball game, popcorn at the movies, or nachos at the bar, simply because it's a comforting part of Americana. If you notice yourself trafficking in rationalizations and cop-outs ("there was nothing healthy on the menu"), please give this topic some sincere reflection and take decisive action. Remember, your ancestors worked unimaginably hard to survive, creating amazing opportunities so that we might enjoy healthy, happy, active and long lives. You deserve nothing less than the very best your genes have to offer.

The most common retort I hear when I bang the drum to emphasize clean eating is, "Hey, everything in moderation." Sage advice indeed, but Mark Twain put this proverb into the ideal perspective when he said, "Everything in moderation, including moderation." As the Korgs demonstrated in Chapter 2, we live in a world where extreme measures are necessary just to avoid serious disease (remember, some three quarters of today's American population will eventually die of largely preventable heart disease or cancer), let alone enjoy optimum health, fitness, energy levels, and body composition. Grok struggled to survive; we struggle to stay healthy in the face of modern temptations and today's convenience-oriented food culture.

I support enjoying the occasional indulgence, but why not make it from the list of the highest quality primal-approved foods? Take a glance at the label of a Milky Way compared to the label of a high-antioxidant, organic dark chocolate bar with no additives, chemicals, chemically altered fats, or fillers (and check the disparity in carb count). This sensible and deeply satisfying indulgence can hardly be described as a sacrifice or compromise. You can walk past the candy machine without skipping a beat.

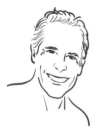

MARK TALK ————————————————————

Now that I've stood on my soapbox to say my piece, I'd like to close this section with a reminder—and a balancing message—to emphasize self-compassion when you pursue lifestyle change. Take the spirit of the 80 Percent Rule to heart and enjoy your pursuit of perfection without becoming too troubled by falling short of whatever lofty goals you envision. Bust loose and have a little fun once in a while, knowing how easy and empowering it is to recalibrate when the cruise, family holiday, or company celebration is over. After all, you deserve it! Ponder this message from popular author Paulo Coehlo: "Diga 'No' sin culpa; diga 'Sí' sin miedo." ("Say 'No' without guilt; say 'Yes' without fear.") This might help you care less about what other people think and care more about honoring yourself.

GOING AGAINST THE GRAIN

Perhaps the most widely accepted health-compromising element of dietary conventional wisdom is that grains are healthy—the "staff of life," as we've been led to believe our entire lives. While grains have indeed enjoyed massive global popularity for the last 7,000 years or so, they are simply not very healthy for human consumption. From 2.5 million years ago, when the first *Homo erectus* arose and steadily evolved into the first modern *Homo sapiens* between 200,000 and 100,000 years ago, and continuing until about 10,000 years ago, humans existed entirely as hunter-gatherers. Early *Homo sapiens* derived their food from 100 to 200 different wild food sources, including animal meats, fruits, vegetables, and nuts and seeds. Cultivated grains were notably absent. Some critics point out that archeological evidence of consumption of wild grains dates back to hunter-gatherer times, but grains, because of the amount of work required to make them digestible to humans, were an insignificant part of the early Paleolithic diet that humans evolved on.

Around 10,000 years ago, forces conspired to create a dramatic shift in the human diet. The widespread extinction of large mammals on major continents, coupled with population increases, forced humans to become more resourceful in obtaining food. Those living by water utilized boats, canoes, nets, and better fishing tools to enjoy the bounty of the sea and lakes. On land, humans refined their toolmaking and hunting strategies to include more birds and small mammals in the food supply.

Escalating competition for animal-sourced food led to agricultural innovations sprouting up independently in the most advanced societies around the world (Egyptians, Mayans, etc.). As grains and, much later, legumes became domesticated, humans derived more and more calories from these high-carbohydrate foods. The transition from hunter-gatherer to an agricultural diet represents an extreme disturbance to human health, for although humans began eating these foods to survive, they are not optimal for long-term health for reasons we will discuss shortly. However, consuming grains did allow humans to successfully reach reproductive age, the ultimate goal from a genetic perspective, so there was no selection pressure causing adaptation at the genetic level. There was no "survival of the fittest" advantage for those humans who were better suited to tolerate grains. I think I can safely assume that most of you have farther-reaching goals than simply surviving to reproductive age. We all want to live long, healthy, vibrant lives, and the plain truth is that eating grains, even supposedly healthy whole grains, runs counter to that goal.

> *We all want to live long, healthy, vibrant lives, and the plain truth is that eating grains, even supposedly healthy whole grains, runs counter to that goal.*

Loren Cordain, Ph.D., author of *The Paleo Diet*, explains:

"For better or for worse, we are no longer hunter-gatherers. However, our genetic makeup is still that of a Paleolithic hunter-gatherer, a species whose nutritional requirements are optimally adapted to wild meats, fruits and vegetables, not to cereal grains. There is a significant body of evidence that suggests that the human genetic makeup and physiology may not be fully adapted to high levels of [cultivated] grain consumption. We have wandered down a path toward absolute dependence upon [cultivated] grains, a path for which there is no return.

Culturally, the cultivation of grains is the key variable that allowed modern civilization to develop and expand. Unburdened from having to hunt and gather, large populations could live permanently in proximity, and labor could specialize for the first time. This led to continued exponential advancements in knowledge and modernization. [Grains] have allowed man's culture to grow and evolve so that man has become earth's dominant animal species, but this preeminence has not occurred without cost.... Agriculture is generally agreed to be responsible for many of humanity's societal ills, including whole-scale warfare, starvation, tyranny, epidemic diseases, and class divisions."

Dr. Jared Diamond, evolutionary biologist, physiologist, Pulitzer Prize-winning professor of geography at UCLA, and author of *Guns, Germs and Steel*, goes so far as to say that agriculture was "the worst mistake in the history of the human race" and that "we're still struggling with the mess into which agriculture has tumbled us, and it's unclear whether we can solve it."

The flourishing of agriculture paralleled a reduction in average human life span, as well as body and brain size, increases in infant mortality and infectious diseases, and the occurrence of previously unknown conditions such as osteoporosis, bone mineral disorders, and malnutrition. As cultural and medical advancements have eliminated most of the rudimentary health risks faced by early humans (predator danger, minor infections turning fatal, etc.), we can now live long enough to develop, suffer, and die from diet-related diseases, including atherosclerosis, hypertension, and type 2 diabetes. (It used to be called *adult-onset diabetes* until millions of kids started developing it in recent years!)

> *The wise man sees in the misfortune of others*
> *what he should avoid.*
>
> —Marcus Aurelius

The Base of the Disease Pyramid

Grains offer the great majority of their calories in the form of carbohydrates, so they cause blood glucose levels to elevate quickly. As you already learned, high-carbohydrate foods such as sugar and grains (and, to a lesser extent, legumes) shock our delicate hormonal systems, which are better adapted to what today would be considered a low-carbohydrate, high-fat hunter-gatherer diet.

Please realize that you are mismanaging your *Homo sapiens* genes by consuming a high-carbohydrate diet, even when you take care to emphasize whole grains over refined grains or sugary foods. Yes, brown rice and lentil soup burn more slowly and have more nutrients than white bread or a candy bar, but all forms of carbohydrate are converted into glucose upon ingestion, and they stress the body's all-important insulin-regulation mechanism accordingly. After consuming that bagel, scone, muffin, French toast, or bowl of cereal (all derived from grains) and a glass of juice (full of sugar) for breakfast, your pancreas releases insulin into the bloodstream to help regulate blood glucose levels. Even after the routine meal just described, many Americans become temporarily diabetic by medical standards, with blood glucose levels soaring to clinically dangerous levels. You know the drill by now. After your meal, insulin is released into the bloodstream to promote the storage of glucose as muscle glycogen or direct its conversion to fat. Experience this often enough and you will gain weight and develop insulin resistance and Metabolic Syndrome.

If, instead, you were to have a Primal Blueprint breakfast consisting of a delicious cheese-and-vegetable omelet with some bacon and avocado, you would enjoy a moderated insulin response and high satiety, leading to balanced energy levels for hours after your meal instead of a sugar high and subsequent energy crash. Furthermore, with blood glucose levels balanced, you would be able to burn either energy from your food or from stored body fat until your next insulin-balanced meal.

Gluten, Lectin—Immune Affectin'

Certain proteins found in grains (and to a lesser extent in certain legumes and dairy products), known as *lectins*, can compromise gastro-intestinal and immune function by damaging the delicate brush borders that line your small intestine. Brush borders (named for their resemblance to paintbrush bristles; also known as *microvilli*) are where most of the nutrients from the food we eat are absorbed. They contain digestive enzymes that help break down carbohydrates, and they allow appropriate forms of nutrients (glucose, amino acids, fats, vitamins, and minerals) to be absorbed into the bloodstream from the intestine.

Lectin damage to brush borders allows larger, undigested protein molecules to infiltrate the bloodstream. The ever-vigilant immune system sees these unfamiliar protein molecules (not necessarily lectins, but anything you ingest that was supposed to be fully processed in the digestive tract

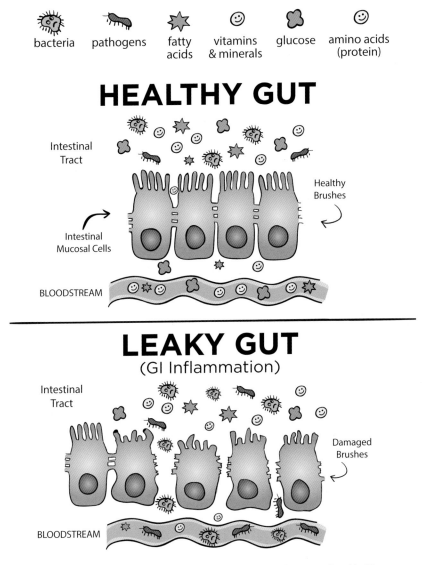

bacteria   pathogens   fatty acids   vitamins & minerals   glucose   amino acids (protein)

HEALTHY GUT

Intestinal Tract

Healthy Brushes

Intestinal Mucosal Cells

BLOODSTREAM

LEAKY GUT
(GI Inflammation)

Intestinal Tract

Damaged Brushes

BLOODSTREAM

Systemic Inflammation • Immune System Issues • Food Intolerances • Poor Health

Damaging the delicate intestinal lining with gluten and other lectins sets the stage for assorted autoimmune and inflammatory health conditions.

before entering the bloodstream) and sets up a typical immune response to deal with them. Unfortunately, these undigested protein molecules can resemble molecules that reside on the outside of healthy cells, including viruses and bacteria. The presence of lectins and other unwanted agents (you could technically classify this stuff as fecal matter!) in the bloodstream leaves your immune system confused as to whom the real enemy is. An autoimmune response (your immune system mistakenly attacking healthy cells) ensues, something experts believe is the root cause of many common diseases such as rheumatoid arthritis, lupus, Hashimoto's thyroiditis, multiple sclerosis, and a host of other conditions.

It should be clarified that certain types of lectins have health-boosting properties for immune function and cancer protection. The lectins discussed in context of this chapter should, according to Sarah Ballantyne, Ph.D., author of *The Paleo Approach*, be called "toxic lectins." The most notorious type of toxic lectin is gluten, a large, water-soluble protein that creates the elasticity in dough. Gluten is found in most common grains such as wheat, rye, and barley, and also to a lesser extent in legumes. Researchers now believe that as many as a third of us could be classified as gluten-intolerant or gluten-sensitive. The most sensitive folks will react to gluten with a perceptible inflammatory response—perhaps a disturbance in the digestive tract like bloating, a flare up of arthritis or skin conditions like acne, and long-term issues like dermatitis, acid reflux, reproductive problems like polycystic ovarian syndrome, assorted other autoimmune conditions, and celiac disease. Even if you aren't in the severely intolerant category, I and other evolutionary health experts contend that *all* of us are intolerant to gluten, even if it's at a subclinical level with no obvious symptoms.

It is very *au courant* in health circles to experiment with gluten-free diets. While I wholeheartedly support that trend, be aware that individuals who realize they are gluten intolerant and switch to a gluten-free diet that is still high in other grains, legumes, and dairy may not fare as well as someone who goes primal and eliminates or greatly restricts these foods. This is because unfamiliar proteins similar to gluten are present in other grain foods (e.g., barley has hordeum, rye has secalin, oats have avenin). Furthermore, with a gluten-free but still grain-heavy diet, you still suffer from the pro-inflammatory effects of excess insulin production, which will exacerbate the severity of your allergic response to lectins and gluten. In my own case, it was only when I ditched grains from my diet entirely that I noticed a complete disappearance of my daily minor digestive complaints and the mild but annoying arthritis in my hands. Many other primal converts similarly report improvements in a variety of physical symptoms and ailments after cutting out grains.

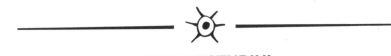

LECTIN LECTURIN'

Just how evil are lectins? This is currently a hot topic in paleo/primal circles because research shows that lectins are often destroyed in the processes of cooking and digestion. The degree to which lectins are problematic clearly varies widely by the individual, which is why strict restriction experiments (21 days minimally; ideally longer) are so important. I remain of the opinion that lectins are problematic for most, if not all, people on some level. I'm particularly concerned about those with mild subclinical inflammatory reactions to lectin ingestion. Without the noticeable adverse effects, there may not be sufficient motivation to consider eliminating them; but there could be a pretty wonderful upside to ditching grains and experiencing a breakthrough in general health that one didn't even know was possible!

If you love your breads and pastas and cereals and don't seem to notice any digestive or immune challenges related to consumption, you might want to consider the rationale that these foods have poor nutrient density in comparison to primal foods, and they contribute to the hyperinsulinemia (chronically excessive insulin production) that remains the most pressing health concern in the modern diet. Just for fun, since you have nothing to lose, consider a 21-day restriction period where you ditch all grains and take note of any changes to your baseline sense of health, immune function, energy levels, appetite, moods, and cognitive performance. It's quite possible that going grain-free (and getting insulin moderated accordingly) will give you a little bump in the aforementioned subjective evaluators. On the quantifiable side, you could run your bloodwork before a 21-day restriction period and then again after and expect to see improvements in blood glucose, triglycerides, and other important inflammatory and cardiac risk markers.

Phytates... to Abate

Whole grains contain high levels of phytic acid, or phytates. These are indigestible antioxidant compounds (also found in legumes, nuts, and seeds) that bind to important minerals such as iron, calcium, magnesium, and zinc in the digestive tract and make them more difficult to absorb. Phytates offer some health benefits (they have antioxidant—"phyto"— and anti-inflammatory properties) when consumed in moderation, but can lead to nutrient depletion when consumed in excess.

Mineral deficiencies are common in underdeveloped nations that depend almost entirely on grain for their sustenance. (Humans across the globe obtain an average of 48 percent of their calories from grains, according to Worldwatch.org; the most impoverished nations get up to 80 percent of total calories from grains.) Obviously, in countries with abundant access to nutrient-dense foods (even fast food hounds get some dosages of tomatoes and lettuce, apple pies have apples, etc.), widespread nutrient deficiencies are rare; but an overreliance on grains and legumes hinders the intake of additional nutritious foods and potentially delivers excessive phytates. This is particularly true for vegetarians who might consume proportionally more whole grains than do omnivores. It should be noted that cooking, soaking, sprouting, or fermenting grains (and legumes) reduces their phytic acid content considerably. However, enough phytates remain to bind to minerals and lead to nutrient depletion, especially when consumed regularly and in large quantities, as with the Standard American Diet.

Some experts believe that excessive phytate consumption from a grain-based diet, combined with other stressful modern lifestyle practices, is contributing to the high levels of osteoporosis in aging females. For example, the chronic overproduction of the stress hormone cortisol has a catabolic (breakdown) effect on the body, including the inhibition of calcium uptake in the skeleton. Dietary phytates also inhibit calcium absorption. This might explain why those with grain-based diets and high-stress lifestyles experience an increased risk of osteoporosis. Excess phytate intake also interferes with vitamin D metabolism and promotes related deficiencies of vitamins A, C, and B12.

We must emphasize the "excess" when talking about the health hazards of phytates. According to Chris Kresser, author of *Your Personal Paleo*

Code, humans can tolerate a moderate amount of phytic acid with no ill effects—around 100 mg to 400 mg per day. If you are eating primally, you will certainly ingest phytates in the nuts you consume, and that is nothing to worry about. Recent studies of the gut microbiome suggest that phytates can play a useful role in building a healthy intestinal tract. Overall, the health risks of phytates are much less of a concern than the health risks of lectins and gluten, which promote intestinal damage, systemic inflammation, compromised immune function, and digestive disturbances. They are simply one more reason why you are likely to benefit from removing grains from your diet.

Say Good-Bye to Fatigue, Illness, and Suffering

> *High insulin levels promote fat storage and disease. Moderated insulin levels (typical of Primal Blueprint eating) stimulate fat burning and good health. It's that simple.*

The single most important requirement to improve your fat metabolism and succeed with long-term weight management is to **reduce the total amount of insulin you produce**. High insulin levels promote fat storage and disease. Moderated insulin levels (typical of Primal Blueprint eating) stimulate fat burning and good health. It's that simple. At the risk of sounding overly dramatic, we must understand that the reasonable, "evolutionary" rationale that is challenging conventional wisdom about grains is going to battle against billions of dollars in corporate interests and government propaganda pushing us to conform to dietary habits that we are not suited for, that do not nourish us, and that are downright destructive to human health.

If you are one of the fortunate folks who are less sensitive to glutens, other lectins, and phytates than most, you might take exception to my wholesale damning of foods that are a dietary centerpiece across the globe. Perhaps you can try eliminating grains for 21 days and taking note of any general improvements in your health and wellbeing. I'll bet your energy will be more regulated after meals, your digestion and elimination will improve, symptoms of minor illnesses or inflammatory conditions will subside, and you will be more successful controlling your weight. And here is the bottom line: whether the results you experience are more subtle or are truly dramatic, there simply are no good reasons to base your diet on grains—and a lot of reasons never to eat most grains again.

> *More die in the United States of*
> *too much food than of too little.*
>
> —John Kenneth Galbraith

SUGAR

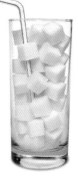

The great dangers and damages caused by excessive sugar consumption are widely accepted and publicized these days. When it comes to dropping excess body fat, even conventional wisdom is admitting that dietary sugar, not dietary fat, is what is making us fat. Science also confirms that sugar (and wheat, by the way) has addictive properties similar to those of hard drugs. You already learned how sugar drives excess insulin production/fat storage, causes cravings, and disturbs your appetite, satiety, and fat-storage hormones (locking you into a carbohydrate-dependency/fat-storage pattern), suppresses immune function, is pro-inflammatory, and causes oxidative damage to important cells and organs throughout the body. It also overstimulates the HPA axis (the fight or flight response), because an insulin-driven blood glucose dive is perceived as a stressful event by the body, prompting the release of cortisol to boost flagging energy levels. When this happens over and over again throughout the day, you get the chronic overproduction of stress hormones that leads to burnout.

Our genetic addiction to sweets is a survival mechanism. When our ancestors discovered sugar (typically during narrow ripening seasons for wild fruit), reward systems in the brain encouraged them to gorge on it and fatten up in preparation for the winter's diminished food supply. Today we don't really need to fatten up for winter, but we still have those same neurological reward pathways giving us pleasure for eating sugary foods. Furthermore, unlike our ancestors, thanks to the grain-based, processed-food-heavy, sugar-laden Standard American Diet, we have to work to *not* eat sugar… and we are destroying our health like at no other time in the history of humanity. (Note, in case my position on this isn't crystal clear: since all forms of carbs are quickly converted into glucose upon ingestion, a grain-based diet—even a whole grain-based diet—might as well be called a sugar-based diet.)

The problem with a sugar-based diet is that glucose molecules are toxic in the bloodstream. Blood-borne glucose molecules are literally "sticky," like the sugary or starchy foods from which they originate. Hence, they are prone to bind with important structural protein molecules throughout the body and generate reactive oxygen species (ROS—aka "free radicals" that contain oxygen molecules) in cells. The process of glucose molecules sticking to and damaging important structural proteins is called *glycation*.

Generally, glycation triggers an inflammatory process that eventually causes tissues to become stiff and inelastic. Consider the wrinkled skin commonly associated with aging (but greatly exacerbated by glycation), the oxidation and inflammation that lead to heart disease, neurodegenerative diseases such as Alzheimer's (senile plaques and neurofibrillary tangles reveal damage caused by glycation), and the frequency of kidney and vision problems among diabetics (who expose themselves to high blood glucose due to poor insulin regulating mechanisms). These examples highlight the fact that longer-lasting cells in the body are more susceptible to glycation damage: aorta (half-life = 100 years); elastin and collagen cells in your skin (half-life = 15 years); as well as pancreatic cells that control insulin release, brain cells, retinal cells, and renal (kidney) cells. Glycation also suppresses the internal production of antioxidants, leaving you more susceptible to free radical damage from exercise, stress, breathing polluted air, or simply living a busy life.

No discussion of sugar would be complete without mention of high fructose corn syrup (HFCS). Fructose has long been considered a superior sweetener to table sugar (sucrose), since it is the primary sugar in fruit and generates a lower insulin response than other types of sugar. (Fructose must be converted into glucose in the liver before it can be utilized in the bloodstream, thus muting both the glucose and insulin spikes.) Unfortunately, the fructose that sweetens most processed foods and beverages today—HFCS—is derived from corn, not fruit. This inexpensive and extremely sweet chemically processed agent is found in the vast majority of sodas, energy drinks, bottled teas and juices, baked goods, desserts, and snack foods.

Once you begin to read food labels, you will probably be shocked at how many products on grocery store shelves contain sugar, often in the form of HFCS. Industrial food is manufactured to be satisfying (in the short term) and addictive. Sweetened beverages are especially problematic because they have a lower satiety factor than solid foods, enabling the consumption of massive carbohydrate calories in a few Big Gulps (pun intended). One study even revealed that drinking sweetened beverages with meals led to a higher food intake, while another indicated that drinking liquid calories instead of solid causes hunger to occur more quickly in the future.

It has been well-established that HFCS is even more lipogenic (fat-promoting) than glucose, since it is readily converted into either glucose or triglycerides in the liver. Diets high in HFCS have been shown to substantially increase triglyceride levels, increase risk of obesity (particularly in kids, since their soda consumption is so excessive in relation to their body weight), and contribute to the development of serious health problems such as type 2 diabetes, Metabolic Syndrome, and non-alcoholic fatty liver disease (NAFLD).

Many health-conscious consumers believe that honey or agave nectar are superior alternatives. Unfortunately, honey has a similar effect on blood sugar levels as table sugar, while agave has a higher fructose concentration than even HFCS (and thus prompts undesirable triglyceride production). Plus, because they all contain fructose, honey, agave nectar, and HFCS will all be especially problematic for those individuals with fructose malabsorption. There's no free ride here!

Artificial sweeteners are to be strictly avoided also, not only due to the health risks of ingesting chemically processed substances, but because they trick the brain into thinking you have just consumed a very sweet food or drink. As a result, your confused hormone response system stimulates an inappropriate insulin release and the "high-low, high-low" cycle begins. Some research suggests that your brain will seek even more "replacement" calories in reaction to being tricked with a sweet food that provides no caloric energy. Supporting this theory are the ever-increasing obesity rates despite widespread use of non-caloric artificial sweeteners in beverages and other foods, which, absent any other variables, should predict a collective decrease in caloric intake and obesity.

All forms of natural and processed sugars and sweeteners have a deleterious effect on your insulin system and general health. The less you eat sweeteners of any kind (yes, even the somewhat less objectionable stevia), the less you will crave them. Try cutting way back on sweets and sodas for even a couple of days and notice how your energy level, appetite, mood, and concentration all regulate nicely. Be prepared—some people do initially experience symptoms like irritability, fatigue, low energy, and headaches if they are used to eating a high-sugar (including high-grain) diet; but once you come out on the other side, you will notice your sugar cravings are much diminished. See if you can maintain this sugar restriction for 21 days to begin to reprogram your genes to not need or want sugar. Although it can be hard at first, it becomes much easier as your body acclimates to its new diet and you begin to reap the rewards of a low-sugar lifestyle. If you can do away with sweet desserts altogether, you'll be well on your way to eliminating the addiction.

BAD OILS
Refined High Polyunsaturated Vegetable Oils

Conventional wisdom has for decades been unwisely steering people away from saturated fats in favor of widespread consumption of refined high polyunsaturated vegetable/seed oils like canola and others (corn, soybean, cottonseed, safflower, sunflower, peanut, etc.—read labels, they're everywhere!) that are easily oxidized and quickly go rancid (on the shelf and in your body!), particularly when heated during cooking. Oxidized vegetable oils have a pro-inflammatory effect on your system, leading directly to assorted health problems and a dis-

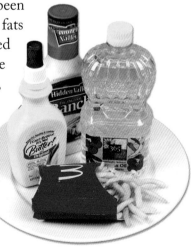

ruption in healthy immune and hormone function. Dr. Cate Shanahan, a prominent paleo-friendly family physician who wrote the acclaimed books *Deep Nutrition* and *Food Rules*, cites research saying that 40 percent of restaurant calories come from refined vegetable oils, since most meals and cooked in this sludge. Dr. Andrew Weil writes that, "Soybean oil alone is now so ubiquitous in fast foods and processed foods that an astounding 20 percent of the calories in the American diet are estimated to come from this single source."

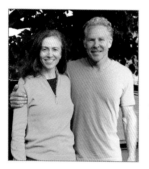

Dr. Cate Shanahan knows her stuff. She's one of the few primal/paleo experts with a hands-on influence in the mainstream medical world. When she says consuming vegetable oil is like getting dosed with radiation, it's time to pay attention—and toss every last offensive item in your home into the garbage immediately.

Ingestion of oxidized vegetable oils is especially destructive to the endocrine system, promoting symptoms such as compromised fat metabolism, diminished energy levels, and sluggish thyroid function. Heavy consumption of these refined oils in the modern diet is implicated as a leading contributor to insulin resistance, obesity, diabetes, heart disease, cancer, immune problems, arthritis, and other inflammatory conditions. Strictly avoid the following categories of refined vegetable oils, replacing them with the approved fats and oils discussed in the previous chapter.

Canola Oil: Canola oil is touted as great for cooking and eating due to its high monounsaturated fat content. Unfortunately, canola oil is a heavily refined, genetically engineered product derived from the rapeseed plant. This plant is believed to be toxic to humans and animals, and particularly harmful to respiratory

The rapeseed plant that canola oil is made from starts out looking pretty. The end result is free radicals and oxidative damage.

function. Most canola oil is put through a deodorizing process that converts some of its natural omega-3s into harmful trans fats. The popularity of canola oil today is a classic example of conventional wisdom taking facts (canola has a high monounsaturated fat content; monounsaturated fats are healthy) out of context or otherwise distorting them at the expense of our health.

Other High Polyunsaturated Vegetable and Seed Oils: These oils are popular in bottles—touted as cooking oils—and are also found in all manner of packaged, frozen, and restaurant foods. Most restaurants, from greasy fast food joints to fine steakhouses, are cooking your food in refined vegetable oil, most likely rancid due to reuse when making multiple batches of French fries, for example. Refined vegetable oils are highly sensitive to heat, light, and oxygen, and indeed can easily go rancid at room temperature, making them an especially poor choice for cooking.

Margarine: Margarine is comprised of offensive ingredients and processed with chemical additives at high temperatures. While most all margarines today have the "trans fat-free" distinction proudly adorning the label, they are almost always made from refined vegetable oils that are extremely unhealthy. Research strongly suggests an increased risk of cancer and heart disease from margarine use. The science is so compelling that even mainstream media has "rediscovered" the benefits of natural saturated fats like butter, and is finally criticizing the flawed thinking that led to the rise of refined polyunsaturated oils like margarine and imitation buttery spreads and sprays. An iconic *TIME* magazine cover from 2014 carried the simple headline: "Eat Butter."

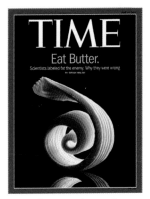

Headline and caption notably lacking in subtlety... it's about time.

Vegetable Shortening: Similar to lard in appearance but chemically produced to create a trans fat. The brand name Crisco is an acronym for "crystallized cottonseed oil." Bad stuff—stay away!

Partially Hydrogenated Trans Fats

Perhaps the most overtly offensive and dangerous elements of the modern diet are toxic chemically altered vegetable oils, commonly called partially hydrogenated fats or trans fats. These agents are created through a high-temperature chemical process that adds hydrogen atoms to mono- or polyunsaturated oils to make them more saturated than they were originally. This "transition" of their molecular makeup gives them the name "trans fats." This process is done to many packaged, processed, and frozen foods—at great expense to our collective health—mainly in order to improve shelf life, and also to alter the texture of food as desired for the end product.

To clarify, a partially hydrogenated oil is a trans fat, but there is another form of trans fat—CLA (conjugated linoleic acid), found in dairy products and grassfed animal products—that is not offensive to health. Naturally occurring CLA trans fats have a slightly different chemical makeup than industrially manufactured trans fats, and these differences distinguish naturally occurring, healthy CLA (made when an animal consumes polyunsaturated oils from grass and converts them during digestion in a process called biohydrogenation) from unhealthy industrially manufactured trans fats.

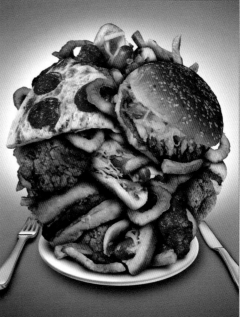

If you see the term "trans fats" bantered about to convey unhealthy oils, it's referencing the partially hydrogenated type of trans fats, not CLA fats. Likewise, the term "hydrogenated" on a food label mostly likely refers to the more common partially hydrogenated oil. Fully hydrogenated oils are actually less health-offensive than partially hydrogenated because they are rendered fully saturated and thus more resistant to becoming rancid and oxidized.

Partially hydrogenated trans fats are found in many leading-brand processed food products in the supermarket including frozen dinners; sweets and desserts; packaged snacks (e.g., crackers, chips, bars, and cookies); deep-fried foods; pastries and baked goods (e.g., donuts, croissants, and cupcakes); peanut butter; soups; and even grain products (e.g., bread, cereal, pasta, and rice mixes). A commonly cited estimate is that 40 percent of all products in a typical supermarket contain these evil fats. Fortunately, the dangers of chemically altered fats have become a hot topic in recent years; witness the highly publicized ban on these fats in New York City restaurants that began in 2007 and has been modeled elsewhere. Today, consumer awareness has helped liberate many processed food products of these offensive agents, but they are generally are still full of sugars, grains, preservatives, and other chemicals.

Partially hydrogenated trans fats are easily oxidized to form free radical chain reactions that damage cell membranes and tissues throughout the body. Because your brain, nervous system, and vascular system consist primarily of fat-based membranes, any dysfunction in these critical areas can be devastating. These fats are not recognized as foreign by the body, so they are incorporated into cell membranes and asked to function as natural fats. Of course, they don't function normally; they just take up space usually reserved for healthy fats and wreak havoc on cellular function. Many scientists consider the cell membrane to be the brain of the cell (as opposed to the more common assumption that the nucleus runs the show) because the membrane receives feedback from the outside environment (e.g., ingested nutrients such as glucose entering the bloodstream, the presence of a virus attacking healthy cells, or increased blood flow due to exercise stimulus) and takes consequent action (e.g., triggers the expression of certain genes or the release of certain hormones).

When you have cell membranes comprising natural molecules and you replace them with synthetic dysfunctional molecules, such as partially hydrogenated fats, the intricate signaling system is compromised. Plain and simple, the routine and prolonged ingestion of these toxic fats is a major contributor to the alarming increase in a variety of adverse health conditions and serious diseases of modern living. Many experts believe there is a direct connection between consuming processed foods and obesity (beyond their direct contribution to caloric excess), theorizing that insulin resistance could be exacerbated by dysfunctional fat molecules accumulating in cell membranes. Research also suggests that consumption of trans and partially hydrogenated fats is a direct instigator for inflammation, aging, and some cancers.

The New England Journal of Medicine reviewed numerous studies and reported a strong link between trans fat consumption and heart disease (including the strong tendency for trans fats to significantly raise LDL cholesterol levels and lower HDL levels). Scientists at the Harvard Medical School estimate that partially hydrogenated fats may be responsible for as many as 100,000 premature deaths each year in the United States. The United States Academy of Sciences says that there is "no safe level" of partially hydrogenated trans fat consumption in the American diet. The good news is that when you change your diet to eliminate these toxic agents, over time your cells will repair or replace these dysfunctional molecules with healthy ones.

Interesterified Fats

When partially hydrogenated trans fats started to become vilified, the food industry faced a big problem. These chemically altered fats play a major role in processed foods being shelf stable and having a pleasing texture. Luckily for processed food manufacturers—and unluckily for health-conscious consumers—another type of chemically altered fat has risen to take the place of partially hydrogenated trans fats. Known as interesterified fats, they are produced by chemically or enzymatically breaking the bonds of triglyceride molecules and then strategically reforming them to make blended, not-found-in-nature fat formulations.

Foods that are now proudly labeled "trans fat free" are instead being made with interesterified fats, which evidence suggests are no less dangerous—and in fact might be more dangerous. An increasing number of well-controlled scientific studies show that consuming interesterified fats raises LDL, decreases HDL, and increases levels of blood triglycerides at levels equal to or greater than the effects of consuming trans fats. One small study also found that people who consumed interesterified fats had 40-percent-higher levels of post-meal blood glucose than they did after eating meals containing more trans fats. Emerging research also demonstrates that interesterified fats are pro-inflammatory.

While there isn't nearly as much research on interesterified fats as there is on trans fats, because they are a newer addition to the food supply, researchers have already raised enough alarming red flags that I strongly advise avoiding foods with interesterified fats. Unfortunately, the FDA does not require food manufacturers to label them. The best way to avoid these dangerous fats, of course, is to avoid eating processed packaged foods. The next best option is to carefully read labels and look for key words like *high stearate* or *stearate rich* instead. Note that these are different than *stearic acid*, which is a naturally occurring fatty acid found in many foods. Stearic acid is used in to manufacture interesterified fats, but it is not itself dangerous.

OTHER FOODS TO AVOID
Grains... Oh, Did I Already Mention Them?

Wheat, corn, rice, oats, barley, millet, rye, breakfast cereals, pastas, breads, pancakes, rolls, crackers, pastries, cupcakes, and the like. I consumed grains with reckless abandon as a major percentage of my dietary calories for some 40 years. It wasn't until I completely eliminated grains from my diet that my nagging, lifelong digestive and inflammatory issues completely disappeared. I've met very few people who consume a grain-based diet and also claim to enjoy ideal weight, experience perfectly satisfactory and steady energy levels, and never feel digestive distress.

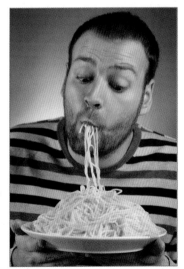

Whatever your perceived sensitivity level, or lack of sensitivity, to grains, it's worth completing the aforementioned 21-day exclusion period to get a glimpse of a potential upside from eliminating grains from your diet. Chances are, even if you are at a decent launching point now, you will experience a noticeable stabilization of daily energy levels, mood, concentration, and appetite, along with improved immune function and a reduction in minor

Ah, imagine what life would be like without pasta! Or instead of imagining, just live life without pasta and feel the difference!

digestive distress. The degree to which grains are tolerated definitely varies on a person-by-person basis (although I contend that they are toxic on some level for all people); but you owe it to yourself to figure out where you are on the spectrum and to see how great you can feel when you fill your plate with primal foods that are nourishing and are guaranteed not to be secretly wreaking havoc on your body.

Legumes

Alfalfa, beans, lentils, peanuts, peas, and soy products are classified as legumes. While legumes can serve as a decent source of protein, fiber, potassium, and antioxidants, they also provide significant levels of carbohydrate and those pesky anti-nutrient lectins. As *Paleo Diet* author Dr. Loren Cordain explains, "Most legumes in their mature state are non-digestible and/or toxic to most mammals, even when eaten in moderate quantities." The fact that legumes need to be altered for human consumption through cooking, soaking, or fermenting should be a good clue that they don't need to be centerpieces of the diet, and that folks with poor gut health or heightened sensitivity to lectins ought to avoid them. And to tiptoe into a sensitive subject, the beans that are consumed liberally by many world cultures (kidney, pinto, black beans, lentils) come with the annoying byproduct of flatulence caused by the fermentation of indigestible carbohydrates in the gut.

While soy has achieved great popularity as a healthy alternative to meat, unfermented soy products contain compounds that may interfere with thyroid hormone production and have a demonstrated estrogenic (feminizing) effect in certain tissue. Some soy products have decent nutritional value, and certain fermented products may be less objectionable (tempeh, natto, etc.). However, they should still be consumed judiciously.

Overall, legumes are far less offensive than grains (lower anti-nutrient levels, better nutritional value), but due to their high carbohydrate

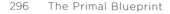

content and potential to compromise gut health, they can be classified as "unnecessary" by Primal Blueprint standards. If you enjoy ideal body fat levels and have a need for supplemental carbohydrates to replenish regularly depleted muscle glycogen, legumes may be just fine. If you are looking to maximize the nutritional value of your diet, reduce excess body fat, and ensure optimal gut health, it's probably best to make an effort to minimize your intake of legumes.

I understand that many people have a strong affinity for legumes and that legumes enjoy a reputation as a healthful food category, particularly among vegetarians who otherwise have limited protein options. It will not be a disaster if you occasionally dip your vegetables in hummus at a dinner party, fry some tempeh with vegetables for a main course, or enjoy side dishes of peas, lentils, or steamed beans. (Consider eating your beans cold for a serving of resistant starches, prebiotics that feed beneficial gut flora.) However, emphasizing legumes in your diet is an inferior strategy to having vegetables, fruits, nuts and seeds, and animal foods as your primary meal and snack choices.

Finally, a cautionary word on the ever-popular peanut. Peanut butter is a staple of most Americans' diets, but unfortunately the peanut is probably the most health-compromising legume. Research suggests that the lectin found in peanuts—agglutinin—is particularly resistant to breakdown by heat or digestion, making it is more likely than other lectins to reach the small intestine intact and do damage. Furthermore, peanuts can be contaminated with a fungal toxin known as aflotoxin, which is linked to a variety of health problems, including liver cancer. Thus, I advise you to eschew peanuts and peanut butter in favor of actual nuts and nut butters that are more nutritious and delicious without the potential toxic effects.

Processed Foods

Anything with chemical additives or that's been heavily altered from its natural state requires little discussion. Realize that you have been pummeled with marketing messages your entire life that entice you to consume branded, boxed "edible foodlike substances"—as *Food Rules* author Michael Pollan likes to say. This has contributed directly and tragically to obesity, illness, and death in your family and community. Knowing what

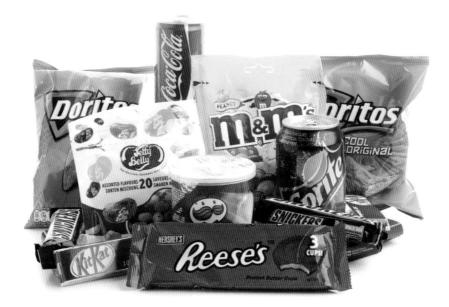

our ancestors didn't eat is perhaps more important than knowing what they did: Grok never touched refined sugar, refined high polyunsaturated vegetable oils, processed foods, or anything with hormones, pesticides, antibiotics, herbicides, fungicides, preservatives, or other chemicals. I might include grains and legumes on this list, too.

BUT SOMEBODY TOLD ME CAVEMEN DID EAT PIZZA!

Evidence exists that certain human populations during hunter-gatherer times consumed wild grains or legumes in small amounts. Amazingly, this aside to the evolutionary story—that prehistoric humans did eat some grains here and there—has been used to challenge the entire premise of the Paleolithic diet. I hear critics say things like "Our ancestors ate whatever they could to survive, and there's proof this included grains!" and then extrapolate that we have a free pass to eat grains with the wild abandon that we do today. Obviously, grains were an insignificant element of the hunter-gatherer diet and the evolution-

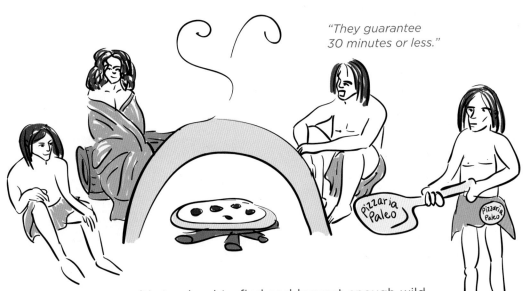

"They guarantee 30 minutes or less."

ary process; it's too hard to find and harvest enough wild grains to account for significant caloric or nutritional intake in comparison to the most prominent hunter-gatherer food sources. Yes, humans are able to consume and digest grains and legumes to ward off starvation (and survive long enough to hunt and gather more nutritious food). Likewise, we can also consume soda, M&M's, and potato chips and obtain some caloric energy to burn for a busy day at the office, but that doesn't mean we are designed to thrive on these foods.

Alcohol

Primal Blueprint veterans know that alcohol was previously categorized as a "sensible indulgence" in Chapter 3 of the original *Primal Blueprint* book, right along with dark chocolate. I lauded red wine as the best alcohol choice for its antioxidant benefits, and expressed my enthusiasm (in the book and also occasionally on MarksDailyApple.com over the years) for enjoying a glass or two of fine red wine with dinner and during evening leisure time. Granted, I also offered pretty strong caveats that alcohol consumption can really mess up weight-loss goals, and furthermore

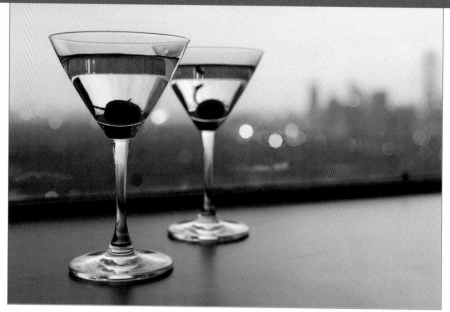

that irresponsible drinking can increase the risk of cancer, auto accidents, divorces, bar fights, and other folly. Even so, it seems like the prevailing vibe I've been giving off is that the Primal Blueprint gives carte blanche to alcohol consumption.

At the nine PrimalCon weekend retreats we conducted all over North America from 2010-2014, we featured a red wine and chocolate evening party to cut loose after the busy, active daily agenda. At these and other paleo social gatherings I've attended over the years, I noticed that many individuals have loose and varying interpretations of the word "moderation" when it comes to alcohol consumption, if you get my drift. After seven years of reflection, research, feedback from primal enthusiasts, and some self-experimentation, I've decided to present a significantly more sobering message about alcohol… so here it is repositioned in the "Avoid Poisonous Things" chapter! After all, we mustn't forget that alcohol literally is a poison. Oh, and wine's antioxidant and flavonoid benefits come from the grapes, not the alcohol; I understand you can obtain grapes from elsewhere than a wine bottle.

Regarding weight management, alcohol calories (which have zero nutritional value) are known as the "first to burn," meaning you will process ingested alcohol calories first and inhibit the burning of other fuels until the alcohol has been metabolized. The "buzz" sensation comes from alcohol's immediate effect on the brain and other tissues. Then, since alcohol is a toxin, the body works quickly to metabolize the alcohol through oxidation. This detoxifies and removes the alcohol from the bloodstream before it damages organs and tissues.

Alcohol contains seven calories per gram in the form of ethanol, which is classified as another form of energy next to carbohydrate, protein, and fat. When alcohol is ingested, an insignificant amount is converted in the liver into fat, and the rest is converted into acetate. Acetate is then released into the bloodstream and burned for immediate energy. When alcohol is consumed in conjunction with carbohydrates, such as in mixed drinks like daiquiris or margaritas, carbohydrate metabolism is put on hold while the alcohol calories are burned first. When carbohydrate metabolism is compromised in this manner, the ingested carbs—and also any fat you might ingest along with the carbs—are more likely to be converted into triglycerides in the liver. Therefore, alcohol earns the distinction of being "lipogenic" (fat-forming) although not in the way that many people mistakenly believe, which is that alcohol calories are somehow converted into sugar, or converted into fat, by the body.

As the "first to burn" calorie source, alcohol inhibits fat metabolism, makes carbs more likely to be converted into fat, and can stimulate increases in appetite.

Alcohol is also believed to partially inhibit gluconeogenesis, which can result in declines in blood glucose and consequent cravings for sugar in conjunction with alcohol consumption. According to Enoch Gordis, M.D., Director of the National Institute on Alcohol Abuse and Alcoholism (NIAAA), the stupor commonly associated with drunks could often be more due to hypoglycemia (low blood glucose) than to the effects of alcohol. A pattern of frequent alcohol consumption can also result in decreased insulin sensitivity and elevated levels of the key appetite-stimulating hormone ghrelin. Yep, getting the munchies in correlation with alcohol intake is validated by science!

Alcohol can have a pro-inflammatory effect on digestive organs, disrupting healthy digestion and nutrient assimilation. It may promote leaky

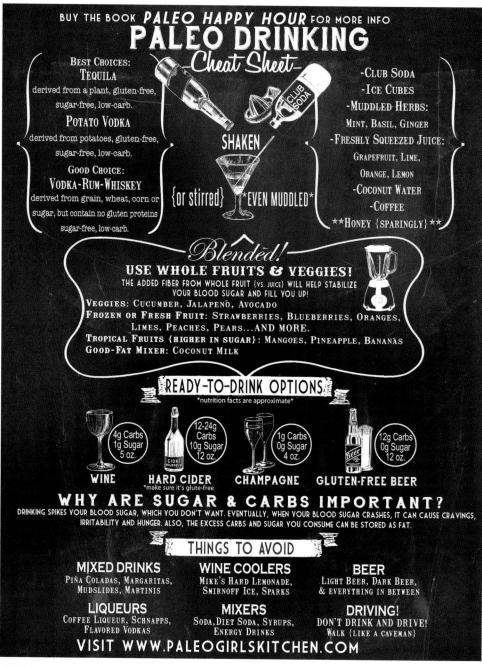

BUY THE BOOK *PALEO HAPPY HOUR* FOR MORE INFO

PALEO DRINKING
Cheat Sheet

BEST CHOICES:
TEQUILA
derived from a plant, gluten-free,
sugar-free, low-carb.

POTATO VODKA
derived from potatoes, gluten-free,
sugar-free, low-carb.

GOOD CHOICE:
VODKA-RUM-WHISKEY
derived from grain, wheat, corn or
sugar, but contain no gluten proteins
sugar-free, low-carb.

SHAKEN

{or stirred} *EVEN MUDDLED*

-CLUB SODA
-ICE CUBES
-MUDDLED HERBS:
MINT, BASIL, GINGER
-FRESHLY SQUEEZED JUICE:
GRAPEFRUIT, LIME,
ORANGE, LEMON
-COCONUT WATER
-COFFEE
HONEY {SPARINGLY}

Blended!
USE WHOLE FRUITS & VEGGIES!
THE ADDED FIBER FROM WHOLE FRUIT {VS. JUICE} WILL HELP STABILIZE
YOUR BLOOD SUGAR AND FILL YOU UP!

VEGGIES: CUCUMBER, JALAPEÑO, AVOCADO
FROZEN OR FRESH FRUIT: STRAWBERRIES, BLUEBERRIES, ORANGES,
LIMES, PEACHES, PEARS...AND MORE.
TROPICAL FRUITS {HIGHER IN SUGAR}: MANGOES, PINEAPPLE, BANANAS
GOOD-FAT MIXER: COCONUT MILK

READY-TO-DRINK OPTIONS
nutrition facts are approximate

4g Carbs 1g Sugar 5 oz.	12-24g Carbs 10g Sugar 12 oz.	1g Carbs 0g Sugar 4 oz.	12g Carbs 0g Sugar 12 oz.

WINE   **HARD CIDER** *make sure it's glute-free*   **CHAMPAGNE**   **GLUTEN-FREE BEER**

WHY ARE SUGAR & CARBS IMPORTANT?
DRINKING SPIKES YOUR BLOOD SUGAR, WHICH YOU DON'T WANT. EVENTUALLY, WHEN YOUR BLOOD SUGAR CRASHES, IT CAN CAUSE CRAVINGS,
IRRITABILITY AND HUNGER. ALSO, THE EXCESS CARBS AND SUGAR YOU CONSUME CAN BE STORED AS FAT.

THINGS TO AVOID

MIXED DRINKS
PIÑA COLADAS, MARGARITAS,
MUDSLIDES, MARTINIS

WINE COOLERS
MIKE'S HARD LEMONADE,
SMIRNOFF ICE, SPARKS

BEER
LIGHT BEER, DARK BEER,
& EVERYTHING IN BETWEEN

LIQUEURS
COFFEE LIQUEUR, SCHNAPPS,
FLAVORED VODKAS

MIXERS
SODA, DIET SODA, SYRUPS,
ENERGY DRINKS

DRIVING!
DON'T DRINK AND DRIVE!
WALK {LIKE A CAVEMAN}

VISIT WWW.PALEOGIRLSKITCHEN.COM

*A little selectivity with your alcohol consumption can help mitigate many of the negative effects, especially if you are sensitive to leaky gut issues or concerns about managing body composition. The infographic from the book **Paleo Happy Hour** is a big help!*

gut syndrome in sensitive individuals by altering the gene expression of the protein molecules involved in the formation of the all-important "tight junctions" in the intestines. Furthermore, it can deplete zinc, a crucial nutrient for healthy intestinal function. Alcohol can also affect body composition by altering the healthy balance of sex hormones in both males and females. Alcohol is known to be directly toxic to the testes, lowering testosterone levels in males. Frequent consumption can disturb hormone functions in the hypothalamus and pituitary glands, damage sperm, and compromise fertility. In premenopausal females, frequent alcohol consumption can cause an assortment of reproductive problems, including abnormal menstrual cycles, delayed ovulation, and infertility. These negative effects are more strongly associated with alcoholism, but reproductive issues can also occur in "social drinkers."

Alcohol can also compromise athletes' peak performance and recovery in assorted ways. It can mess with your deep sleep cycles and the critical hormonal processes (especially the release of human growth hormone during deep sleep) that repair and rejuvenate your body for the next day. All-time triathlon great and current coach Mark Allen culled alcohol research applicable to athletes and reports that alcohol metabolism preoccupies the liver, hindering the liver's crucial role in processing nutrients for performance and recovery (including interfering with testosterone production); it interferes with water balance in cells, which hampers ATP production; and it compromises your ability to perform in the heat.

Back to what's often the primary concern of lifestyle change—losing excess body fat: alcohol ingestion detracts from fat-loss goals by contributing empty calories (that you will burn before tapping into stored body fat), interfering with other ingested calories (promoting the conversion of ingested carbs into fat), and increasing appetite. These effects are significant even with what's commonly considered to be "moderate" drinking, such as one or two glasses of wine or one or two beers daily. And believe me, we hear from many primal-aligned eaters who are frustrated with lack of fat reduction but cop to a significant amount of daily alcohol consumption. If you insist upon consuming alcohol and want to do the least damage to your fat-loss goals, consume it alone, in a sensible and moderate manner (I meant "alone" without other calories, silly).

If you decide to drink alcohol, consider navigating to the least objectionable options. Red wine by itself (without a side order of carbs) is a sensible choice. The antioxidants and flavonoids in red wine help counter the oxidation of small, dense LDL cholesterol that characterizes cardiovascular disease. However, recent research suggests that the highly touted benefits of the antioxidant found in red wine, grapes, some berries, dark chocolate, and specialized sup-

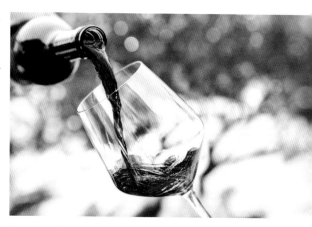

I now enjoy a glass of naturally produced red wine perhaps once or twice a month instead of my more habitual evening consumption prior to 2014.

plements might be exaggerated. A study published by Johns Hopkins on citizens of European countries with high wine consumption found no correlation with disease protection or longevity. While there is no doubt that consuming antioxidant-rich foods offer health benefits, it may not be a worthwhile rationalization for enthusiastic alcohol consumption.

The recent advent of so-called organic/naturally produced/"paleo" wines offers some interesting drink for thought because their less-offensive production methods may mitigate of some of the adverse health effects of alcohol consumption, from hangovers to leaky gut irritation. As with the industrialized production of grains, modern wine production techniques result in an end product quite disparate from the simple, organic fermented grape juice wines that our ancestors enjoyed. Today's industrialized wines are higher in alcohol content, sugar content, and also filled with chemicals and additives to improve texture, color, and flavor. The FDA has approved 76 chemicals and additives for use in winemaking. Conventionally produced wines also often contain fungicides, mycotoxins, and phthalates. Yep, this is true even for expensive wines. Furthermore, the only governmental requirement for wine labels is to list the percentage of alcohol content.

It's very likely that in sensitive people, the industrialized production methods and resultant extra stuff in your wine can be a significant contributor to negatives like headaches, sleep disturbances, and leaky gut symptoms reported by sensitive drinkers. Could it be that it's not the alcohol in the wine per se that's giving you the hangover, but the chemicals? It's worth trying a naturally produced wine and determining for yourself. Todd White, proprietor of Dry Farm Wines, produces products that contain only grapes and the wild yeasts that live on the grapes themselves. There is great momentum toward natural wines in Europe, but America is lagging behind a bit. You can visit dryfarmwines.com and learn more about wines produced organically, without irrigation (which increases yield and sugar content of the wine, but dilutes the quality and washes away nutrients).

Tequila is also primal friendly, since it's derived from a plant and free from gluten and sugar. Beer is less advised because it is made from gluten-containing grains, and anyone sensitive to gluten may have negative reactions to most beers. (There are an increasing number of gluten-free beers coming to market now, but that won't necessarily help those who are sensitive to other components of grains.) Other alcoholic beverages that are less offensive for leaky gut and fat-loss goals are the hard liquors such as vodka, rum, and whiskey, hard cider, potato vodka (yep, made from potatoes and thereby gluten-free), and champagne.

RETHINKING ALCOHOL IN MY LIFE
—HOW ABOUT YOURS?

While the glass or two of red wine I'd enjoy with dinner most every day for years was an enjoyable and comfortable ritual, I started to get the sense that even my moderate consumption might be compromising my sleep. Oh, I would fall asleep easily—almost "pass out"—at 9:30 or 10:00 P.M., but I would commonly awaken at 2:00 or 3:00 A.M. My mind would start racing, I'd notice a slightly elevated heartbeat, and it could take an hour to fall back asleep. I never awoke with anything like a hangover, but I had a sense that the effects of the alcohol—especially because I was metabolizing at rest instead of while moving around being active—might be interfering with my efficient cycling through the phases of sleep, from light REM cycles to the deepest restorative cycles.

As you learned from my distressing health history eating a grain-based diet, I have a very sensitive digestive tract, with an increased susceptibility toward intestinal permeability—aka leaky gut syndrome. The anti-nutrients in whole grains are the worst offenders here, but sensitive folks can also experience an inflammatory autoimmune response to legumes, casein proteins in dairy, and even alcohol. Research is clear that drinking enough to get you to .08 blood alcohol (four to five drinks in one hour for most) allows endotoxins to leak into the bloodstream and generate a rapid inflammatory response. Other research shows that even moderate wine consumption (one to three glasses per day) aggravates leaky gut in sensitive patients and can result in small intestinal bacterial overgrowth (SIBO), a common cause of bloating, gas, intestinal pain, diarrhea and constipation.

In 2014, I decided to experiment with a 45-day abstention from alcohol. I immediately noticed an improvement in my sleep cycles and a complete resolution of my occasional gut issues. Furthermore, if I challenged my gut with, say, a bite or two of bread dunked in olive oil at a restaurant, or fish tacos with corn tortillas now and then, or even an occasional alcoholic drink, I was much more resilient against the familiar digestive distress of my past. You may not have the sensitivities that I do, but we must admit that alcohol is one of those areas where it's easy to overindulge without noticing (or not have a reference point of total sobriety to which you can compare your sleep, muscle recovery, or digestive function).

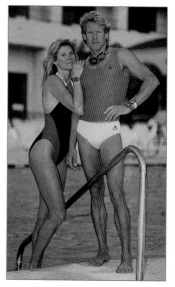

Hanging out at a "bar" with Carrie! (circa neon-teen ninety)

I don't want to discourage you from enjoying your life, and we all realize what a central role alcohol plays in modern culture and social interaction. After all, if it weren't for alcohol, I never would have met my wife Carrie. Just kidding—we met at the SportsClub LA fitness center, but I think you get the point: the Primal Blueprint doesn't need to be handing out free passes for alcohol consumption. And furthermore, I trust you will make responsible decisions in all areas of life (more on that with Law #8—Avoid Stupid Mistakes), including alcohol consumption.

Well, you just absorbed a pretty heavy hit here on the subject of alcohol! As I've pledged throughout the book, I want to stand first and foremost for enjoying life and communicating a refreshing alternative to the pain, suffering, and sacrifice that we've long associated with getting and staying lean, fit, and healthy. Furthermore, my strategy is to arm you with the information and tools to make sensible, health-promoting decisions and to understand the consequences of your lifestyle decisions. This is different from taking a "my way or the highway" angle or using a shaming approach (as seen on TV!) to get you to toe the line.

So, if you are a connoisseur of wine or fine tequila and greatly enjoy this element of your life within sensible parameters, I toast you. If you like Sunday afternoons of beer and football on the coach, we can still be friends and you can keep your primal card. Since alcohol is such a centerpiece of social gatherings, the idea here might be to reflect on whether you really require alcohol to have a good time, or are you perhaps just bowing to prevailing cultural norms without sufficient reflection? It seems a significant percentage of alcohol consumption is driven by peer influence, the need to slide smoothly into a social situation, fit in, and collectively loosen up. Rest assured, ethanol is not mandatory to achieve this. Brad Kearns, my Primal Blueprint Publishing sidekick and *Primal Endurance* co-author, explains that among the reasons he is a non-drinker is because, "I'm already weird and loosened up at parties."

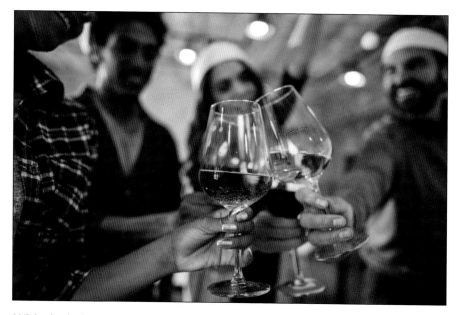

With alcohol as a cultural centerpiece, it's easy to default to drinking automatically per social cues. Primal enthusiasts looking to drop excess body fat and optimize health might benefit from deeper reflection on their alcohol consumption habits.

If you take away the social and cultural noise and reflect on your ultimate goal of living a happy, healthy life, maybe you will land in a perfectly optimal consumption pattern of two glasses a week or teetotaling so people can enjoy the real you at gatherings, or whatever. Just like with your diet and exercise habits, an intuitive and mindful (instead of robotic) approach can be highly effective here. And on that note, remember that having some self-compassion is important here. Using alcohol to unwind from stress might not get as high a score as a meditation session, but go ahead and do what you gotta do today and reflect on the payoff (or perhaps lack of payoff) you get from your behavior. Similarly, if you overdo it on rare occasions (or less than rare occasions), reflect on your behaviors with an open heart and compassion. Instead of beating yourself up and allowing downward spirals to happen (not just with alcohol but with whatever else), resolve to do your best and strive to make continual progress, even through small steps, to engage in lifestyle behaviors that promote optimal gene expression.

CHAPTER SUMMARY

In modern life, poisonous things come in wrappers, bottles, or boxes and compromise health insidiously over decades. Make a sincere effort to reject the powerful manipulative forces of corporate advertising and social influences pushing you in the direction of poor food choices, and cultural norms favoring unhealthy dietary habits. The big three foods to avoid are sugars, grains, and processed high polyunsaturated vegetable/seed oils. These modern toxins stimulate excess insulin production, promote a carbohydrate-dependency/fat-storage pattern, are pro-inflammatory, cause oxidative damage, suppress immune function, and are nutritionally inferior to plants and animals.

1. Grains: While grains (wheat, rice, bread, pasta, cereal, corn, etc.) have been presented as healthy staple foods for thousands of years of civilization, our genes are maladapted to ingesting them. They promote wildly excessive insulin production in comparison to a hunter-gatherer diet, leading to difficulty burning stored body fat (and hence lifelong weight gain) and serious long-term health problems, including heart disease and diet-related cancers.

In addition to stimulating excess insulin, grains offer minimal nutritional value in comparison to primal foods. Objectionable compounds in grains compromise health mildly to severely, depending on your sensitivity. Lectin proteins, particularly gluten, can promote intestinal permeability (leaky gut), leading to or exacerbating assorted autoimmune and inflammatory conditions. When consumed in excess as with a grain-based diet, phytates can inhibit the absorption of minerals. The whole grains that are lauded for superior nutritional value and lower glycemic response than refined grains are still vastly inferior to primal foods and also stimulate excessive insulin, inflammation, and fat storage. Furthermore, whole grains have higher levels of anti-nutrients than refined grains, potentially exacerbating the aforementioned conditions. Even individuals who are not highly sensitive to gut-disturbing properties of grains are much better served nutritionally and health-wise by comprising their diets of delicious primal-approved options.

2. Sugar: Sugar drives excess insulin production/fat storage; disturbs your appetite, satiety, and fat-storage hormones (locking you into a carbohydrate-dependency/fat-storage pattern); suppresses immune function; is pro-inflammatory; causes oxidative damage to important cells and organs throughout the body; and overstimulates the fight or flight response. Furthermore, sugar has addictive properties, making it difficult to transition sugar out of the diet.

Glycation is the process of glucose molecules binding to and damaging important structural proteins in cells throughout the body, especially the longer-lasting cells (cardiac, skin, retinal, kidney, pancreas, brain). Sweetened beverages are particularly problematic, because they have a lower satiety factor than solid foods, making it easy to ingest massive amounts of sugar. High fructose corn syrup (HFCS) is a heavily processed sweetener that is more easily converted into fat (lipogenic) than other sugars. Artificial sweeteners still stimulate an insulin release and additional cravings for sugar. "Natural" sweeteners such as honey, agave nectar, and maple syrup are not processed to the same degree as HFCS, to be sure, but they too have the same insulin-promoting effect and all the baggage that comes with that.

3. Refined High Polyunsaturated Vegetable/Seed Oils: In recent decades, we have unwisely transitioned from saturated animal fats to refined vegetable/seed oils. Unlike more temperature stable saturated fats, high polyunsaturated vegetable/seed oils undergo oxidative damage during their processing and are vulnerable to further oxidative damage when heated during cooking. Oxidized pro-inflammatory vegetable/seed oils directly disturb healthy cellular, immune, endocrine, and hormone function. Dr. Cate Shanahan says they are "no different than eating radiation." Strict avoidance of canola oil and other vegetable and seed oils, margarine, and vegetable shortening is critical to health.

Partially hydrogenated trans fats and interesterified fats are chemically altered molecules found inheavily processed foods are highly toxic to the body and are a major contributor to inflammation, accelerated aging, and many cancers. They promote rampant oxidation and free radical damage in the body and disturb the healthy composition and function of cell membranes. Consuming these fats has also been linked to a number of cardiovascular disease risk factors. Interesterified fats are another form of chemically altered fats that are just as objectionable as trans fats, but unfortunately don't require FDA labeling and can confuse consumers accordingly.

5. Other Foods: Legumes have superior nutritional value and fewer anti-nutrient concerns compared to grains, but they still stimulate excess insulin production and can cause problems for those with lectin sensitivity. They are deemed "unnecessary" in the Primal Blueprint picture because, like grains, they displace other healthier options from your diet.

Heavily processed "edible foodlike substances" are typically made from grains and sugars—zero nutrition, major health objections. Be a conscientious consumer of processed packaged foods; always read labels carefully for hidden sugars and dangerous fats that will often be disguised under oblique names.

Alcohol, originally categorized by Primal Blueprint as a "sensible indulgence," has been repositioned as the "poisonous thing" that it is. While little elaboration is necessary on the dangers of irresponsible alcohol consumption, even moderate alcohol consumption can disrupt fat-reduction efforts (it's the "first to burn"), promote leaky gut and related autoimmune conditions, and also hamper sleep, recovery, and sex hormone synthesis.

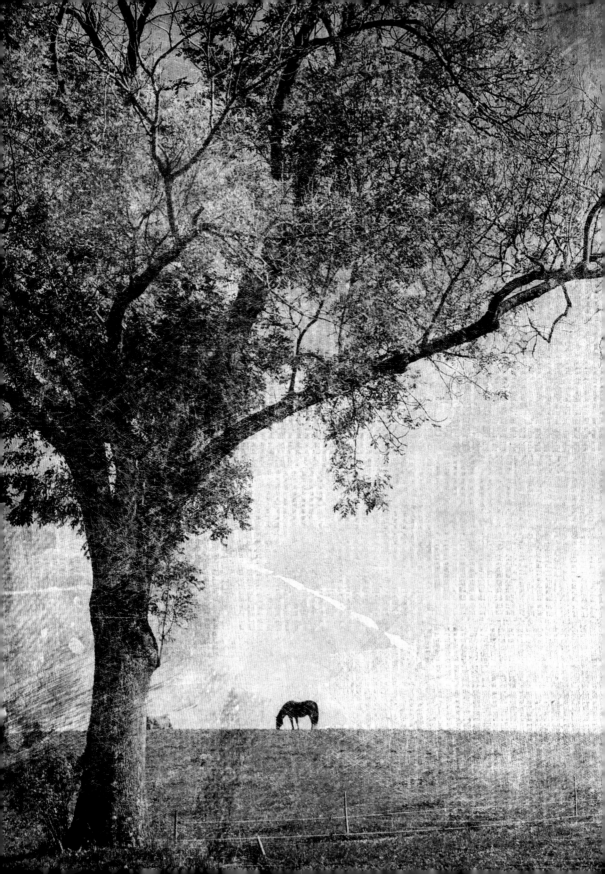

CHAPTER SEVEN

THE PRIMAL BLUEPRINT EXERCISE LAWS

Move, Lift, and Sprint
for Functional, Full-Body Fitness

IN THIS CHAPTER

I detail the rationale behind and the benefits of the three Primal Blueprint exercise laws: Law #3, Move Frequently; Law #4, Lift Heavy Things; and Law #5, Sprint Once in a While. Following these laws will enable you to approximate Grok's active lifestyle and develop a broad and highly functional state of fitness. Primal Blueprint Fitness develops a versatile and diverse set of abilities that allow you to enjoy an active, high-energy lifestyle and to tackle varied athletic challenges safely and competently. The Primal Blueprint exercise laws will also help delay the aging process by preserving lean muscle mass, which correlates with enhanced organ function, a concept known as *organ reserve*.

I contrast the benefits of Primal Blueprint Fitness with the many drawbacks and health risks associated with conventional wisdom's fitness recommendations and with the narrow, specialized athletic goals that many people pursue but that are minimally functional and often compromise general health. (Endurance athletes and bodybuilders often fall in this category.) A chronic pattern of slightly-too-difficult workouts promotes carbohydrate dependency, compromises weight-loss efforts, hampers immune and endocrine function, and even elevates disease risks.

Moving more during daily life is a critical, but it's an often-overlooked element of a total fitness routine. Even fit folks can suffer from the "active couch potato syndrome," where excessive periods of inactivity (commute, work, digital leisure time) can overwhelm the benefits of regular workouts. Furthermore, there are assorted flexibility/mobility practices like Pilates, tai chi, and yoga, as well as properly conducted stretching exercises, that enhance health, reduce injury risk, and complement focused fitness and athletic goals.

Lifting heavy things entails conducting brief, intense sessions (lasting just 10 to 30 minutes) that build explosive strength, promote the release of anti-aging hormones, and avoid the catabolic effects of prolonged sessions that leave you exhausted and depleted. And few things are more primal than Law #5—run for your life once in a while! Brief, intense sprints (on foot, or other maximum efforts that are low or no impact, such as on the bike or in the pool) trigger optimal hormone balance, lean muscle development, accelerated fat metabolism, and incredible fitness breakthroughs.

I discuss the best strategic approach for conducting workouts for each of the three Primal Blueprint laws, including pointers on form for running and cycling. I also describe the benefits of going barefoot. Specific workout suggestions for strength training and sprinting are provided in the Bonus Material at the end of this book and online at MarksDailyApple.com, including a free downloadable ebook called *Primal Blueprint Fitness*.

*Those who think they have not time for bodily exercise
will sooner or later have to find time for illness.*

—Lord Edward Stanley
Three-time United Kingdom Prime Minister
(1799-1869)

T he movements that dictated how our genes evolved were simple: squat, crawl, walk, run, jump, climb, hang, carry, throw,
push, pull, a bunch of other actions we probably don't even
have names for, and most of all just moving, plain and simple.
This primal "training program" helped Grok survive the rigors of a hostile environment, explore new territories, track and hunt, find and exploit
new types of food, build shelters, and basically become exceptionally fit,
even ripped, by today's standards.

Becoming super fit is as simple as blending lots of low-level movement (cardiovascular activity through both structured aerobic workouts and walking around more in daily life, along with complementary
flexibility/mobility practices) with intermittent bouts of higher-intensity efforts. There is little need for the incredible complexity of today's
fitness scene—the expensive gym equipment, obsessively detailed and
regimented training programs, and fancy contraptions such as cyclome-
ters, GPS units, calorie-burning meters, and body sensors. These gadgets,
while possessing a high cool factor, can also lead you astray from the
benefits of having a simple, varied, and intuitive approach to exercise.

Unfortunately, commuting, work, digital entertainment, and modern
comforts promote prolonged periods of inactivity, hindering our opportunities to obtain even the bare minimum requirements for daily movement. While making a concerted effort to lodge a respectable number of
cardio workout hours each week is laudable, it's not enough to counteract
the massive sedentary forces we face. So the directive to "move frequently"
involves a multi-tiered approach: conduct your regular cardio workouts,

Pursue challenges that turn you on instead of worrying about what the magazines say is the 'best' workout, or the marketing hype that glorifies extreme events.

making sure you remain at or below your aerobic maximum heart rate (more on this later); avoid prolonged stillness at all costs by taking brief walks, trying out a standup desk, and adding movement habits like taking stairs instead of elevators, habitually parking at the far end of parking lots, and doing errands on foot; and add complementary movement practices such as Pilates, yoga, tai chi and expert-guided mobility exercises to help you move functionally and safely. (Again, more on this later.)

Beyond the challenges of sedentary modern life, conventional wisdom has brainwashed us to believe that a lean, fit body comes from either lucky genes or following a regimented, overly stressful exercise routine. It's no wonder that many well-meaning fitness enthusiasts have become either exhausted or totally turned off to getting fit. Millions more stick with flawed approaches that leave them disappointed and discouraged when they fall far short of their ultimate peak performance potential and ideal body composition.

You can get extremely healthy and fit on a few hours a week of basic walking/moving around and comfortable cardio workouts, one abbreviated strength workout a week lasting 10 minutes, another longer strength session of up to 30 minutes, one sprint session every 7 to 10 days (lasting perhaps 15 or 20 minutes, but with only a few minutes of hard effort in total), and regular efforts to integrate flexibility/mobility exercises (perhaps while relaxing in front of the TV at home). That adds up to only a few hours dedicated to exercise out of the 168 at our disposal each week.

Amazingly, you don't have to endure the fatigue and exhaustion that so many have suffered when following conventional wisdom's recommendation to adopt a consistent and unnecessarily complex exercise program. You don't even have to be consistent; in fact, it's better if you are *inconsistent* with your workout routine. Heck, the old saying "All you need is a pair of shoes" doesn't even apply—you don't even need shoes! (See the "Happy Feet" section later in the chapter.)

THE PRIMAL BLUEPRINT FITNESS PYRAMID

Functional fitness, stress/rest balance, anti-aging benefits

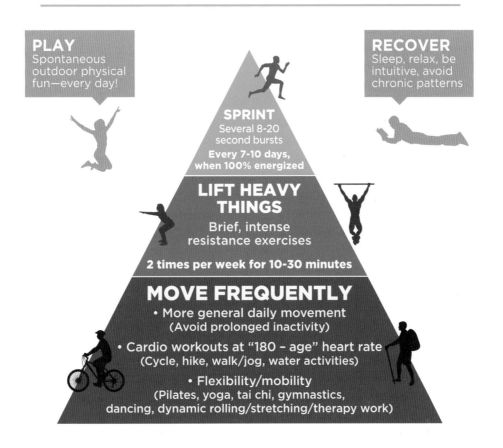

PLAY
Spontaneous outdoor physical fun—every day!

RECOVER
Sleep, relax, be intuitive, avoid chronic patterns

SPRINT
Several 8-20 second bursts
Every 7-10 days, when 100% energized

LIFT HEAVY THINGS
Brief, intense resistance exercises
2 times per week for 10-30 minutes

MOVE FREQUENTLY
- More general daily movement (Avoid prolonged inactivity)
- Cardio workouts at "180 – age" heart rate (Cycle, hike, walk/jog, water activities)
- Flexibility/mobility (Pilates, yoga, tai chi, gymnastics, dancing, dynamic rolling/stretching/therapy work)

If you are currently racking up a dozen or more hours of chronic cardio each week, or hitting the gym most every day for prolonged strength training sessions where you cycle through repeated stations or exercises until you reach failure with high reps and light weights, I encourage you to reframe your perspective from "more is better" to "brief and intense is better." If you find yourself bouncing off the walls with extra energy because your new primal schedule is too easy, *make your hard workouts even harder*—not longer or more frequent. Remember, the goal is to trigger optimal gene expression, not fill in all the blanks of your logbook and teeter on the edge of injury and burnout.

> *Reframe your perspective from "more is better" to "brief and intense is better."*

For those interested in the effects of primal exercise on weight loss, I must first remind you of my critical assertion that 80 percent of your body composition success is determined by how you eat. Reprogramming your genes through dietary modification is the best way to become fat-adapted so you can derive most of your energy from stored (or ingested) fat, instead of the disastrous dynamic in modern life where the population is dependent upon regular feedings of high-carbohydrate meals for energy. When you moderate insulin production and upregulate your fat-burning genes, you will trend toward your ideal body composition over time. The details of your exercise program—what we commonly believe to be the most significant factor in weight-loss success or failure—are actually much less influential than you might think. Reducing excess body fat is predominantly about hormone optimization through a low-insulin-production diet.

Science is now validating the idea that calories burned during exercise minimally contributes to your fat-loss goals; rather, exercise stimulates a commensurate increase in appetite, so you eat more calories when you burn more calories.

When you exercise the Primal Blueprint way, you will indeed fine-tune your fat-burning system, but only if you are also eating right. Your low-level movement—while it doesn't burn a ton of calories—will greatly enhance your ability to metabolize fat both during exercise and at rest. Meanwhile, brief, intense strength and sprint sessions elevate body temperature and stimulate an increase in fat metabolism, not only during the workout

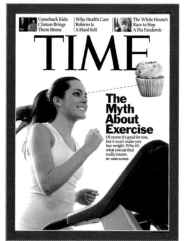

"The Myth About Exercise" TIME Magazine cover story details why the oversimplified "calories in, calories out" equation for weight loss is flawed.

but also for many hours afterward. Eating primally moderates insulin production, boosts fat metabolism, and normalizes appetite. Put everything together and you reprogram your genes to become a fat-burning beast around the clock—the only reliable method for reaching and maintaining your ideal body composition. The primal approach stands in sharp contrast to conventional wisdom's "calories in, calories out" model where you hope the 600 calories burned during your 50-minute step aerobics class will somehow lead to weight loss. Recall that Kelly Korg ingested nearly double that on her quick visit to Jamba Juice!

PRIMAL BLUEPRINT FITNESS

With a balanced approach patterned after Grok and designed to promote optimal gene expression, you will develop a broad range of skills and attributes (strength, power, speed, endurance) that allow you to do pretty much whatever you want (or, in Grok's case, survive the various challenges of primal life) with a substantial degree of competence and minimal risk of injury or burnout.

By breaking free from the cycle of using carbs to fuel stressful, prolonged, sugar-burning chronic cardio workouts, you can easily get into the generally accepted favorable body fat percentage range of 10 to 18 percent for men and 14 to 24 percent for women. This is true no matter who you are or how plump your family tree is. The Primal Blueprint Fitness strategy will not just lower body fat levels but tone your entire body and also give you some noticeable definition in your arms, legs, and core. When you expand your horizons beyond "jogging at a strenuous pace for five songs," your body will begin to show the effects all over, most notably by correcting the common trouble spots of excess butt, hip, thigh, and abdominal fat.

For the competitor, you can expect to branch out beyond your

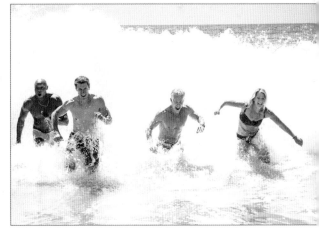

bread-and-butter skills to become a more complete athlete. Those who rely on bulk to hoist mucho plates or post up under the basket will become leaner and improve their power-to-weight ratio (how strong you are in relation to your body weight). This translates into more pull-ups, a higher vertical leap, and more quickness on your first step. Those who tend to be slight of frame and lacking in raw power will add a bit more muscle and improve pure strength and explosiveness, expanding their repertoire not only to outlast the competition but also to out-power them. And all of us who move frequently will elevate our health and fitness status out of the narrow competency of being able to perform magnificent athletic feats and into the realm of being truly healthy, functional, and poised for longevity.

Power-to-weight ratio is a critical Primal Blueprint Fitness benchmark because it has a strong functional component. A skinny dude like the late Bruce Lee was by reasonable definition more powerful than Hulk Hogan because of having a superior power-to-weight ratio. Decathletes like American Brian Clay (5'11", 185 pounds; 180cm, 84 kg), 2008 Olympic decathlon gold medalist (and primal/paleo eating enthusiast!), or the remarkable current Olympic champion and world record holder Ashton Eaton (6'1", 185 pounds; 185 cm, 84 kg), are great examples of balanced all-around performers. The demands on the decathlete to sprint, hurdle, high jump, pole vault, and throw the shot, discus, and javelin at levels respectable to individual event specialists blow away the vein-popping magazine cover models, who might look really impressive but would be seriously outmatched in any sort of athletic contest.

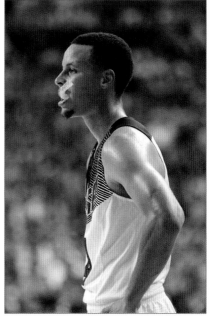

Natursports / Shutterstock.com

NBA Most Valuable Player Stephen Curry displays a wonder of never-before-seen athletic skills on the basketball court. Enjoy the show!

Beyond the reputation that decathletes enjoy for being the greatest all-around athletes in the Olympic realm, basketball stars like Stephen Curry and LeBron James blend an incredible array of skills—speed, endurance, strength, agility, and explosiveness—to perform seemingly superhuman feats. (Ever try a 360-degree slam dunk, even on a low basket? It ain't easy! I miss occasionally...) The popular CrossFit movement envisages the ultimate athlete as a combination gymnast, power lifter, and sprinter. The ideal exercise practices, and the body that you aspire to build, come down to personal preference within the broad guidelines of the Primal Blueprint. Do the exercises that turn you on the most—in your mind, your heart, and your genes!

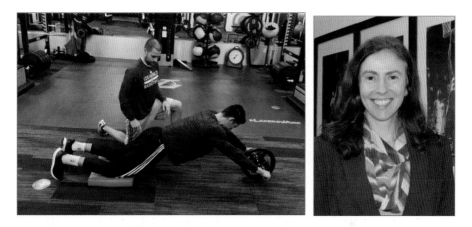

P.S. Speaking of the NBA, primal/paleo-style eating is really catching on. Numerous players are now embracing primal habits, including LeBron James, who dropped excess body fat and toned up with a summer-long strict ketogenic eating pattern in 2014. The Los Angeles Lakers have implemented a program overseen by Dr. Cate Shanahan to get players eating primal-aligned meals on road trips. Tim DiFrancesco, Head Strength & Conditioning Coach, inspires Lakers players to train, eat, and even sleep per primal guidelines.

I know you would probably like me to provide a specific, day-by-day workout plan to reach your Primal Blueprint Fitness goals, but the fact is, it is better to make sure your workout decisions align with your energy and motivation levels than to follow a strict schedule. Your most urgent priority is to simply move around more each day—no pressure, no stopwatch, no formality needed. Just avoid prolonged periods of inactivity.

Supplement basic movement with structured cardio sessions, but make absolutely sure that during these workouts you maintain a comfortable heart rate at or below your aerobic maximum of "180 minus age" in beats per minute. (See the sidebar "The Maffetone '180 – Age' Formula" later in this chapter.) Exceeding aerobic maximum heart rate and drifting into chronic exercise patterns is an extremely common mistake among everyone from novices to elite athletes. We'll spend ample time discussing this important matter to make sure you are comfortable slowing down and building aerobic fitness without compromising your health.

> *Instead of following a strict schedule, align your workout decisions with your energy and motivation levels.*

Perform complementary movement exercises that build flexibility, balance, range of motion, and coordination to support functional movement and prevent injury. Put your muscles under load with strength training sessions once or twice a week, but keep them brief and intense. Sprint once in a while when you are super motivated and energized. Don't forget to include play as part of your fitness regimen too.

A whimsical, intuitive, unstructured approach to fitness might feel uncomfortable if you are accustomed to flawed conventional wisdom that values consistency, gadgetry, and judging your fitness progress by the obsessive tracking of quantifiable data such as miles covered, calories burned, weights and reps, time in target heart rate zone, or placement in the race. If you have a techie bent and enjoy tracking your fitness output, that's great. Just remember that your mind and body will thrive with an intuitive approach and likely struggle with a regimented approach.

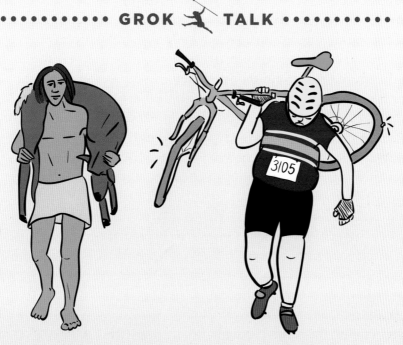

"That was fun!"   "That was fun?"

Grok and his hunter-gatherer pals knew nothing of the superficial silliness that frames the fitness industry today. Our hunter-gatherer ancestors' motivation to exercise was completely pure: to meet basic needs of food and shelter, to satisfy the innate human desire for adventure, competition, and play, and to explore the boundaries of the human spirit, regardless of what measured results came of it. I urge you to determine the success of your fitness program by how much fun you are having and how much personal growth you experience from striving for your goals. Pursue challenges that turn you on instead of worrying about what the magazines say is the best workout or about the marketing hype that glorifies extreme events, such as the marathon or ironman triathlon as ultimate athletic accomplishments. In my opinion, both are far too difficult for almost all of the entrants and their real life daily responsibilities.

Organ Reserve: The Key to Longevity

Keep in mind that the benefits of a sensible exercise program extend far beyond competitive success and looking good. The more lean muscle you maintain throughout life, the better your organs will function, up to an obvious point of diminishing returns; for example, a bodybuilder has heaps of excess muscle that serve little or no functional purpose and require a lot of caloric energy to sustain. Optimal organ function correlates with maximum longevity and excellent health.

Organs, like muscles, adhere to the natural law "use it or lose it." When you hit the deck for 50 pushups, the conscious decision to engage these muscles in a work effort calls your heart, lungs, liver, and other organs into action. Blood chemistry changes as you burn glycogen and fat, process oxygen, and produce metabolic byproducts (e.g., lactic acid) at an accelerated rate. You are asking your organs to keep up with your active lifestyle, in the process strengthening them to better withstand the demands of daily life and the natural aging process.

In contrast, when your activity diminishes, as in the classic paradigm of aging, muscles and organs can atrophy. Their function decreases because they are given no reason to remain at 100-percent efficiency. An unfit person has lower bone density, less lung capacity (the quantity of air you can exchange on each breath), and less stroke volume (the amount of blood your heart pumps with each beat) than a fit person. Today, the aging process should really be called the "process of physical decline largely due to inactivity and lifestyle habits that result in mismanaged genes."

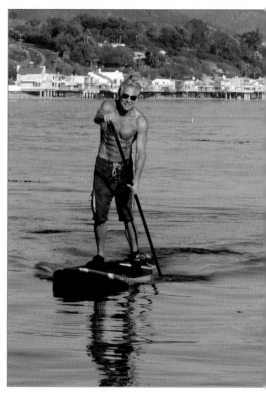

My ability to perform an extreme and narrow fitness feat like run a 2:18 marathon is gone, but my more balanced fitness regimen today promotes organ reserve and longevity.

Because all of your organs and body systems work synergistically, you are vulnerable to your weakest link. For example, an unfit accident victim or a surgery patient who loses excessive blood and has a heart operating at only 45 percent of potential capacity will often fare differently than a fit person with superior heart function suffering the same trauma. Bones break more easily among the unfit. Pneumonia is a common cause of death among the elderly due to the inability of their weakened lungs to help clear the germ-laden mucus effectively through coughing. When you keep your muscles fit throughout life, your organs come along for the ride. Yes, chronological aging will eventually cause your muscles and organs to wear out after 120 years or so, but this seems like a more appealing process than the distorted one that prevails today. Use it or lose it!

> *Walking is the best possible exercise.*
> *Habituate yourself to walk very far.*
> —Thomas Jefferson

PRIMAL BLUEPRINT LAW #3: MOVE FREQUENTLY

In a modern world with tremendous momentum toward sedentary living (how's that for an oxymoron that's actually true?), honoring Law #3 requires the three-pronged approach of moving more in daily life, conducting cardio workouts at aerobic heart rates, and performing complementary flexibility/mobility exercises. Devoted fitness enthusiasts tend to fixate on the accumulation of impressive and prolonged structured workouts, but the truth is that short-duration activity sessions really do add up and make a significant contribution to your aerobic conditioning and overall health. Grok and company didn't worry about issues like coordination, range of motion, and flexibility because their regular everyday movements would have supported these areas of functionality. Today, most of us are woefully deficient in frequent, varied movement and spend excessive time sitting still. When we do get moving, it's often a narrow activity like running or moving through a sequence of weight machines. This makes flexibility/mobility exercises a critical element of law #3.

If you can manage truly active days, a single long hike on the weekend, and a few shorter walks or cardio machine sessions during the week, and you complement those with a fairly small amount of time devoted to complementary movement practices, you will dramatically reduce your risk of heart disease (in comparison to being sedentary), support efficient metabolism, better control your weight, and, in conjunction with the strength and sprint workouts, achieve the broad athletic competency that characterizes Primal Blueprint Fitness.

As you broaden your perspective about fitness, your top priority is to find more ways to move. No matter how deskbound your job is, you can make some inroads in this area. How about taking phone calls or conducting in-person meetings on the move? How about climbing a couple flights of stairs to deliver a message to your coworker in person instead of phoning? If you take your kids to the playground, don't just park yourself on a bench, get up and walk around the perimeter or, better yet, get out there and play with them (and fulfill Primal Law #7 at the same time!). Walk your dog every day—he lives for it! When you watch a TV show, get up and do some air squats during the commercials. (Does anyone watch commercials anymore?) It doesn't really matter what you do, as long as you are moving frequently and in a varied manner to stimulate different muscle groups.

One reason we might not move more during the day is that the modern workplace culture equates being productive with being glued to a task, grinding away for hours at a time without a break. Plenty of science validates that cognitive function is improved when you take frequent breaks from tasks requiring stationary concentration. This is why casino card dealers work under high-pressure circumstances for 40 minutes followed by 20-minute breaks, repeated throughout their 8-hour shift. The harder you work—and I mean delivering either physical or mental effort—the more important it is to break from peak cognitive focus for some gentle movement. If you are a physical laborer, your breaks might be to stretch and move your body in different ways, including compensatory movements if you do a repetitive task.

The specifics of expert recommendations vary on this subject, but it's safe to say that for every 2 to 3 hours of peak cognitive focus, you need 15 to 20 minutes of devoted break time. Ideally these breaks will involve deliberate movement or even light exercise (such as the kind I will present shortly in the complementary movement section), as well as sunlight or fresh air. If you work at a desk job, I also strongly encourage you to integrate a standup experience into your workday. You don't need to invest in an expensive rig (although those are great if you can afford them). If you just elevate your computer keyboard and monitor on some boxes, you are in business. You may not be able to go for long periods at first, so feel free to lower back down to sitting position and just strive for variation of any form during your work day. Nutritious Movement™ expert Katy Bowman and I present a comprehensive multimedia educational program on the topic of standup desks and creating variation in your workplace called *Don't Just Sit There* that you can find at PrimalBlueprint.com.

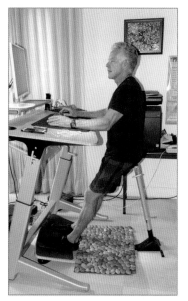

My Focal standing desk with special pogo-stick-style Mogo seat allows me to alternate from standing (notice the cool pebble mat for a nature texture on my feet) to getting a little support from the seat. The decades-long tightness in my hip flexors was significantly alleviated after only a few weeks of using this set-up.

I truly believe that simply introducing more general movement throughout the day in 5-, 10-, or 15-minute increments is one of the greatest changes you can make for your overall health and fitness. Walking is the most obvious choice, but you can also count stretching, calisthenics, a yoga sun salute or tai chi sequence, ascending and descending stairs, pedaling a lonely stationary bike for a few minutes, throwing down some breakdancing skills in the lunch room, and whatever else you fancy to get your body out of stagnant, inactive patterns and into activity and variation patterns. Making a commitment to moving more will improve musculoskeletal health, increase fat burning, help regulate appetite hormones, improve attention and mood, and fight fatigue. This is a crucial even for those of you who consider yourself already active but who nevertheless spend many hours a day sitting still. Plain and simple, being sedentary for long periods wreaks havoc on your body, even if you start your day with a five-mile run or end it with 50 laps in the pool. Sure, Grok probably spent considerable time lounging around conserving energy, but he certainly never spent eight hours in a chair, hunched over his keyboard with terrible posture.

You have to stay in shape. My grandmother,
she started walking five miles a day when she was 60.
She's 97 today and we don't know where the hell she is.
—Ellen DeGeneres

While frequent everyday movement should be a priority throughout your day, it is also important to log some time doing deliberate cardio-vascular workouts at a comfortable pace. For those heavily indoctrinated into the conventional wisdom that medium-to-difficult-intensity cardio is the path to health, fitness, and weight control, consider again the premise of the Primal Blueprint. It's clear that our ancestors were lean, strong, and extremely active, and they were most certainly capable of running long distances at a respectable pace similar to today's gung-ho endurance athletes. However, our ancestors did this very rarely, because the risks of failure were so severe. Imagine Grok chasing some game animal all-out for a few hours in the hot desert sun and—oops—not succeeding in killing it. He's squandered valuable energy reserves (increasing glucose metabolism by a factor of 10) yet has no food to replace that energy. He has suddenly become some other animal's potential prey because he is physically exhausted. Instead, it's more likely that Grok relied on superior tracking ability (using his highly evolved brain) and walking or slow jogging (using his superior fat-burning system), rather than literally chasing down his prey.

I'm particularly concerned about the vast numbers of fitness enthusiasts in the gyms and on the roads who generally take their pace to slightly uncomfortable in order to get that sensation of "getting a workout" and experiencing that invigorating pulse of stress hormones—the endorphin high—upon completion.

•••••••••• GROK TALK ••••••••••

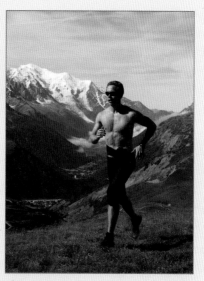

It's important to acknowledge the addictive nature of the so-called runners high or endorphin rush that happens when you trigger the fight or flight response from prolonged vigorous workouts. When you push your body beyond a comfortable aerobic endurance effort, you stimulate the release of assorted feel-good hormones and neurotransmitters like cortisol, dopamine, serotonin, epinephrine, and norepinephrine—the cocktail recipe for the endorphin rush. This is a genetically hard-wired mechanism to support survival by dulling sensations of fatigue and pain when you are immersed in what's perceived to be a life-or-death effort.

When these powerful chemicals linger in your bloodstream after that vigorous long-distance run, hike, or bike ride, you experience a state of bliss akin to the effects of prescription painkillers. Remember, the term endorphin literally means endogenous (internally manufactured) morphine. Slowing down to promote aerobic fitness and protect health requires you use some significant restraint and let go of the instant gratification provided by the endorphin rush.

"But This Feels Too Easy!"

A key factor in promoting optimum health according to the Primal Blueprint is to make sure that you conduct the vast majority of your cardiovascular workouts at or below your **maximum aerobic heart rate**. Your maximum aerobic heart rate is the point where you reap maximum aerobic benefits (i.e., maximum fat burning) with a minimum amount of anaerobic stimulation. Don't confuse aerobic maximum with your absolute maximum heart rate, which is the fastest your heart can pump when delivering a brief, all-out effort; aerobic maximum is considerably lower than absolute maximum. If you increase your effort beyond aerobic maximum heart rate, you start burning an increasing percentage of glucose instead of fat, and you stimulate more stress hormone production due to the difficulty of the effort.

Your maximum aerobic heart rate can be calculated using Dr. Phil Maffetone's simple formula of "180 minus age" to identify the upper limit, in beats per minute, to achieve an aerobic workout. For example, a 44-year-old exerciser would conduct aerobic workouts at a heart rate of 136 or below. Aerobic (meaning literally, "with oxygen") exercise is comfortable and energizing, and it improves your ability to burn fat both during exercise and at rest. During properly paced aerobic workouts, your heart and other energy systems work a little harder to handle the extra fuel and oxygen delivery demands, but not so much that you are physiologically overstressed. The specific biochemical signals created by this low-level aerobic activity produce numerous health and fitness benefits as follows:

Improved Fat Metabolism: You train your body to efficiently utilize free fatty acids for fuel, a benefit that is realized 24 hours a day, with a higher metabolic rate and a preference for fat over glucose (provided you eat primally). Low-level aerobic exercise also helps balance blood glucose levels and regulate appetite.

Improved Cardiovascular Function: You increase your capillary network (blood vessels that supply the muscle cells with fuel and oxygen), improve the functionality of your muscle mitochondria and also manufacture additional mitochondria (the "energy powerhouses" of the cell), increase the stroke volume of your heart (more blood pumped with each beat), and also improve oxygen delivery by your lungs.

Improved Musculoskeletal System: You strengthen your bones, joints, and connective tissue so you can absorb increasing stress loads without breaking down. This is critical to your ability to perform and recover from your high-intensity primal strength and sprint sessions.

Stronger Immune System: You enhance the function of your immune system by stimulating beneficial hormone secretions and by building a more efficient circulatory system.

Increased Energy: You finish workouts feeling energized and refreshed, rather than slightly fatigued and depleted (as you typically do when you follow a chronic cardio schedule of moderate-to-difficult-intensity workouts conducted too frequently).

Those with competitive endurance goals might not be satisfied to putter along exclusively at a slow pace and believe they can take down the competition with that approach. And it's true that intense workouts that approximate the challenge of your competitive goals deliver outstanding fitness benefits. However, whether you are a casual fitness enthusiast or an elite athlete, you must establish a strong base of low-level aerobic conditioning before you can actually benefit from stressful, higher-intensity workouts. The tertiary benefits of low-level work (better balance, strong postural muscles, increased mitochondrial development and capillary profusion, and strengthening of bones, tendons, and ligaments to prevent injury) might not be as readily apparent as the direct competitive application of beating your personal record at a time trial, but one cannot happen without the other.

This concept of "base first, then intensity" has been proven successful by the training regimens of the world's greatest endurance athletes of the last 50 years, beginning with the pioneering work of New Zealand running coach Arthur Lydiard. Lydiard's prize students, including 1960 and 1964 Olympic track gold medalist Peter Snell (today one of the world's leading exercise physiologists), showed that long-duration, low-intensity training, coupled with intense interval training and adequate rest (rest was another far-out concept for the '60s), could lead directly to Olympic gold medals and world records at races as short as 800 meters (which last less than two minutes).

When I completed my career as an elite marathoner and triathlete and transitioned into a career as a personal trainer, my training regimen shifted dramatically. I was still out there moving for several hours a day, but I went from busting my brains out with super-fit training partners to moseying along with a succession of clients on my daily calendar. Unlike many of today's fitness trainers who stand there and count reps, I got outside with my unfit to moderately fit clients and did their workouts with them. Bike rides that I previously hammered at 20-plus mph for hours were now conducted at 13 mph. The long, hard trail runs of my marathon days were replaced with easy jogs where my heart rate barely exceeded 100 beats per minute (only 50 percent of my max). With a young family and a career filling my days, I rarely had time to do my own specific workouts. I made the most of what free time I had by conducting short, extremely intense interval sessions once or twice a week—on cardio equipment like my beloved VersaClimber or running a few quick repeats around the track. Usually these sessions lasted around 20 minutes until my next client came strolling in.

When I jumped into the occasional long- or ultra-distance endurance race, the results were shocking to me. My "by chance" regimen of very, very slow workouts coupled with occasional very short, intense workouts was effective beyond my wildest dreams. I was able to place among the top competitors in the world in my age group and very close to the standards set by top professionals of that era. Indeed, the Primal Blueprint parameters literally took shape in my mind as I blew by my rivals (who were putting in big chronic cardio miles, just like I used to) despite what most experts and prevailing conventional wisdom would have deemed ridiculously inadequate preparation.

If you try out this aerobic base building and almost certainly have to slow down significantly to stay in your aerobic heart rate zone, try not to become frustrated at your leisurely pace or to feel that you're not really benefitting from the workouts because the effort feels much easier than what you are used to doing. It's important to understand that the efficiency of your aerobic system—your ability to burn fat during sustained exercise—is by far the most important predictor of performance.

Building a strong aerobic base gives you a higher platform from which to launch all competitive efforts that extend beyond your aerobic maximum and into the higher heart rate zones. For example, if you can run 9-minute miles comfortably at aerobic heart rates, you may be able to drop to a 7:30 per-mile pace in a competitive effort. What's more, when you are delivering a maximum competitive effort anywhere from a few minutes up to the all-day ultraendurance events, most of your energy production comes from your aerobic system because it is completely engaged, in addition to the anaerobic energy production that happens when your heart rate elevates. Dr. Maffetone asserts that a competitive effort of two hours is 99 percent aerobic, and only 1 percent anaerobic—a concept that is confirmed in exercise physiology texts.

When you have the patience and discipline to keep your workouts aerobic for months and months, you will experience a gradual and steady improvement in your aerobic function—you'll go faster (running, pedaling, rowing, or whatever) at the same maximum aerobic heart rate.

•••••••••• GROK 🎿 TALK ••••••••••

Emphasizing aerobically paced exercise not only makes you go faster, it's healthier. Your body burns fat much more cleanly than it burns glucose. Glucose is the quickest and easiest fuel to burn, but it burns dirty—producing more free radicals and causing oxidative damage in your body. When you burn fat—by exercising at a slower pace and eating the right foods—you utilize oxygen and mitochondria to minimize oxidative damage.

Becoming aerobically efficient is like having a powerful, clean-burning solar power plant for your energy needs. Being aerobically deficient and carbohydrate dependent is like operating with a dilapidated coal power plant, spewing smoke and generating inflammation and free radicals.

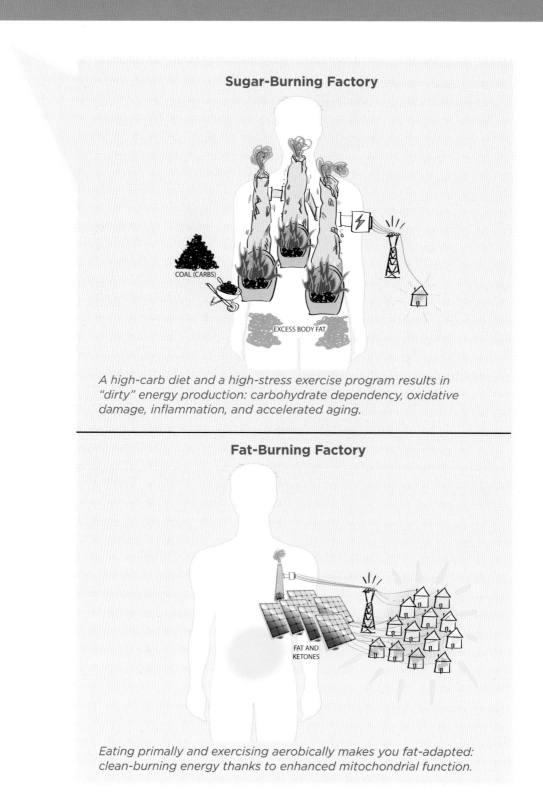

Sugar-Burning Factory

COAL (CARBS)

EXCESS BODY FAT

A high-carb diet and a high-stress exercise program results in "dirty" energy production: carbohydrate dependency, oxidative damage, inflammation, and accelerated aging.

Fat-Burning Factory

FAT AND KETONES

Eating primally and exercising aerobically makes you fat-adapted: clean-burning energy thanks to enhanced mitochondrial function.

Doing cardio workouts at 180 minus age or below often requires a significant adjustment in mindset to reject the "no pain, no gain" mentality toward workouts. You should feel very comfortable at this heart rate and embrace a rhythm of workouts that are not strenuous or stressful. At 180 minus age heart rate, you can easily converse without getting short of breath, and you finish feeling refreshed and energized instead of slightly fatigued and hungry, as you might after more strenuous workouts.

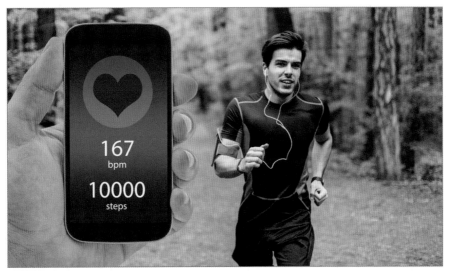

Because it's so easy to exceed maximum aerobic heart rate without feeling any strain, it's absolutely essential to use a wireless heart rate monitor. This dude is jeopardizing a promising modeling career with his chronic cardio ways generating oxidative damage, and eventually wrinkles...

Because the 180 minus age level is so comfortable, it's critical to monitor your heart rate during workouts with a wireless chest strap and watch. You simply cannot trust perceived exertion to keep you aerobic, because you don't really feel any significant strain even as you drift 5, 10, or 15 beats above your aerobic maximum. Many people find when they first start conducting cardiovascular workouts at or below their aerobic max that they have to go considerably more slowly than they had been. Rest assured that this is normal. If you discipline yourself to slow down accordingly, you will progress steadily over time. Your progress can be tracked by conducting the Maximum Aerobic Function (MAF) test frequently—I'll detail this shortly.

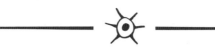

THE MAFFETONE "180 – AGE" FORMULA

Quantifying maximum aerobic heart rate (defined as the point where maximum aerobic benefits occur with a minimal amount of anaerobic stimulation) is not an exact science, and there is a range of opinion on the matter from leading exercise physiologists, coaches, and elite athletes. Some believe that max aerobic heart rate correlates with a laboratory-defined state called ventilatory threshold (VT), a point where increased effort 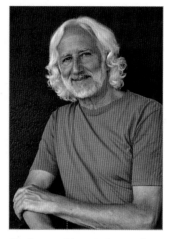 would cause a non-linear spike in ventilation, glucose metabolism, lactate accumulation, fight or flight hormone release, and the recruitment of oxidative fast-twitch (type IIa) muscle fibers. VT studies suggest this occurs in well-trained athletes at around 77 percent of maximum heart rate, and around 75 percent of max in lesser-trained athletes.

After extensive research on the matter, the Primal Blueprint position is to strongly support Dr. Phil Maffetone's "180 minus age = maximum aerobic heart rate" formula. The Maffetone formula has been field tested by thousands of athletes over decades, can be calculated without laboratory testing and without needing an accurate maximum heart rate value, and is on the conservative side in comparison to the VT calculations. Training with a conservative number still supports excellent aerobic development and lessens the risk of the disastrous chronic cardio patterns that occur when one routinely exceeds aerobic maximum.

Keep in mind that as you improve your fitness, your speed at maximum aerobic heart rate will improve, but there is never a justification to increase your maximum aerobic heart rate beyond your 180 minus age calculation. What this means is that while a fitter athlete performs at a higher level than a novice at the same heart rate, the relative difficulty of the workout is similar with all exercisers. It feels comfortable!

The Maffetone formula offers some adjustment factors to the calculation based on your current state of health and fitness. Take 180 minus your age as your baseline number, and then adjust it accordingly if appropriate:

1. Subtract 10: Recovering from illness, surgery, or disease, or taking regular medication.
2. Subtract 5: Recent injury or regression in training, get more than two colds annually, allergies, asthma, inconsistent training, or recently returning to training.
3. No Adjustment: Training consistently (4x/week) for two years, free from aforementioned problems.
4. Add 5: Successful training for two years or more, success in competition.

Regarding the low end of the aerobic zone, it's really nothing with which to concern yourself. Even a leisurely walk is delivering a training effect that will make a significant positive contribution to your overall aerobic conditioning.

The best thing about heart rate training is that it individualizes your experience to ensure you get an optimal workout. This critical "individual" element—one that can make or break your entire exercise program— has long been ignored by group class instructors and social groups working out together. Generally speaking, asking a class or group of workout partners to keep pace together is a recipe for failure *for all but the fittest members of the group.* As a final note, occasionally exceeding 180 minus age when you feel great and want to really go for it is just fine—as long as you adhere to a pattern of mostly aerobically paced workouts and you get adequate rest and recovery after occasional challenging workouts or races.

A Case Against Chronic Cardio

In contrast to the comprehensive benefits of frequent, comfortably paced exercise, getting more serious about working out can really mess you up if you have a flawed approach. Conducting cardiovascular workouts that are too hard (above maximum aerobic heart rate), last too long, and are done too frequently with insufficient recovery between them adds up to a disastrous pattern I call "chronic cardio." I'd estimate that the vast majority of folks you see working out on cardio machines, jogging through the neighborhood, or keeping pace in the group class are exceeding 180 minus age (often by a wide margin) for the duration of nearly every session.

While a workout that exceeds 180 minus age by 5, 10, or 15 beats might not feel at all difficult at the time, a sustained pattern of chronic cardio—even when you are just a few beats over your aerobic maximum—can lead to numerous problems with metabolism, physiological stress management, immune function, and general health. A routine of chronic cardio requires large amounts of dietary carbohydrates each day to support it. While the risks of excess fat storage and hyperinsulinemia (overproduction of insulin) are moderated somewhat by a heavy exercise schedule, they are still significant because you are teaching your body to prefer glucose for fuel, not only during workouts but around the clock. (More on this topic shortly.) Chronic exercise patterns are also believed to promote increased laziness throughout the day, both consciously

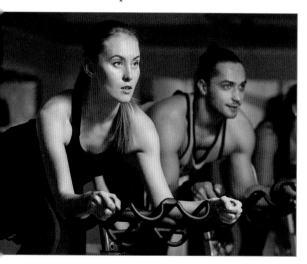

("Hey I did my workout, I think I'll just drive the half-mile to the mailbox.") and subconsciously, where you tend to be less active and burn fewer calories as a reaction to the stress of chronic cardio.

The real kicker is that for all your hard work, chronic cardio is unlikely

Group energy, pumping music, and vigorous effort can yield an endorphin buzz and a sense of accomplishment, but a chronic cardio pattern can destroy your health. Just you wait, she'll get wrinkles like the dude on page 335

to actually help you lose weight. Fat burns well in the presence of oxygen (i.e., when you are in your aerobic zone), but as exercise intensity increases, your body's preferred fuel choice shifts from primarily fat at lower intensities—at heart rates up to 180 minus age—to an ever-increasing percentage of glucose, which is quicker and easier to burn when oxygen is lacking due to your quickening pace. Workouts have a powerful effect on your metabolic function at rest, so burning sugar during workouts teaches your body to prefer burning sugar at rest. Furthermore, when you frequently deplete your energy reserves with a pattern of chronic workouts, your brain learns to overeat, especially quick-energy carbs, as a genetically programmed survival adaptation against the life-or-death risks of starvation or depletion of physical energy. If you are looking to reduce body fat primarily through vigorous cardiovascular exercise (as conventional wisdom recommends), you are quite likely to fail unless you slow down your pace and alter your diet to limit your carb intake.

Chronic cardio—a program I followed for nearly 20 years as a marathoner and later as an ironman triathlete—is bad for your health, period.

Besides the weight-loss issues, chronic cardio increases the production of the prominent fight or flight hormone cortisol. Cortisol is great in short bursts to elevate your physical and cognitive function per your hard-wired fight or flight response. When you engage in chronic cardio, you call upon the fight or flight response too frequently and for workouts that are too long in duration. When cortisol is chronically elevated, you break down hard-earned muscle tissue, suppress immune function, suppress key anabolic hormones such as testosterone and human growth hormone, promote sugar cravings and fat storage as previously mentioned, and ultimately head down the road to fatigue, illness, injury, and burnout.

Over the long run, chronic cardio increases systemic inflammation in the body, leading to elevated disease risk, increased oxidative damage, and accelerated aging. Realize that inflammation is the body's response to a stressor; again, great in the short term and destructive in the long term. It's ironic that many people in their forties and fifties start engaging in chronic-style marathon or triathlon training in hopes of improving health and delaying the aging process when, quite often, it has the exact opposite effect.

CHRONIC CARDIO DRAWBACKS —POCKET REFERENCE

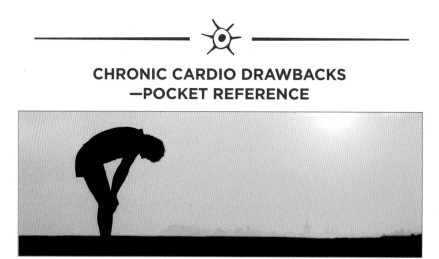

Strike this pose in yoga class—okay. Strike this pose after routine training session—not okay.

A consistent schedule of frequent, sustained, medium-to-difficult-intensity (above your 180 minus age aerobic maximum) workouts can overstress the body and lead to these negative consequences:

Hormone Imbalance: Chronic cardio causes a prolonged elevation of cortisol and other stress hormones and a corresponding suppression of testosterone and growth hormone. This compromises optimal fat burning and muscle development, and suppresses immune function and sex drive. When cortisol and other fight or flight hormones are stimulated too frequently, the end result is burnout. Yes, you get the "runners high" when cortisol, dopamine, serotonin, epinephrine, norepinephrine and the other powerful endorphin rush chemicals are flowing through your bloodstream, but chasing this high too often will lead to burnout.

Injuries: Recurring muscle fatigue, repetitive impact, restrictive footwear, and inflammation from excessive catabolic hormones released in response to chronic cardio traumatizes joints and connective tissue.

Metabolism: Burning more sugar (while exercising above a heart rate of 180 minus age) leads to eating more sugar leads to producing more insulin leads to storing more fat.

Stress: Excessive and prolonged stimulation of the fight or flight response increases systemic inflammation and oxidative damage, compromises immune function, increases disease risk, and accelerates aging.

One Trick Pony: Chronic cardio compromises development of power, speed, strength, and lean mass, and leads to muscle imbalances and inflexibility. Total fitness is sacrificed in favor of narrow, minimally functional aerobic endurance.

I am fully aware of the many loud and passionate voices extolling the psychological and lifestyle virtues of devoted endurance training, and I agree that pushing and challenging your body with inspiring competitive goals supports mental, emotional, and also physical health (albeit with the significant caveats already discussed). An exercise physiologist friend of mine countered my "case against cardio" position recently by reminding me that Hawaii Ironman finishers are vastly healthier than the average population. While true, let us not forget, in the words of Jay Leno, the "average" we are dealing with: "Today there are more overweight people in America than average-weight people. So overweight people are now average. Which means you've met your New Year's resolution."

Furthermore, I'll assert that an old has-been like myself (goals: eat primally, with no processed carbs; nail a couple brief, intense strength workouts each week, in the gym or outdoors; conduct one all-out sprint workout per week; and hang with the young guns for a two-hour Ultimate Frisbee match on weekends) possesses superior health and total body fitness to one-dimensional, routinely overstressed physical specimens that strut in their Speedos down the main drag of Kailua-Kona, Hawaii, every October during Ironman week. Seriously, they really do strut around shirtless and in Speedos. There is even a very popular annual "Underpants Run" before the Ironman that started as a parody of the unchecked Speedo scene in Kailua-Kona.

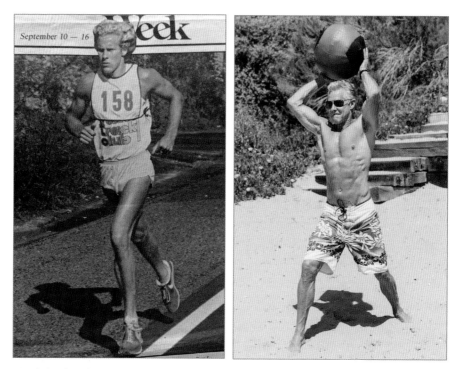

Back in the day I was good for one thing: endurance. Ask me to do a few deadlifts or dig a hole (to install a ladder to wash basement windows perhaps?) and I was headed for delayed onset muscle soreness. Today, even with a few decades of aging (check that hair color—still blond, right? Right?), I'm fitter by every possible measure except the finish line clock at an endurance race.

If you start to feel good during a marathon,
don't worry, that will pass.

—Don Kardong
U.S. Olympic marathoner and author

Yes, today's ironmen can dispose of me in short order in a long-distance swimming, cycling, or running race (it would've been a different story back in the day, but I digress…), but their endurance superiority comes at great cost. Collectively, they tend to suffer from recurring fatigue and adrenal burnout, frequent overuse injuries, frequent minor illnesses from suppressed immune function (I get a cold maybe once every five years; a fair number of ironman triathletes get five every year), and, last but certainly not least, high overall life stress scores—something often touted as the number one heart attack risk factor.

Having spent many years immersed in the type A community of driven fitness enthusiasts and competitive endurance athletes, I am aware that many heads will nod in agreement with my message—and then turn around and plug along with their familiar exhausting training regimens. If serious exercise is a centerpiece of your life, I don't wish to deprive you of your passion. That's right, go ahead and hammer that 3-hour group ride or that 10-mile trail run with the big boys and girls, but only do these things once in a while. This will produce far superior fitness benefits and eliminate the risk factors of repeating highly stressful workouts too frequently.

Complementary Flexibility/Mobility Practices

The various sedentary elements of modern life, especially folding into a sitting position for hours on end, cause an assortment of both minor and serious health problems: musculoskeletal weaknesses and imbalances, hormone dysregulation (especially relating to fat metabolism—sitting promotes insulin resistance), diminished cognitive function, chronic pain and obesity, and even distortion in the shapes of cells and tissues that have been squooshed and immobile too frequently. These problems can be partially—even largely—addressed by increasing everyday movement in assorted ways. However, because our sedentary tendencies are so severe, and because when we do exercise it is often in narrowly-focused, chronic patterns, we can greatly benefit from exercises specifically designed to improve balance, flexibility, coordination, and range of motion in problem areas like the neck, upper and lower back, hip flexors, hamstrings, and calves.

Dr. Kelly Starrett, former elite athlete turned physical therapist, CrossFit superstar, and author of the best-seller *Becoming a Supple Leopard: The Ultimate Guide to Resolving Pain, Preventing Injury, and Optimizing Athletic Performance*, is a fervent advocate of mobility exercises to improve functional health. Mobility exercises are similar to stretching, but instead of involving only muscles, they also target the tendons, ligaments, and fascia that support the entire musculoskeletal system. One of my favorite mobility exercises is to do a handful of mini-lunges—great for counteracting the shortening of the hip flexors caused by sitting for long periods.

A big difference between mobility work and traditional stretching is that mobility stretches are generally held for two minutes (or even longer—Dr. Starrett likes to put his CrossFit athletes through a 10-minute squat test!). Holding positions for a while help identify areas of weakness or imbalance. If you find yourself shaking or aching in the lower back or the calves when trying to hold a deep squat, you can work diligently to make those problem areas more mobile and durable.

As always, performing a static stretch on a cold muscle is not recommended, so brief cardiovascular warmups are advised before getting into any serious mobility work. You can also tack mobility work onto the end of a cardio or strength workout when you are nice and warm and loose. Dr. Starrett has an extensive series of mobility WODs (workouts of the day) posted on YouTube that you can check out.

Practices like yoga and Pilates also develop mobility and flexibility, with the added benefit of strengthening a variety of muscles, notably the core. Core strength is essential to maintaining proper posture, which in turn helps circulation and breathing, relieves back and neck pain, supports your joints, and protects against muscle injuries. Yoga and Pilates also have meditative elements; participants focus on breathing and promoting calmness, which can contribute to emotional and mental wellbeing and counteract the stress that pervades modern life. Tai chi and qigong similarly focus on breathing and slow, deliberate movement involving the whole body and can confer both physical and mental benefits as well.

The more you sit—or on the other end of the spectrum, the more you perform repetitive movement exercise like running—the more important it is that you add complementary movement practices into your routine. Mobility work helps develop proper alignment and strengthens small stabilization muscles and connective tissues. For endurance athletes, attention to complementary movement practices helps preserve good technique even as you fatigue from sustained effort. You may have run plenty of miles in preparation for a marathon race, but if your hip flexors blow out at mile 20 (thanks to your sedentary patterns outside of workouts and insufficient mobility workouts), all that conditioning can go to waste because of your inability to exhibit efficient technique down the home stretch.

Preserving form under fatigue is a critical performance marker that is often overlooked in the quest to accumulate as much volume as possible in your desired sport. Experts like Dr. Starrett also recommend adding self-myofascial release (deep tissue massage) using foam rollers, lacrosse balls, or other tools to help relax muscles, improve range of motion, and reduce post-workout soreness. Spending a few minutes "rolling out" at the end of a busy day or after a tough workout helps stimulate the calming, relaxing parasympathetic nervous system. Yes, even when you get in there deep and get that good hurt going! Self-myofascial release is a great way to speed recovery and help you unwind to facilitate a good night's sleep.

I recommend performing some basic stretching and mobility exercises daily. For example, when you take that 15-minute break and walk away from your computer, walk a bit to warm up and then choose a couple exercises that counterbalance the muscles that have been contracting and shortening while sitting at your desk. For example, in the *Don't Just Sit There* book and video series, Katy Bowman demonstrates exercises like "wall angels" and "pelvic slides" to regain mobility in the muscles and joints especially traumatized by prolonged sitting.

Formal practices like yoga and Pilates are a wonderful to obtain expert guidance and comprehensive, long-duration sessions that are difficult to do on your own. Keep in mind that it's possible to overdo it even with yoga or Pilates and drift into a chronic pattern. Hitting that sunrise power yoga class five days a week can be an invigorating and addicting way to start your days, but it can qualify as chronic cardio due to the difficulty of the sessions and insufficient recovery between them. Resolve to move more in ways that are fun and invigorating for you. Don't worry if you only have five minutes to spare—every little bit counts when it comes to battling against our high-tech, increasingly inactive lifestyles.

Effective Stretching

Due to the sedentary elements of modern life, we can surely benefit from sensible stretching practices that help us transition from an inactive state to activity (e.g., a workout in the morning or after a long sedentary period), prepare us for and protect against injury before intense activity, and finally to help the body return gracefully to a rested state after a vigorous workout. That said, a flawed approach to stretching can compromise performance and recovery, and actually increase injury risk. Here are some recommendations for effective stretching:

Dynamic Stretches: Stretching while moving your muscles through an intended range of motion, such as the series of running warmup/technique drills pictured on page 358.

Functional, Full-body Stretches: Examples include the Grok Hang and the Grok Squat detailed in the coming sidebar. Here, simply elongating or compressing your body through natural range of motion, such as lowering to the ground for a squat or hanging from a bar, provides a safe and effective stretch.

Post-workout Static Stretches: The best time for static stretches isolating certain muscle groups is after a vigorous workout when you are warm and loose, and may need to work through some tightness that developed as a consequence of your effort.

What you want to particularly guard against is doing static stretches to cold muscles, especially where you apply extra force. A classic example is the hurdlers stretch where your rest a straightened leg on an elevated surface and apply downward pressure to stretch the hamstring. Recent research suggests that such static stretches may cause a *neuromuscular inhibitory response* in your muscle such that it gets weaker (by up to 30 percent) for up to 30 minutes after the stretch.

Dynamic stretches like the sprint warmup sequence pictured on page 358 generally involve simulating the desired movements of your upcoming workout with an exaggerated range of motion. Moving through a specific range of motion helps protect against that undesirable neuromuscular inhibitory response caused by applying too much stretch for too long to a muscle. You still have to be sensible about controlling the resistance with your dynamic stretch, but you can easily feel that point where you experience resistance at the limit of your flexibility when you are doing a quad pull or a mini-lunge, for example. With any stretch, even a simple hang or squat, avoid introducing any pain or sharp, localized discomfort. Skip or adapt any prescribed stretch that doesn't feel right. Be sure you are balanced before commencing a stretch, and ease into and out of all stretching positions.

If you are engaged in a chronic training pattern and overworking tired muscles, the ensuing soreness and tightness might make you feel like stretching frequently. I have a better idea: *chill out* and let your muscles recover! Muscle tissue repair is best accomplished through extra rest and sleep, gentle movement, and good nutrition (especially avoiding inflammatory foods like grains, sugars, and refined vegetable oils). If you are exercising primally, your muscles should feel supple and strong nearly all of the time. Sure, you'll occasionally get sore and stiff after challenging workouts; this is nature's way of telling you to get some rest.

IF YOU DON'T KNOW SQUAT, TRY HANGING WITH GROK

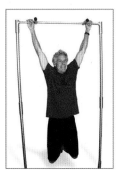

My two favorite stretches are timeless, all-purpose classics: the **Grok Hang** and the **Grok Squat**. The Grok Hang offers a safe, full-body stretch that leaves you feeling exhilarated every time. It's also an effective strengthening exercise—as primal as they come. It's as simple as grabbing hold of a bar or tree branch (with overhand grip) and hanging for as long as you can support yourself.

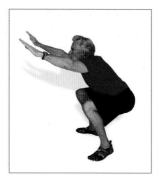

The Grok Squat involves squatting down to the ground, lowering your torso between your bent knees, taking care to keep your spine straight and elongated, until your butt is nearly touching the ground and arms are extended in front of you. This natural movement provides a safe, gentle, efficient post-workout stretch for your feet, calves, Achilles, hamstrings, quadriceps, buttocks, lower and upper back, and shoulders. For thousands of years, people have squatted as a natural "sitting" position in the absence of chairs (to say nothing of Barcaloungers!). For Grok—and millions of people today in the less developed world—squatting is the default position for resting, socializing, eating meals, and even eliminating.

Try a Grok Squat for 20 seconds, and notice what a comprehensive effect you get from such a basic movement. If it's first thing in the morning or you're a little stiff from some intense activity or other stressor (e.g., traveling), simply lowering into the position provides a good stretch. When I'm feeling warm and loose, I'll gently rock back and forth and/or extend my arms out farther to obtain a deeper stretch. I recommended maintaining a straight back as you lower into position, but I allow myself a little spinal curvature at the bottom (to get a specific stretch on my lower back muscles) because I am experienced doing so. As a general rule, all of your stretches should be performed with a straight and elongated spine. One caution: if you haven't done this for a while, are overweight, or have joint issues, you can begin to ease into this stretch (and keep yourself from going too low or falling over) by holding on to a post or another stationary object.

While the Hang and the Squat are both technically static, and I've cautioned against the dangers of static stretching, these stretches are safer because they are regulated by your own bodyweight.

PRIMAL BLUEPRINT LAW #4:
LIFT HEAVY THINGS

The popular conventional wisdom concept of following a strength-training routine that calls for prolonged strenuous workouts several days a week is deeply flawed. Your body thrives on intuitive, spontaneous, and fluctuating workout habits—not ego-driven regimentation organized around an arbitrary time period of seven days that has no special relevance to your fitness progress. When your muscles are challenged beyond what they are used to, the signals generated by the effort prompt genes to make those muscles stronger; it is the challenge that is important, not the strict adherence to a regimented program. Workouts should be high-intensity and brief in duration to elicit the most desirable hormonal response. Just as with chronic cardio, when you conduct strength training sessions that last too long and are done too frequently with insufficient rest, you drift into a chronic exercise pattern that is destructive to health. Furthermore, a chronic workout pattern promotes mediocrity, because your workouts are too long and too frequent to develop the raw power and explosiveness that the "lift heavy things" law is all about.

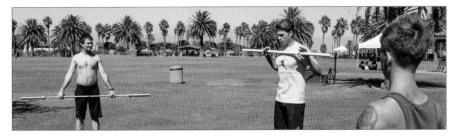

Lifting "heavy things" has broad meaning here. Besides actual weights, machines, and resistance equipment, you can challenge your bodyweight against gravity.

Regarding the particulars of how to balance upper- and lower-body efforts, "push and pull" workout groupings, light weight with high reps or heavy weight with low reps: *it doesn't matter that much!* The idea is to challenge your body on a regular basis with brief, intense workouts involving full-body, functional movements. The specifics of your workout are based on personal preference. You can do just fine using a park bench and monkey bars, frequenting a fancy gym with a high-priced personal trainer, or getting busy in your garage with a few basic weights, elastic tubing, or creative "primal" implements such as kettlebells, slosh tubes, and sandbags. Check out MarksDailyApple.com for hundreds of interesting and challenging resistance workout ideas.

> *Challenge your body on a regular basis with brief, intense workouts involving full-body, functional exercises. The specifics of your workout are based on personal preference.*

Personally, I'm a devoted gym rat, but my faithful appearance at the local gym a few days a week has a heavy social element. Some days I'll be in there for an hour and 15 minutes, shooting the breeze, preening, and trash-talking with my pals, interspersed with some embarrassingly low-effort exercises where I barely sweat. Other days, when I'm feeling fired up, I'll push it hard for 25 minutes of maximum effort sets with short rest. After these workouts, I have trouble slipping my sweatshirt on and sticking my key in the ignition to drive home, but I am exhilarated, and recovery is quick. These hard days are few and far between, but they make a big difference. Overall, once you get the Primal Blueprint eating strategy dialed in, you see that it does not require that much time to maintain excellent all-around functional muscle strength and a lean, toned physique. It's simply a matter of establishing a reasonable baseline commitment of regular workouts, with the occasional super effort that stimulates a fitness breakthrough.

A high-intensity, short-duration workout will stimulate the release of adaptive hormones—particularly testosterone and human growth hormone—that get you lean, energetic, and youthful. Work hard and complete your session in less than 30 minutes, even (or especially) if you are an experienced lifter. That's right—go against the conventional wisdom of long, drawn-out workouts of the same old sets with the same weight and repetitions. Even a 10-minute session can produce excellent fitness benefits.

Always align the difficulty of your sessions with your energy level, and don't push yourself beyond what you are motivated and inspired to do. On the other hand, if you feel energized and ready to ramp it up a notch, go for it!

I suggest you shoot each week for one comprehensive 30-minute session and another abbreviated session lasting 10 to 15 minutes. If you are a "more is better" person, I'll argue in favor of increasing the intensity of these sessions rather than adding additional workouts. Feel free to experiment with the types of exercises that are most fun for you and with a routine that fits most conveniently and comfortably into your daily lifestyle. If you like altering your routine per the popular buzzword "muscle confusion," that's fine. If you are a creature of habit and prefer to do the same workout over and over, that's fine too—as long as it adheres to the "brief, intense, full-body functional movements" description.

The Bonus Material at the end of this book offers descriptions and photographs of what I call the Primal Essential Movements—four simple, safe, bodyweight resistance exercises (pushups, pull-ups, squats, and planks) that can get you super fit in less than an hour a week. Realize that this concept of sporadic, intuitive exercise means you have permission to take—and will, in fact, greatly benefit from—vacation time for your muscles. The more extreme your goals and training regimen are, the more discipline required to balance your overall stress levels on both a micro (daily or weekly) and macro (annual) scale. As I discovered for myself (the hard way), trusting the body's need for balancing rest and intermittent stress can lead to results that are superior—in terms of weight loss or peak competitive performance—compared to the die-hard trainaholics who never miss a workout and never get sufficient rest.

To make sure you are adhering to the Primal Blueprint philosophy, I suggest paying close attention to your energy level and even your emotional state in the hours after a strength workout. After even my toughest sessions, I feel alert, energized, and positive—basically a natural buzz—for hours afterward. My muscles, while certainly not eager to repeat the workout in the immediate future, feel pleasantly relaxed, loose, and warm. In contrast, if your muscles feel stiff and sore after strength sessions, or you feel like taking a nap, raiding the fridge, or snapping at your loved ones, back off on the duration and possibly even the difficulty of the workout. If you routinely experience next-day muscle soreness after your workouts, you are probably going too hard. Once in a while you will feel a little stiff, but you don't have to exhaust yourself to that extent to get and stay strong and explosive.

Strength Workout Specifics

Your strength sessions should generally start with a brief three- to five-minute warmup using light weights or calisthenics specific to the muscle groups you'll be working that day. A few sets of easy pushups and some jumping jacks might be sufficient. For the main set, emphasize exercises that engage a variety of muscles with sweeping, real-life movements (squats, pull-ups, pushups, etc.) instead of a series of isolated body part exercises. (This includes those ever-popular, narrow-range-of-motion ab machines!) Remember that you are striving to achieve a good power-to-weight ratio and balanced, functional, total-body strength. Follow an intuitive and fluctuating approach focused on maintaining a proper balance of stress and rest.

This approach is a simpler and safer alternative to popular routines designed to pack on more muscle than your body is naturally suited for or to produce disproportionate muscles ("Develop huge guns in six weeks!") in the interest of vanity over functionality. For example, I like to run on an inclined treadmill for a few minutes in stocking feet, without letting my heels touch the ground. This offers a real-life functional test for my calves and works the small muscles, tendons, ligaments, and connective tissue in my lower extremities that are otherwise artificially protected and unchallenged in high-tech running shoes. I gradually incline the treadmill to reach from two to five degrees and then steadily increase the speed, making sure my heels don't bear weight or provide propulsion.

Keep in mind that I just made this exercise up one day, and you may or may not like it. However, I think it offers an important counter to the time spent working out and walking around in overly cushioned and arch-supported running shoes. Contrast the broad benefits of this exercise with something like donkey calf-raises. This narrow-range-of-motion exercise (sit with a weighted bar across your knees and lift your toes off the ground repeatedly) has minimal functional benefit; besides, I'll stack my calves up against any bodybuilder's!

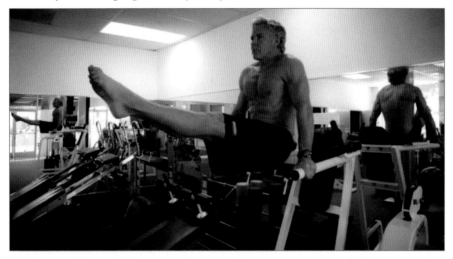

Because Primal Blueprint Fitness workouts are intended to recruit as many muscle fibers as possible and to build functional strength rather than sheer bulk, I wouldn't worry about following some predetermined and deliberate effort-recovery cycle. Instead, try to be slightly explosive with most of your movements. By that I mean you should apply a controlled dynamic force to each repetition such that you complete it at a speed that allows you to maintain form and a reasonable pace for the number of reps you intend to complete. Do that and, believe me, you'll slow down naturally on that final rep or two! This method will fully load the muscle and trigger the biochemical signal to grow stronger.

Much has been written about breathing while lifting weights, some of it relevant (to protect your back from damage) and some of it conjecture. When you apply force, you should generally be either exhaling or holding your breath. This will form a sealed air space in the transverse abdominal muscles of your lower core that protect your lumbar spine. While some camps caution against holding your breath, there is no scientific support to affirm this is harmful. In fact, I find I can bang out two or three reps in a row more effectively when holding my breath and then can catch my breath during a recovery phase. There are many excellent resources—

from certified personal trainers, magazine articles, books, video websites like CrossFit.com, articles on MarksDailyApple.com, and even your imagination (observing certain obvious safety rules, such as spine stability)—to help you create an ideal total body routine for your needs. The possibilities are nearly limitless as long as you honor the strategic rules of Primal Blueprint-style training.

> *My own prescription for health is less paperwork*
> *and more running barefoot through the grass.*
>
> —Leslie Grimutter

PRIMAL BLUEPRINT LAW #5: SPRINT ONCE IN A WHILE

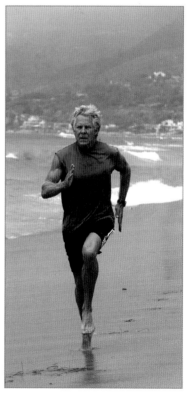

Obviously, Grok's life featured the occasional brief all-out sprint, not for sport but rather to kill or avoid being killed. These bursts of speed were enhanced by fight or flight adrenaline-like chemicals flooding the bloodstream. When Grok survived a run to safety from a charging bear, the resulting biochemical signals prompted a cascade of positive neuroendocrine, hormonal, and gene expression events, the net effect of which was to build stronger, more powerful muscles and an ability to go a little faster the next time.

Modern research confirms the Primal Blueprint premise: the occasional series of short, intense bursts can have a more profound impact on overall fitness—and especially weight loss—than can cardiovascular workouts lasting several times as long. Sprinting elicits a spike of adaptive hormones into the bloodstream, delivering a potent anti-aging effect in the spirit of "use it or lose it." Sprinting improves resilience to physical (muscle contractions) as well as psychological fatigue, allowing you to go longer and faster during sustained efforts at lower intensities. Sprinting, especially high-impact sprints (running), strengthens muscles, joints, and connective tissue. Finally, sprinting can help accelerate fat loss because the intensity of the effort has an extreme impact on your metabolic function for many hours after the workout. Sprinting has been found to elevate your metabolic function up to 30 times higher than resting baseline, a measurement known as Metabolic Equivalent of Task (MET). Thirty MET workouts send a strong adaptive signal to your genes to shed excess body fat, because excess weight is a tremendous hindrance to sprinting performance. Again, this is a survival mechanism to prepare for future (perceived as life-or-death) maximum physical efforts.

The profound benefits of sprint workouts really hit home for me back in the early 1990s when I'd take my personal training clients to the Santa Monica College running track. We'd often share this beautiful facility with some of the world's greatest Olympic sprinters. These physical specimens were a sight to behold. Obviously, they were blessed with remarkable genetic gifts, but it was also clear they were training and living in a manner that brought out the best of their genetic potential. In getting to know some of these athletes and their coaches, it became apparent how remarkably different their training methods were from the prevailing templates of the fitness and nutrition industry.

These Olympians were not out there all day circling the track to exhaustion. Their workouts consisted of minimal amounts of very slow jogging, casual stretching (between competition-specific drills), unhurried efforts to fuss with their equipment (e.g., starting blocks or resistance tools), and, finally, a brief series of explosive

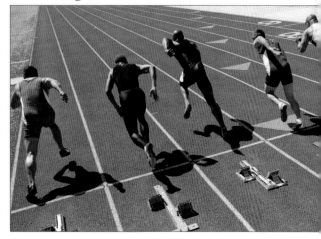

efforts—lasting seconds, not hours. Their banter during these sessions was light; they were always smiling, laughing, joking, and clowning around in between the intense focus of their main sprint sets.

They also spent some serious time in the gym working very hard with weights, but these track and gym sessions were interspersed with frequent easy or rest days, including occasionally sleeping in until double figures and taking daily naps. Their training diets were not laden with tofu, frozen yogurt, and energy bars; they were more likely to feast on chicken and ribs after a workout. Carl Lewis, considered by many to be the greatest Olympic athlete of all time, with nine sprint and long jump gold medals to his credit, reportedly trained only an hour per day at his peak. Three-time Olympic gold medalist and multiple-world-record-holding Jamaican Usain Bolt emphasizes often in his interviews and autobiography how "lazy" he is in training. Maybe he's actually onto something, since he is the fastest human in history.

Introducing sprinting into your exercise routine is not as easy as lacing up a pair of shoes and heading out the door to go jogging. Sprinting is a physically stressful activity that requires a significant fitness base, muscle strength, and flexibility. To reduce injury risk, beginners are advised to choose exercises that are low or no impact. Sprinting up a steep hill (and walking down to commence repeat efforts) offers a lower-impact option than flat running, while stationary cycling presents a no-impact option. I don't recommend outdoor cycle sprints (except for expert riders) due to the danger factor. You can also choose cardio machines (VersaClimber, elliptical, StairMaster, etc.), but I prefer running because the weight-bearing nature (and thus the increased degree of difficulty) of the activity offers maximum benefits, such as improved bone density and greater stimulation for muscle gain/toning and fat loss. If you are unfit, inexperienced, or have joint issues, cycling or using an elliptical machine might be the best way to start.

For running sprints in particular, you'll want to start the first few sessions gently, gradually increasing the speed and intensity of your sprints over time. You also need significant recovery time after sprint workouts. I recommend conducting a sprint workout approximately once every 7 to 10 days, and only when you have high energy and motivation levels. That's right, even as few as two to three sprint sessions per month can produce outstanding fitness benefits and break you out of chronic cardio ruts that may have lasted years.

Running yields the greatest benefits but comes with a higher risk of injury if you are out of practice (say, if you haven't chased down any animals or scored any touchdowns in the last few decades). Novices can start with three to four sprints of 15 seconds, short of full speed, with long rest periods (up to 60 seconds) in between efforts. You will likely experience some muscle soreness in the days after these efforts, but your body will quickly adapt to your new workout routine. You can then build up to a workout that includes six all-out sprints of 8 to 20 seconds (running) or up to 30 seconds per sprint for low- or no-impact sprint workouts (e.g., stationary bike).

All you really ever need to do is six reps, and never longer than the aforementioned times. If you try to sprint for 30 seconds, it's not really a sprint—you can't sustain a true maximum effort for that long running (you can go a bit longer on low-impact sprinting since it's less strenuous). And if you try to do more reps, you'll introduce a fatigue factor to the workout that is not advised. Instead, focus on delivering sprints of *consistent quality* during the workout. This means a similar time and similar perceived exertion for each effort (your perceived exertion should be just below "all-out"—where you feel powerful and in control of your technique, not strained or flailing.) If you are running sprints across an athletic field and the first effort takes 17 seconds, successive efforts should be pretty close to the same time. If you have to try significantly harder to hit 17 seconds, or if you drift up to 20 seconds at the same perceived exertion, it is time to end the workout. As fitness progresses, strive to increase speed before considering increasing the number of reps.

I also recommend supplementing your sprint workouts by conducting technique drills and wind sprints during other workouts. If you devote a few minutes during other workouts to getting your muscles and joints more resilient for sprinting, you will progress quickly and minimize injury risk. Wind sprints entail running slower and shorter efforts than during a formal sprint workout, but taking care to exhibit good technique. A handful of efforts lasting just five to seven seconds, performed at say 85-90 percent of maximum effort, makes for a good wind sprint set. This might be a warmup to a main set of faster running on sprint day, or they can be thrown into a more casual workout another day. Wind sprints and technique drills like exaggerated knee lifts, exaggerated leg turnover, mini-lunges, or hamstring "kickouts" are only moderately strenuous and will condition your muscles, tendons, and joints to perform better and recover faster during your formal workouts.

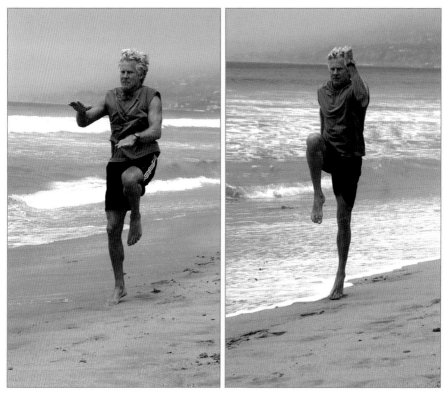

"High knees" and other drills help reinforce good technique and prevent injuries by condition muscles and joints for high-impact sprint workouts.

You should never push your body through an intense workout if you have any symptoms of fatigue, stiffness, soreness, compromised immune system, or another malaise. As discussed with strength training, your sprint sessions should be intuitive, intermittent, and spontaneous—just as they were in primal life for Grok. The occasional sprint workout will elicit the most desirable gene expression effects—much more so than workouts performed come heck or high water just because it's Tuesday.

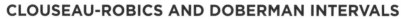

CLOUSEAU-ROBICS AND DOBERMAN INTERVALS

While I've discussed the fight or flight response in the negative context of excessive aerobic exercise or hectic modern life, you should realize that eliciting a stress response is desirable with your sprint workouts. The difference here is that the brief, intense stress is exactly what your genes crave to build fitness and strength and to optimize metabolic function.

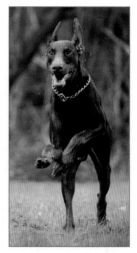

Imagine if every so often someone rudely interrupted your jog around the track by turning a vicious Doberman loose. I guess now you'd run as fast as possible, right? Or, like Inspector Clouseau, say you hired a martial arts master as a personal assistant to launch surprise attacks when you least expect it. Preposterous as it sounds, this type of sporadic, intense, "life-or-death" stimulation just might produce far superior fitness benefits than filling in all the blanks in your training log.

Sprint Workout Specifics

Your sprint efforts should last between 8 and 20 seconds running, and up to 30 seconds for low- or no-impact activities. Choose your duration, recovery interval, and number of repetitions by your ability level. Sprints of 8 seconds or less are fueled by pure ATP in the muscle cell. Sprints of 8 to 20 seconds are fueled by lactate. Maximum efforts between 20 and 30 seconds are fueled by glucose. (Glucose fuels maximum efforts up to two minutes; after that you burn a mix of glucose and fat.) While the scientific particulars may only be relevant to athletes trying to hone sport-specific skills and mimic competitive circumstances (track-and-field events of varied distance, football, soccer, etc.), you might like to vary your routine over time to include short, medium, and longer sprints.

Longer sprints—up to 20 seconds—with short rest develop your anaerobic lactic acid buffering system (a desirable ability for a half-mile or mile race), while the shorter sprints with long rest periods develop your pure speed and explosiveness (such as for a 100-meter race). All types of sprint training will stimulate your fat-burning systems, lean muscle development, and beneficial hormone flow, particularly the release of testosterone and human growth hormone. In this case, even though you will not be burning fat during the actual sprints, your body will become more efficient at burning fat to recover over the long term.

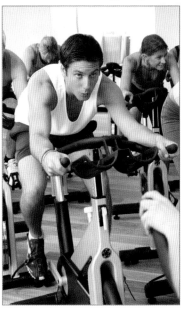

Because the weight-bearing aspect of running makes it significantly more difficult than cycling, running sprints should be shorter than cycling sprints. I prefer gradually ramping up my speed, going all out for about 15 seconds once I hit my sprinting pace, and then taking a full rest period of around 40 seconds between efforts. I'll complete six of these efforts, typically on grass or at the beach on hard sand or even in soft sand. Sometimes I'll get lucky and discover a clean path of deeper soft sand freshly upturned by the beach tractor—begging to be blemished by my footprints! The high-resistance sand sprinting stimulates different muscle groups, as I have to lift my knees higher to generate maximum turnover.

Ideally, you should sprint on a stable natural surface, such as a grass athletic field or the beach. Use a running track or cement road if you can't find a suitable natural surface. While I like uneven surfaces to develop balance and foot strength for walks and hikes, don't risk it for sprinting. Use a smooth, straight, safe course with excellent footing. It can take a long time to acclimate to running sprints, so be patient with your progress. As you gain more competency, you can also aspire to minimize your dependency on bulky running shoes and run your sprints barefoot or in

Vibrams. Again, be patient as you transition toward the advanced exercise of barefoot sprinting.

On other days, my cycling sprints might consist of six 30-second all-out sprints with 2-minute recoveries. Regardless of your specific workout choice, your entire sprint session—including brief warmup and cooldown periods—will require less than 20 minutes. The Sprint Workout Suggestions in the Bonus Material section offer several options for novice, intermediate, and advanced workouts, including an exciting plyometric workout, a stadium steps workout, and a couple of low- or no-impact sprint options, such as sprinting up steep hills or on a stationary bike.

Proper Running and Cycling Form

In order to prevent injury and ensure your movements are as efficient and powerful as possible, proper form is key. You must respect these important basics:

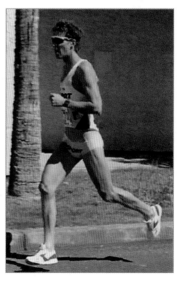

Running: Torso faces forward at all times, shoulders and pelvis square to your forward direction. Refrain from side-to-side swiveling of the hips or the shoulder girdle. Arms and hands are relaxed as pumping is initiated from the shoulders. Elbows are bent at 90-degree angles. Don't let arms or hands cross the centerline of your body. Focus on fast turnover by striding in a motion similar to pedaling a bicycle. Lift foot quickly off the ground in a dorsiflexed position (toes pulled up, foot flexed), drive knees high, and then initiate the next stride quickly. Your heel should nearly kick your butt during the recovery phase of the stride. Envision your foot clearing the height of your opposite knee on each stride.

Triathlon legend Andrew MacNaughton let his moods dictate his workout decisions—a sage approach that took him to the top of the sport.

When you experience the inevitable tightening up midway through your sprint, focus on keeping your face, arms, and hands loose and relaxed. Notice in videos or photographs of Olympic sprinters how their jaws are slack and their hands are soft and open. Be aware of your breathing rhythm and resist the temptation to hold your breath or pant shallowly. Take deep, powerful breaths by focusing on a forceful exhale.

Cycling: Strive for a rhythmic cadence in a range of 80 to 100 revolutions per minute. Most recreational cyclists pedal at far too low a cadence, putting excessive strain on the muscles instead of balancing the cardiovascular and muscular load with an efficient cadence. Focus on applying circular force to the pedals rather than just stomping down. I highly recommend a clip-in pedaling system to achieve a proper circular stroke. Maintain a level pelvis at all times. Do not rock your pelvis from side to side in an effort to impart more force. Keep your upper body virtually still, with arms, chest, neck, and head relaxed and supple.

Be sure that your seat height is appropriate. A quick test is to place your heel (unclip it from the pedal) on the pedal axle when it's at the very bottom of the pedal stroke. You should be able to extend your leg fully (with pelvis level) and barely touch (or barely miss) the pedal axle. A seat that is too high or too low will stress the knees and also lead to rocking. Resist the temptation to tense your muscles when the effort becomes difficult. Breathe deeply by inflating your diaphragm fully on the inhale. Because you are bent over, you should feel your diaphragm pressing against your rib cage when you inhale; then relax and allow a natural exhale.

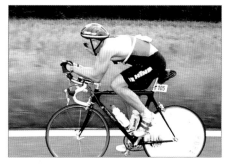
Mike Pigg terrorized the triathlon circuit for a decade with his fluid technique and aerodynamic position.

Happy Feet

One of the most annoying non-primal elements of today's fitness movement is shoes. You heard me, shoes are lame. Sure, typical athletic shoes provide substantial support, cushioning, and general protection, but they also immobilize your feet inside the shoe—much like being in a cast.

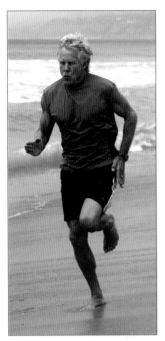

Hence, the complex network of 52 bones (a quarter of the total in your entire body) and dozens of tendons, ligaments, and small muscles cannot work their magic to provide balance, stability, impact absorption, weight transfer, and propulsion.

Constantly wearing shoes during exercise and daily life leads to weakened feet, fallen arches, shortened Achilles tendons and calf muscles, imbalances between the hamstrings and quadriceps, an inefficient gait, and, of course, recurring pain and injury. The 43 million Americans who experience foot problems daily (we will spend an estimated $900 million annually on foot care products) offer another disturbing example of living in conflict with our ancestral heritage.

Granted, shoes are essential for contact sports or activities involving hard surfaces, such as football, soccer, basketball, volleyball, running on the road, and the like. However, for your purposes of conducting basic Primal Blueprint Fitness activities, going shoeless on occasion (and gradually increasing frequency over time) is possible and beneficial. Keep in mind that a lifetime spent in "casts"—desensitizing and weakening your feet for their primary functional purpose—will require that you proceed with extreme caution with your barefoot endeavors. Here again I'll make a concession for modern life (I don't think Grok had any broken glass to worry about on his hikes) by recommending you try gradually integrating minimalist shoes like Vibram FiveFingers into your workout and daily routine.

The Vibram FiveFingers consists of a lightweight, form-fitting rubber sole attached to a nylon-like sock and a hook-and-loop closure system. Vibrams slip onto your bare feet like fingers into a glove (with a slot for each toe) and offer excellent protection from sharp objects and debris.

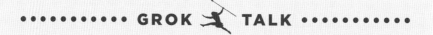

The Vibram company made headlines in 2014 when they settled a class action lawsuit brought by people who became injured wearing the shoes. These poor victims claimed that they relied on misleading claims about how wearing Vibrams can help strengthen feet. Primal Blueprint Law #9—Avoid Stupid Mistakes comes to mind... Looking at the product, it's pretty obvious you are not getting the same support as a padded shoe and that you might wanna proceed in a measured way with a transition to more barefoot time. Duh.

"I ran five miles in these things yesterday and my calves are really sore. It seems like there's no support"

"That's outrageous, egregious, and irresponsible. I think we have a strong case"

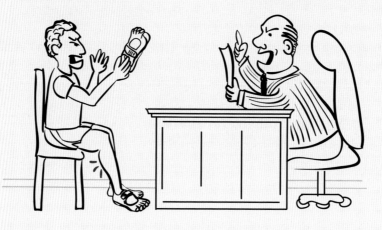

While Vibram offers the most authentic barefoot experience with the individual toe compartments and the form-fitting sole, it's an extreme departure from typical active footwear and can consequently present an injury risk if you are too enthusiastic with your barefoot efforts. With the explosion in popularity of the barefoot movement over the past decade, there are now numerous other minimalist footwear options available. Consider the choices offered by Merrell (merrell.com) and other compa-

The only exercise some people get is jumping to conclusions, running down their friends, side-stepping responsibility, and pushing their luck!

—Author Unknown

nies, where you can choose from models offering a graduated assortment of cushioning and support. More support is important for use on rocky trails. You can also strive to gradually minimize the amount of heel lift in your footwear until you are comfortable in a "zero drop" (heel is not elevated from toe box) shoe that allows for the best range of motion and functionality of your Achilles tendon.

Make an effort to gradually introduce barefoot time into your workouts and everyday life, providing ample time for your feet to adjust and get stronger without undue shock. For example, on my first few long hikes in FiveFingers, I kept my normal shoes in a small pack just in case I needed them. Some mild next-day soreness in your calves and arches is to be expected after your initial barefoot endeavors. This is just a natural part of the adaptation process, just as with strength training. However, make sure you don't experience any pain during your efforts to get your feet more primal. Be particularly careful if you are minimally active or overweight or if you have a history of foot problems or other medical issues. As with most other primal activities, it is better to ease into a new form of exercise than to overdo it.

You can get some low-risk barefoot time by adopting the Eastern tradition of removing your shoes when you enter your house and otherwise using minimal footwear whenever you don't need the protection or decorum of more substantial footwear. Get a pair or two of minimalist footwear, use them first for walking around, then for short workouts, and gradually increase your use as you remain pain-free. Many runners will conduct their distance runs in traditional shoes, then end the session by jogging a mile or two on grass in Vibrams or bare feet. Hopefully one day you'll work up to running some sprints barefoot—it doesn't get any more primal than that!

CHAPTER SUMMARY

1. Primal Blueprint Exercise Laws: Mirroring Grok's active lifestyle is not a complex endeavor requiring the extensive time, money, or specific equipment that conventional wisdom suggests is necessary to achieve fitness. You can get extremely fit in as little as a few hours a week, provided you exercise strategically with a balance of extensive low-intensity movement (blending structured aerobic workouts and increased general everyday activity), periodic high-intensity, short-duration strength-training sessions, and occasional all-out sprints.

Best results will come when your exercise routine is unstructured and intuitive, and workout choices are aligned with your energy and motivation levels. Always allow for sufficient recovery and pursue goals that are fun and inspiring. Weight-loss goals are attainable when you combine primal eating and frequent low-level exercise (fine-tuning your fat-burning system) with occasional brief, intense strength and sprint sessions (to stimulate an increase in lean muscle and metabolic rate).

2. Primal Blueprint Fitness: Primal Blueprint Fitness means you have a broad range of skills and attributes (strength, power, speed, and endurance, with power-to-weight ratio as a critical benchmark) that allow you to do pretty much whatever you want with a substantial degree of competence and minimal risk of injury. In contrast, narrow, specialized fitness goals are popular today (e.g., for endurance athletes and bodybuilders). These goals often compromise functional fitness and general health. By exercising—and eating—Primal Blueprint style, you will develop the unmistakable physique of a well-balanced athlete and eliminate the drawbacks of narrowly focused, overly stressful exercise programs.

3. Organ Reserve: Leading an active lifestyle and maintaining functional lean muscle mass correlates with optimal organ function and longevity, because your organs must keep up with the physical demands you place upon your body. In contrast, inactivity will accelerate the aging process; weak muscles make for weak organs. Maintaining organ reserve with good fitness habits will make the chronological component of aging minimally relevant—organs take around 120 years to wear out naturally!

4. Move Frequently: Primal Blueprint Law #3 is a matter of blending structured aerobic workouts at a comfortable heart rate (not to exceed 180 minus age in beats per minute) with increasing all forms of general everyday movement. This means taking the dog for a stroll around the block, taking stairs instead of elevators, taking frequent breaks from your work desk to walk the halls or courtyard, performing some brief stretches, calisthenics, or yoga moves, and generally doing everything you can to avoid prolonged periods of inactivity and get your body moving.

Structured aerobic workouts such as walking, hiking, easy cycling, cardio machines, or (if you are fit) jogging at a moderate pace offer excellent health benefits, including improved cardiovascular, musculoskeletal, and immune function and fat metabolism. In contrast, chronic cardio (a pattern of sustained workouts that exceed the 180 minus age aerobic maximum heart rate) can deplete the body of energy (leading to increased appetite for quick-energy carbohydrates), inhibit fat metabolism, suppress immune function, promote overuse injuries, and generally result in the condition best described as burnout. Hard to believe, but slowing down workout pace and moving around more in daily life help you reduce excess body fat in ways that more vigorous workouts will not. When you emphasize aerobic, fat-burning workouts, you produce less inflammation and oxidative damage than an overly stressful, glucose-burning exercise pattern generates.

Complementary flexibility/mobility practices such as yoga, Pilates, tai chi and properly executed stretching are recommended to increase flexibility, range of motion, balance, and coordination, to prevent injury, and to counteract the weaknesses and imbalances that arise from both being too sedentary and engaging in chronic cardio patterns. Stretching must be done properly to avoid injury risk: warm up muscles first with brief cardio. Emphasize dynamic (moving through range of motion), functional, full-body stretches on warm muscles.

5. Lift Heavy Things: Best results in strength training come from a sporadic routine of workouts that are brief in duration and intense and explosive in nature. These workouts will stimulate the release of adaptive hormones such as testosterone and human growth hormone, helping improve body composition and delaying the aging process. Exercises should focus on natural human movements (lunges, squats, plyometrics, pushups, pull-ups, planks, and other body weight resistance exercises) instead of isolations on narrow-range-of-motion gym machines. The difficulty of your workouts should be aligned with energy and motivation levels: push hard when you feel like it and take it easy or skip workouts when you are tired. With this approach, you will avoid the risk of injury, exhaustion, and burnout that comes from trying to follow a consistent schedule of exhaustive, long-duration strength training sessions that are done too frequently and are too lengthy to be considered truly explosive. These types of "chronic" strength workouts lead to an overproduction of stress hormones and send you toward burnout in the same manner as does chronic cardio.

Primal-style strength training sessions can be completed in as little as 10 minutes and never longer than 30 minutes. Twice a week is plenty for even experienced strength trainers. When in doubt, go hard or go home!

6. Sprint Once in a While: No workout is more primal than an all-out sprint. Efforts like these fueled human evolution through survival of the fittest! Today you can enjoy excellent fitness, body composition, and health benefits from intense sprinting, modeling the "use it or lose it" principle. All-out sprint sessions should be conducted sporadically when energy and motivation levels are high. Sprint efforts should last between 8 and 20 seconds for running (up to 30 seconds for low- or no-impact activities), with complete rest between efforts to ensure maximum performance. Strive to deliver *consistent quality* of efforts, where each sprint is similar in time and perceived exertion level. Complete four to six sprints in a workout, along with proper warmup and cooldown, Novices can do low-impact options, such as uphill sprints or stationary bicycle sprints. Formal sprint workouts can be supported by brief efforts of technique drills and wind sprints (perhaps thrown into less strenuous workouts) that improve technique and resiliency of muscles, tendons, and joints.

7. Technique: Proper form in running and cycling is imperative. For running, the body should always face forward, the center of gravity should be stable, and wasted motion (e.g., side-to-side movement) should be eliminated. Focus on striding in a circular motion (a la cycling) with center of gravity always balanced over feet. For cycling, ensure proper seat height and apply circular force while pedaling at a rapid, efficient cadence of 80 to 10 rpm.

8. Barefoot: Make a gradual transition to spending more time barefoot or in minimalist shoes during daily life and during workouts. Going barefoot will recalibrate your entire musculoskeletal system so that you walk, stand, and move more efficiently in all manner of daily activity, including appropriate fitness and athletic endeavors. By increasing your barefoot competency, you will reduce the risk of chronic pain and injury to your feet and through your lower extremities, and you will actually improve your technique, balance, explosiveness, speed, endurance, and kinesthetic awareness.

Vibram FiveFingers provide the most authentic barefoot experience. There are numerous graduated options available from other footwear companies that offer a minimalist experience with more protection and less injury risk than cold-turkey efforts. Strive to make a safe, sensible, gradual transition to a more barefoot-dominant lifestyle. By doing so, you will eliminate the hazards of wearing bulky shoes that restrict natural foot motion, weaken stabilizing and propulsion muscles, and increase risk of chronic pain and injury—the very things cushiony shoes are claiming to prevent!

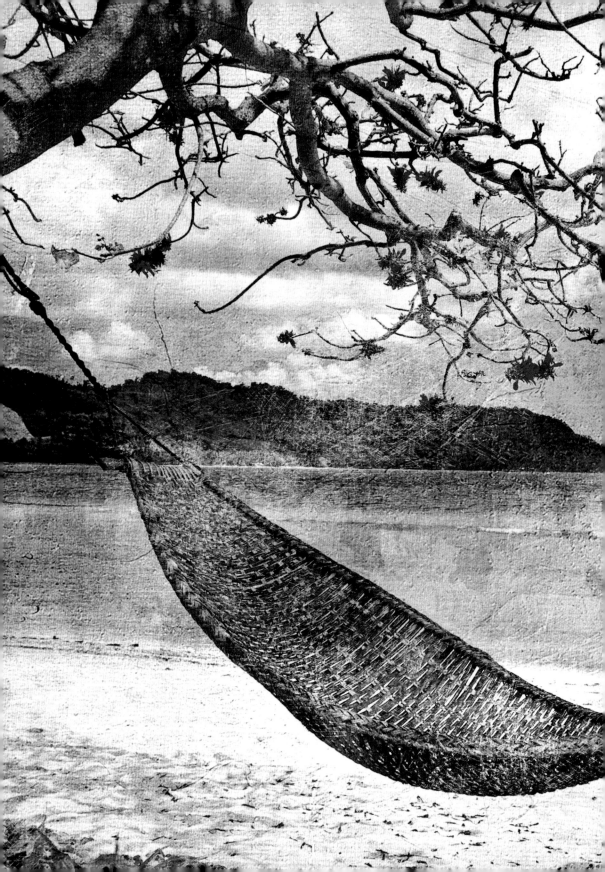

CHAPTER EIGHT

PRIMAL BLUEPRINT LIFESTYLE LAWS

If You Don't Snooze, You Lose

IN THIS CHAPTER

I detail the five lifestyle laws of the Primal Blueprint: Law #6, Get Plenty of Sleep; Law #7, Play; Law #8, Get Plenty of Sunlight; Law #9, Avoid Stupid Mistakes; and Law #10, Use Your Brain. While Grok's diet and exercise patterns were clearly major influences in shaping how his (and our) genes evolved, there were other environmental and behavioral forces that were no less important in perfecting the DNA recipe for a healthy, vibrant human being.

Law #6, Get Plenty of Sleep, delivers obvious benefits but is widely compromised today. Good sleep entails understanding the basic physiology of sleep cycles, establishing consistent habits, minimizing artificial light and digital stimulation after dark, taking advantage of the benefits of napping, and effectively prioritizing your time. Law #7, Play, is a widely neglected lifestyle law that can deliver widespread benefits and make you quantifiably more productive when balanced effectively with work. Law #8, Get Plenty of Sunlight, is an area where conventional wisdom has let us down, scaring us into avoiding the outdoors due to misinterpreted risks of skin cancer. Obtaining optimal levels of vitamin D, synthesized from sun exposure on your skin, is critical to cellular health and cancer prevention.

Law #9, Avoid Stupid Mistakes, explains how our obsessive desire to control or eliminate all sources of potential danger has made us lazy and inattentive. Cultivating the skills of vigilance and risk management is essential to avoid self-inflicted trauma and unnecessary suffering. Law #10, Use Your Brain, is about pursuing creative intellectual outlets unrelated to your core daily responsibilities and economic contribution. Finding more stuff to do with your brain may seem counterintuitive to many of us who feel our brain function and mental energy is maxed out each day. However, the unrelenting pace of modern life and intense pressure to achieve and consume strongly conflict with our genetic makeup and can lead to feelings of restlessness and discontent. Making time for hobbies and personal growth challenges will keep you feeling refreshed and excited about life.

I am two with nature.

—Woody Allen

PRIMAL BLUEPRINT LAW #6: GET PLENTY OF SLEEP

For billions of years, nearly all life forms on Earth evolved to be biologically in sync with the consistent rising and setting of the sun. This circadian rhythm (from Latin: circa, meaning "around" and dia, meaning "day") governs our sleeping and eating patterns, as well as the precise timing of important hormone secretions, brain wave patterns, and cellular repair and regeneration based on a 24-hour cycle. When we interfere with our circadian rhythm via excessive artificial light and digital stimulation after sunset, irregular bed and wake times, jetlag, graveyard shift work, and alarm clocks, we disrupt some of the very processes we depend upon to stay healthy, happy, productive, and focused.

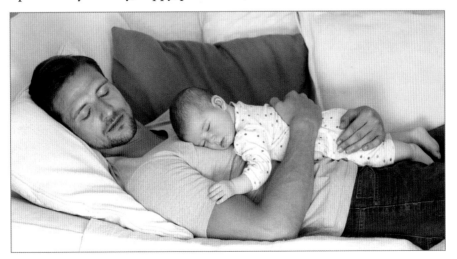

Conventional wisdom usually recommends seven to eight hours of sleep per night, but optimizing sleep is not as simple as that. In *Lights Out: Sleep, Sugar, and Survival*, authors T. S. Wiley (anthropologist and medical theorist) and Bent Formby, Ph.D. (biochemist, biophysicist, molecular biologist) emphasize the importance of syncing your sleep with your circadian rhythm; they recommend getting nine-and-a-half hours per night during the darker months of the year, with less sleep acceptable during the long daylight hours of summer. Obviously, the variation in your sleep duration by season will be more extreme the farther you live from the equator.

In addition to obtaining the requisite number of hours, your sleep must be of high quality—not hampered by a disruptive environment, objectionable medications or foods, or behaviors that elevate stress hormone production (vigorous exercise, digital screen use, or other high stimulation) in the hours before bed. Calm, quiet, dark evenings, and consistent bed and wake times, are critical factors for high-quality sleep.

Sleep was long thought to be a passive state, but we now understand sleep to be a dynamic process. The brain is active during sleep (but responding to internal stimuli, not external), and it drifts in and out of various sleep stages in a cyclical pattern. Our natural sleep cycle oscillates between stages of lighter sleep (Stage 1, the transition from wake to sleep; and rapid eye movement, or REM, when you experience vivid dreams and can be woken easily) and deeper sleep (Stage 2 and slow-wave sleep, together called non-REM sleep, when you are out like a light and experience maximum restorative hormone flow, rebalancing of brain chemicals, and cellular repair in muscles and organs). This cycling of non-REM into REM, back and forth, is repeated throughout the night, with each complete cycle lasting about 90 minutes.

If you divide your night's sleep into three equal time periods, the highest percentage of non-REM sleep occurs in the first third, while the final third of your sleep time is characterized by a lengthening of the REM cycles and a shortening of the deep sleep cycles. The middle third is a balance between the first and the last. Waking up naturally involves letting the cycles play out until finally, after a period of exclusive REM sleep, you wake up effortlessly. REM sleep is characterized by increases in heart rate, respiration, and muscle and brain wave activity, making it easy to rise from this more alert state.

The sleep hormone melatonin presides over you falling asleep and going through the sleep cycles. Melatonin is manufactured in the pineal gland near the center of the brain. As light diminishes, the pineal starts to convert the feel-good hormone serotonin, which has kept your mood elevated all day (and which is why so many of us take SSRI meds—to avoid depleting serotonin), to increasing amounts of melatonin. This process is called dim light melatonin onset (DLMO), and its effects include relaxing brain waves and muscles, lowering your blood pressure, reducing your body temperature, slowing your heart rate and respiration, and ultimately coaxing you toward sleepiness. After sleep, with the morning light stimulating your central nervous system, melatonin production is suppressed and serotonin begins to increase, along with cortisol, to help you transition to a wakeful state. As the hormone balance shifts, you wake feeling mentally and physically refreshed and ready to face the day.

At least, that's how it's *supposed* to work. In our modern world, evenings of artificial light and digital stimulation wildly disrupt these light-sensitive hormones. When your retinas get blasted with artificial light after sunset, melatonin production is suppressed while stress hormone levels are elevated. This gives you that familiar second wind of energy and alertness to crank through your email inbox or Netflix queue. Right at the time when your body should be feeling sleepy, the influx of light-triggered stress hormones keeps you wired, prompts sugar cravings, and, hormonally, kicks you into fat storage mode.

The quality of light matters, too. Light bulbs, computers, televisions, smartphone screens, and other electronic gadgets all emit *blue light*—a vivid hue on the electromagnetic spectrum that can spike cortisol, suppress melatonin, increase insulin production, hamper leptin signaling, and spike ghrelin. Chronic blue light exposure after dark dramatically impacts your sleep quality and makes you more vulnerable to oxidative damage, accelerated aging, and fatigue. It can even increase your risk for certain cancers and degenerative eye disease.

We are all well aware that sleep is an indispensable component of proper immune and metabolic functioning, growth, and tissue and muscle repair; that it's critical for cognitive and social functioning, memory, and emotional wellbeing; and that a good night's sleep feels fantastic. Unfortunately, we are egregiously disregarding the importance of sleep in modern life. Study after study show that an increasing number of Americans are seriously sleep deficient. A 2013 Gallup poll found that American adults get an average of 6.8 hours of sleep nightly, compared to 7.9 hours in 1942, and 40 percent reported getting 6 or fewer hours per night. According to a 2011 survey from the National Sleep Foundation (NSF), over 60 percent of American adults believe they are not getting enough sleep, with about the same number reporting that they have problems sleeping "every night or almost every night." Furthermore, the NSF recently reported that according to their parents, 29 percent of 12- to 14-year-olds and 56 percent of 15- to 17-year-olds get 7 hours of sleep or less per night—much less than their growing brains and bodies need. All in all, the numbers point to a serious sleep problem in this country.

Chronic sleep deficit may lead to weight gain by affecting how your body processes and stores carbohydrates and by altering hormones that affect your appetite and metabolism. It can negatively impact your mood, concentration, and memory retention during the day, making you less productive and more irritable and impatient. Insufficient sleep can also lead to hypertension, elevated stress hormone levels, irregular heartbeat, compromised immune function, and drastically increased risk for obesity and heart disease. Irregular sleep patterns are implicated in some cancers (for example, among night shift workers).

Our natural (or actually I should say, "learned") inclination to be constantly entertained is difficult to balance with our need for adequate restoration. It's not until we are truly exhausted that sleep moves up the hierarchy of wants and needs. It shouldn't be that way. Sure, you can get away with some occasional departures from your routine with no ill effects. Just as with your dietary choices, if you are able to observe a consistent bedtime 80 percent of the time, the 20 percent of the time when you stay up late, wake up super early, or otherwise skimp on perfect rest won't be as dangerously taxing on your body. On the other hand, if you consistently disrespect healthy sleep habits, you create momentum in the wrong direction and will struggle to achieve basic health and fitness goals, especially losing excess body fat.

In today's hectic, overscheduled world, adults (and unfortunately children, too) sacrifice sleep to squeeze in one more activity, a few chores, another hour or two of work, or just one more TV episode. Sleep is easy to forgo because it feels less important in the moment than finishing up that work project, say, and because being tired the next day seems a small price to pay. Of course, the price of chronically skimping on sleep is much greater than that, as you now know. And on the flip side, getting sufficient high-quality sleep can help facilitate all the other things we want to do during the day by sharpening our cognitive faculties, allowing our body to build muscle and recover from illness and injury, and generally warding off the fatigue that makes it hard to get motivated to get going.

If you are not getting enough sleep, it is imperative that you find concrete ways to carve out more sleep time, whether that means signing out of your work email every evening at a certain time, shortening your early morning workouts, or dropping out of that late-night indoor soccer league. I know this is easier said than done for many, and it might mean making some hard choices, but it an absolutely crucial step if you want to take charge of your health. Now is the time to make steps in the right direction.

How to Get an "A" in "Zs"

Here are some important measures you can take to get optimum amounts of high-quality sleep. Visit MarksDailyApple.com for more discussion on this topic, including some helpful tips to beat jetlag.

Minimize Artificial Light and Digital Stimulation after Dark: Limiting your nighttime exposure to bright, artificial lights and digital stimulation should be your first line of defense for improving sleep quality. Ideally, you should shut off blue-light emitting screens—like your smartphone, computer, TV, or tablet—two hours before bedtime (at the bare minimum, one hour). If you must work on a computer or check your email on your smartphone after sunset, download the free software program f.lux (available for all platforms at justgetflux.com) to adjust the color temperature of your electronic screens and synchronize with the ambient light of your environment. If you are an iPhone or iPad user, Apple has gotten wise to the problems of blue light at night and in March, 2016, added to its latest operating system a feature called "Night Shift," which automatically changes the quality of the light emitted from your device at

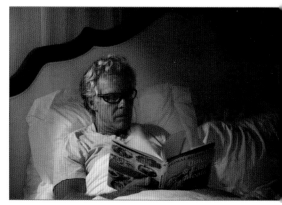

Screens are off in the final hour before bedtime, and I'll wind down with a good book and some mellow yellow lenses before lights out.

night to make it less disruptive to your circadian rhythm. Other devices have similar features. Activate this in your device settings (but still make an effort to power down your electronics well before bedtime).

As much as possible, favor candlelight or firelight soon after sundown, or switch out some of your harsh, regular light bulbs for orange "insect" bulbs (available at hardware/home supply stores) to create a similar effect. Consider getting a pair of yellow- or orange-tinted UV protection glasses to wear indoors at night, which will ensure the light reaching your eyes falls in the red-orange-yellow spectrum (which, unlike blue light, doesn't interfere with melatonin production).

Create an Ideal Sleeping Environment: It's critical to make your bedroom an area of minimal stimulation and maximum relaxation. Your bedroom should be used only for sleeping (well, okay, that other stuff, too), with absolutely no computer, television, work desk, or clutter. Aim for complete darkness, and eliminate nightlights and LED screen emissions, and even small lights from power indicators and phone chargers.

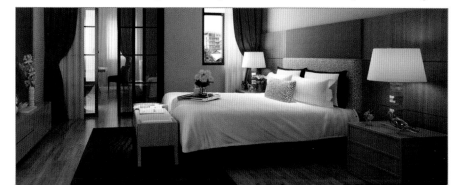

(You can keep a flashlight by the bed for the times you need to get up.) Keep the room temperature in the range of 60-68°F (16-20°C); we're hardwired to sleep in colder temperatures. You should have a clear physical and psychological separation between your bedroom and other areas of the house where you do work or enjoy entertainment. Browse the Internet or page through design magazines to get a feeling for the beauty of contemporary, minimalist bedroom styles.

Follow Consistent Bed and Wake Times: Establish a consistent, circadian-rhythm-friendly routine to optimize hormone flows and ensure that you enjoy sufficient sleep cycles (which might mean gradually altering your bedtime and wake-time to align with the changing of seasons). Remember that melatonin floods your bloodstream on circadian cues triggered by darkness. For 2.5 million years, that meant sunset; today it means *the time that you make it dark*. You experience the highest percentage of deep sleep at the outset of your night. Sorry, but if you miss bedtime, sleeping in to reach your typical hourly total will not completely catch you up.

If you are a night owl, you can probably develop some level of tolerance for a consistent, artificial-light-induced late-night bedtime and an artificially darkened late-morning awakening. If circumstances such as shift work require that your sleep habits depart from the Earth's natural light and dark cycles, make a strong effort to sleep with an eye mask (check mindfold.com for a total darkness sleep mask) in a completely darkened room, since all of your skin cells (not just your eyes) are sensitive and responsive to light.

Wind Down the Night and Ease into the Day: It's important to wind down calmly in the hours preceding your bedtime. Minimize your central nervous system stimulation before going to bed so you can have a smooth, relaxing transition from your busy day to downtime. Take an evening stroll with the dog, enjoy some mellow hobbies like drawing or board games, or chat with loved ones. Reading is a time-tested popular method to wind down, but choose fiction or something light to promote maximum relaxation; stay far away from disturbing news or work-related documents.

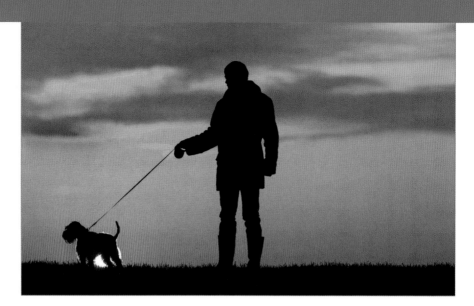

It may also be helpful to decompress your busy brain by jotting down your thoughts before bed. Take 5 or 10 minutes to write out everything from your day—accomplishments, stresses, and concerns—as well as goals or to-dos for the following day. This is especially helpful if you are troubled by a problem. It's easier to arrive at solutions if you don't try consciously to force them. Get your worries down on paper, and then let your sleeping mind do the work for you. You'll wake up feeling clearer and more positive.

No day is so bad it can't be fixed with a nap.

—Carrie Snow
Stand-up comedian

In the morning, awaken gradually and naturally (which means ditching disruptive alarms as much as possible). Staying in bed for a few minutes to read or talk ("Again, your name was… ?"), or starting your day with some light breathing and stretching exercises, is preferable to springing up after a blaring alarm and rushing into action. Resist the urge to check your phone or email first thing in the morning, as exposure to news or personal communication can trigger a stress response and throw you into a reactive, overstimulated mode. A brief warm shower can help stimulate your central nervous system naturally and get blood circulating—a particularly good idea if you are going to exercise soon after awakening.

Enjoying a cup of herbal tea, taking the dog out for a walk, stepping outside for some fresh air, stretching in the morning sunlight, or engaging in another calming ritual can help you welcome the day in a more pleasant way. Hard-core Grok disciples can even try a cold-water plunge upon awakening in the summer months—beats a high-carb breakfast any day as a morning energizer!

Eat and Drink the Right Stuff: Eat your last meal a couple hours or more before bed so digestion does not interfere with your sleep process. Forget the popular magazine blather about dosing with carbs before bed (insulin hampers melatonin release) or eating tryptophan rich foods like nuts or turkey to facilitate sleep. The best sleep aid is to have your digestive system relaxed in the hours before bed. This is especially true for alcohol consumption. Even casual drinkers might unknowingly suffer from compromised sleep cycles due to the delayed effects of metabolizing alcohol consumed earlier in the evening. Consider an abstention experiment (I detailed my own at MarksDailyApple.com) and see if you sleep more soundly. If you have trouble falling asleep or enjoy a bedtime ritual involving tea, chamomile in particular is touted for its mild sedative effect.

Put the Nap Back on the Map

Historically, many cultures across the world have long had a great appreciation for naptime, especially in warm-weather countries in Latin America, Asia, the Mediterranean, North Africa, and the Middle East. Unfortunately, it seems the fast pace of modern life (combined, perhaps, with some weird puritanical guilt factors) prevents napping from being a culturally acceptable lifestyle habit in many places today. Developing a habit of taking downtime when you need it can help you stay happy, productive, and stress-balanced throughout the day. If you have obstacles that hamper your evening sleep, napping can become essential to preserve your health. Even if you have minimal complaints about your nighttime sleep, a routine afternoon nap can help give you a significant productivity boost that you may not even realize you need and deserve.

> *Develop the awareness and the discipline to go down for 20 minutes and perhaps up to 90 minutes when you experience daytime sleepiness.*

The reality is, we are all hard-wired to nap! You have undoubtedly experienced that post-lunch dip in energy levels where you feel sleepy and it's hard to focus on your work. This doesn't happen just because you ate too much; it is a natural part of your circadian rhythm. We all experience a lull somewhere around 2:00 P.M. (We experience a similar dip around 2:00 A.M., but hopefully you don't notice because you are asleep.) In fact, scientists call the period of the early afternoon, between 1:00 and 3:00, the "nap zone," and some cite this as evidence that we are biologically programmed to be biphasic sleepers (to sleep in two distinct periods—a long sleep at night and a nap during the day).

In addition to the circadian rhythm, the sleep-wake cycle is governed by a process called the *homeostatic sleep drive*, or sleep pressure. Scientists believe that sleep pressure is specifically linked to slow-wave sleep—the deep, most restorative sleep. If you are deficient in slow-wave sleep, either because you have not slept well at night or because you have been awake and cranking away on your busy day for many hours, you will experience a lot of sleep pressure urging you to nod off. This could be another reason we desire a nap, especially in the afternoon, as sleep pressure builds throughout the day.

Many experts recommend a nap period of approximately 20 minutes in order to recharge and wake feeling rejuvenated. This is ideal for increasing alertness and improving motor functioning. However, naps of up to 90 minutes can be beneficial, especially if you are running behind on nighttime sleep. That's a wide range, so it really should be left to personal preference how long your nap lasts. Ideally, you can set aside time for whatever duration nap you might need and awaken naturally when the time is right. Obviously, if your evening sleep habits are optimal, you will probably only need occasional 20-minute naps to get an "A" in sleep. If you are perennially exhibiting poor nighttime sleep habits, you may

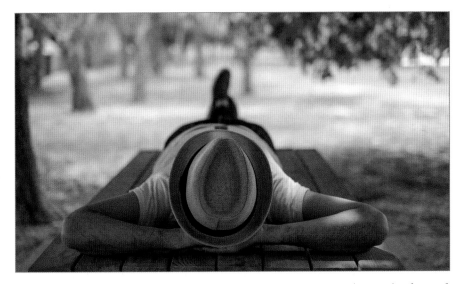

require frequent hour-long power sessions to get your brain, body, and immune system functioning optimally.

If your naps last up to an hour or beyond, chances are you will awaken to that familiar post-nap grogginess, officially called *sleep inertia*. The sensation can be unpleasant, especially as you might be eager to get up and going with your busy day after a nap. People often use sleep inertia as an excuse to skip naps, falsely believing that it can compromise your ability to fall asleep later in the evening. The truth is that sleep inertia isn't bad—it just means you woke up from slow-wave sleep. If you just ride out that groggy feeling you will feel refreshed and ready to go in a matter of minutes. If you are worried about the folklore that suggests napping will interfere with your ability to fall asleep at night, fear not. Naps, even those fog-inducing deep sleep beauties, are unlikely to compromise your ability to fall asleep successfully.

If you plan correctly, you can actually nap strategically to reap specific benefits, according to Dr. Sara Mednick, one of the world's leading sleep experts, a Harvard-trained psychologist currently a professor at UC Riverside, and author of *Take a Nap—Change Your Life*. Dr. Mednick explains that morning naps will contain proportionately more REM sleep than afternoon naps, which will contain more slow-wave sleep. For that reason, morning naps will be better for recharging creative thinking skills and solidifying emotional memories, while afternoon naps are better for reinforcing learning and improving cognitive function. If you time your nap to fall in the perfect "nap zone" and nap for a sufficient duration, you will get the best of both worlds.

Develop the awareness and the discipline to go down for 20 minutes and perhaps up to 90 minutes, any time you experience daytime sleepiness. Even better, prioritize a block of nap time in your daily schedule to improve productivity, alertness, and mental clarity. Even if you are not practiced in napping and feel like you are not able to fall asleep easily, routinely getting away from your normal high-stimulatory environment for a 20-minute rest period in a cool, quiet, dark setting can provide excellent restorative benefits. With practice, you will likely find yourself increasingly able to relax on demand and eventually become a pro at actually nodding off during your nap time. Consequently, you will join other luminaries throughout history known for their ability to unplug: Winston Churchill, John F. Kennedy, Napoleon, Albert Einstein, Thomas Edison, Leonardo da Vinci, and all five Kardashian sisters.

Art is older than production [making things for practical use] for us, and play older than work. Man was shaped less by what he had to do than by what he did in playful moments. It is the child in man that is the source of his uniqueness and creativeness.

—Eric Hoffer
American writer and philosopher (1902-1983)

PRIMAL BLUEPRINT LAW #7: PLAY

Most people pay lip service to the fact that play—activities done just for the enjoyment they bring—is important for happiness and wellbeing, yet compliance with this primal law, even among health-minded people, is low. We have been so heavily socialized into regimented, technological, industrialized life that scheduling time for play (now there's an oxymoron!) is a big challenge. I don't know about you, but I don't think the word *playdate* existed when I was a kid. Oh, we had play dates in my neighborhood, all right—365 of them, to be exact. They lasted from the final school bell till the dinner bell and were not deterred by mud, rain, sleet, or snow (no kidding, I'm from Maine!). We didn't need our moms making transportation arrangements via e-mail or cell phone. We just needed air in our lungs, bike tires, and basketballs.

As the challenges and responsibilities of making a living or managing a family accumulate in our adult years, we collectively adopt the belief that play is for youth. The truth is that play is for everyone, and those absorbed in the incredible complexity and breakneck pace of modern life probably need it most of all. Regularly taking time away from work and domestic duties, school, and other grown-up responsibilities to express the childlike elements of your basic nature through play helps quench your thirst for adventure and challenge (physical and mental), improves health, relieves stress, strengthens your connection with friends and community, and simply enhances your enjoyment of life.

Learning disability specialist Dr. Lorraine Peniston enumerates many research-proven psychological benefits of play, including:

- Perceived sense of freedom, independence, and autonomy
- Enhanced self-competence through improved sense of self-worth, self-reliance, and self-confidence
- Better ability to socialize with others, including greater tolerance and understanding
- Enriched capabilities for team membership
- Heightened creative ability
- Improved expressions of and reflection on personal spiritual ideals
- Greater adaptability and resiliency
- Better sense of humor
- Enhanced perceived quality of life
- More balanced competitiveness and a more positive outlook on life

There is plenty of evidence attesting to the fact that we can be more productive when we carve out time for play in our busy schedules. A New Zealand study reported that following a vacation, people were 82 percent more productive and enjoyed enhanced quality of sleep—but

43 percent of Americans had no vacation plans in 2007 due to work pressures (and it's probably worse now). A 2006 study described in the *Sunday Times* (England) noted that the percentage of married couples citing lack of quality time due to overwork as the basis for divorce had more than tripled in recent years, while the traditional leading reasons, such as violence and infidelity, dropped sharply. Australian research suggests that frequent breaks from a sedentary workday produce numerous health benefits, including weight control and favorable blood levels of triglycerides and glucose. There is also ample evidence that positive experiences such as enjoyable play boost your immune function, perhaps in part because they relieve stress, which is known to suppress the immune system and increase susceptibility to illness. For example, in one study published in *Health Psychology*, researchers found that positive leisure activities were associated with increased immune response, and the effects lasted several days. (On the flip side, negative experiences had the expected immunosuppressive effects, but they lasted only about a day.)

For the majority of us who move far less than we are genetically programmed to, busting loose outdoors, in fresh air and sunlight, for some relatively unstructured physical fun will produce the best physical and psychological benefits. If you are one of the few who have a physically demanding job, mellower pursuits (drawing trees in the park, skipping rocks in the pond) might indeed be the ticket.

> *We don't stop playing because we grow old;*
> *we grow old because we stop playing.*
> —George Bernard Shaw
> **Irish playwright and political activist (1856-1950)**

My favorite activity of the week is a regular Sunday afternoon pick-up Ultimate Frisbee game with other hard-core Malibu locals. Ultimate is a great sport, requiring diverse athletic and strategic skills, and is fun for players of all ages and ability levels. I'd say it's a safe sport, too, except for my freak accident that resulted in a serious knee injury in 2007—possibly attributed to a still-17-year-old brain directing a 54-year-old body to get some big air for a circus catch! Most important, my enjoyment of play time has prompted me to reframe my main reason for exercising: I train primally so I can play hard at whatever I want whenever I choose, whether it's Ultimate, snowboarding, soccer, stand up paddling, or golf.

If you can take the spirit of this message to heart, you can make something happen that will change your life. Let's be clear that I'm not advocating selling the shop and becoming a surf bum. All work and no play makes for a dull boy, but all play and no work makes for a foreclosure. Balance is important in all areas of life, and it's up to you to define your level of work-play balance. It might help to keep this popular sentiment in mind: "No one ever said, 'I wish I'd spent more time at work' on their deathbed."

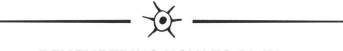

REMEMBERING HOW TO PLAY

Perhaps adults don't play more because they think they don't know how. In childhood, play is natural and easy; children don't overthink it. As adults, we are often uncertain how to proceed. At its essence, play is simply any activity you undertake purely because it is pleasurable. As you can imagine with such a broad definition, innumerable activities can qualify as play, and how you define it for yourself is highly individual. Play activities can be imaginative, creative, and spontaneous, or highly structured and planned. They can involve a lot of physical movement or very little. You can play indoors or outdoors, alone or with others. Play might or might not involve competition and/or cooperation. There are no rules here besides acknowledging that most of us lead largely indoor, sedentary, highly structured lives and might best balance our predictable daily routines with unstructured outdoor physical fun.

Most important of all is to discover what it is that you enjoy. Here are some ideas to get you started:

Follow the leader: If you have kids (or nieces, nephews, grand-children, friends' kids), take them outside or to the park and just do what they do. Swing, do the monkey bars, draw with chalk, blow bubbles, climb a tree, pretend you're a dinosaur, whatever. Let go of any self-consciousness and release your inner child.

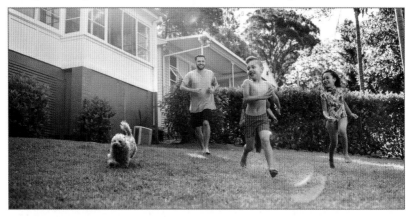

Play a game: There are a million ways to do this. You can start by revisiting simple games from your childhood, like tag or hide-and-go-seek (great fun in the woods!).

Be a groupie: Recreational sports teams, pick-up games, and training clubs (e.g., for cycling or running) are common in most areas, but there are many other kinds of teams and groups, too. Join—or organize!—a local hiking club, or find a nature photography meet-up. Participate in Gishwhes, a massive international team scavenger hunt. Thanks to the Internet, it is easy to find others with similar interests and join a group either locally or virtually.

Just go outside and move: Walk. Run. Pedal. Skip. Wade. Swim. Play fetch with your dog. Splash in puddles. Dig in sand. Find a trail. If you are in a big city, search online for walking tours of your area and play tourist for a day.

Unplug: Go out in nature with no electronics, just for a day or even better for several days. If you're in a city, find a park. If you can, go camping. Even just being in your yard will do. Without your electronics to distract you, your innate ability to create your own fun will kick in.

Take it up a notch: Try something you've never done before, especially if it takes you out of your comfort zone. Perhaps check out one of my favorites, like slacklining or stand up paddle boarding. Try snowshoeing, belly dancing, indoor rock climbing, or aerial yoga. Make it a social event by enlisting adventurous friends to join you.

PRIMAL BLUEPRINT LAW #8: GET PLENTY OF SUNLIGHT

While the dangers of excessive sun exposure are well recognized and heavily promoted by today's medical community, it's important to challenge conventional wisdom's blanket statement to avoid the sun, or lather up with tons of sunscreen. Exposing large skin surface areas to sunlight enables your body to manufacture vitamin D, which helps regulate growth in virtually every cell of our bodies and prevent a variety of diseases. Vitamin D—which is technically a hormone rather than a vitamin—is essential for healthy teeth, nails, and bones, working in conjunction with other fat-soluble vitamins to promote skeletal development. It assists in the absorption of other key nutrients, such as calcium and vitamins A and C, and is a major player in proper immune function. It supports healthy pregnancies and fertility, triggers genes that produce mood-elevating beta-endorphins, stimulates serotonin and the regula-

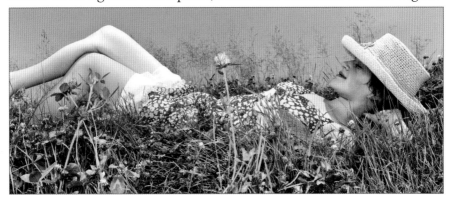

tion of circadian rhythms, and even improves fat metabolism. Vitamin D has also been shown to play a role in the prevention of breast, prostate, ovarian, pancreatic, and colorectal cancers, multiple sclerosis, cardiovascular disease, diabetes, autoimmune diseases, dementia, hypertension, and inflammatory conditions, such as arthritis.

Intriguing new research suggests that vitamin D plays a role in regulating the expression of the p53 gene in skin cells. This is noteworthy because p53 acts as a spell-checker during each of the hundreds of millions of cell replications that occur each day, informing the cell when something has gone awry and instructing it to make necessary changes. Many scientists believe p53 is an important first line of defense against the kinds of mutations that can develop into cancers. The vitamin D regulatory network likely works alongside and in conjunction with p53, and together the two systems protect against cancer, including skin cancer, by suppressing tumor growth and defending against oxidative damage caused by ultraviolet radiation. That's right, that means healthy sun exposure can *prevent* cancer, including malignant melanoma, the most serious form of skin cancer. By contrast, fears about the less serious carcinoma (driven by overexposure of sensitive areas like the face) can be managed by habitually covering up or using a healthy sunscreen.

The bottom line is that generously exposing large skin surface areas of your body to direct sunlight during the times of day and year of peak solar intensity in your area is essential for health. Early humans spent hundreds of thousands of years absorbing powerful equatorial rays over their entire bodies every day. When we first migrated a significant distance away from the equator around 50,000 years ago (leaving the Levant—the present day Middle East—to venture into Europe), we evolved lighter skin pigmentation and hair over a relatively short evolutionary time period. This genetic adaptation enabling more vitamin D production under less intense sunlight was a matter of life or death for our ancestors—and it still is today.

Just as we've suffered devastating health consequences from the relatively recent shift in the human diet away from hunter-gatherer to grain-based, the same dynamic holds for our sun exposure—except this lifestyle alteration has been even more abrupt. Only in the last couple of centuries of industrialization have millions of people in the developed world gone for long periods of time with little to no direct sun exposure. And with an increasing tendency (especially among our younger generations) to stay inside fiddling on digital media instead of romping, frolicking, and otherwise exploring the great outdoors, our already dismal level of sun exposure is declining even further.

The problem is further compounded by the fact that when we do go outdoors, many of us take great pains to "protect" ourselves with high-SPF sunscreens (which are themselves laden with dubious chemicals), and by staying in the shade or covering most of our skin with clothing. It's no surprise, then, that a 2009 study published in the *Archives of Internal Medicine* found insufficient vitamin D levels in a full 77 percent of American participants—and similar figures are estimated for other sun-challenged urban population centers around the world.

Consequently, there has been an alarming increase in health problems related to vitamin D deficiency. The symptoms of vitamin D deficiency are not as overt as the disturbing image of scurvy-stricken sailors staggering around lacking vitamin C (which was, interestingly, partly a result of their high grain consumption), but the health consequences are devastating nonetheless. The risk increases for those with confined lifestyles (spent in the home, office, or auto—a la Ken Korg), those with dark skin living distant from the equator, children with vitamin-D-deficient mothers, the elderly, or people who are house- or hospital-bound. Recent research suggests that vitamin D levels also tend to be low in those with obesity and Metabolic Syndrome.

Dr. Joseph Mercola, Internet health advisor (mercola.com) and author of *The No-Grain Diet*, states:

> The dangers of sun exposure have been greatly exaggerated and the benefits highly underestimated. Excess sun exposure is not the major reason people develop skin cancer (many believe poor diet, exposure to other environmental toxins such as swimming pool chlorine, and insufficient sun are more significant risk factors). [A study from the Moores Cancer Center at UC San Diego suggested that] 600,000 cases of cancer could be prevented every year by just increasing your levels of vitamin D.

Granted, the "fell asleep slathered in baby oil at the beach" burn-and-peel ordeals are indeed bad news. Medical experts suggest that even a few severe sunburn episodes in your early years (who hasn't fallen asleep on the beach or poolside as a teenager?!) can generate sufficient ultraviolet radiation damage to potentially lead to the development of carcinoma (less serious growths that are easily removed from skin surface) or melanoma (a more serious form of cancer) in later decades. But there is a happy medium between too much sun and too little.

Regular exposure of large skin surface areas to sunlight remains the primary way to obtain an ample amount of vitamin D.

Regular exposure of large skin surface areas (torso, arms, and legs) to sunlight during the months and times of day of peak solar intensity at your latitude remains the primary way to obtain an ample amount of vitamin D. For most lighter-skinned people, maintaining a slight tan indicates that you are obtaining optimal sun exposure, while a burn is, of course, unhealthy.

Contrary to conventional wisdom, even the healthiest diets provide inconsequential amounts of vitamin D compared to sun exposure. Vitamin D experts recommend you obtain around 4,000 International Units (I.U.) per day, but the SAD provides only around 300 I.U. per day, and the vaunted glass of milk provides only around 100 I.U. By contrast, 20 minutes of direct summer sunlight onto large skin surface areas can produce around 10,000 I.U. of vitamin D, which can easily be stored in your cells for future use.

In the winter months, when the sun's rays are not intense enough to generate sufficient vitamin D production (this is the case for three to five months per year for locations in North America—you'll know it's downtime for D when you can't get a tan even with prolonged sun exposure), supplements and safe-designated artificial tanning implements can be useful or even essential if you are at high risk for deficiency.

If you have an indoor-dominant lifestyle or even a hint of other afore-mentioned risk factors, you should regularly test your blood for vitamin D. (Make sure it's for "25-vitamin D" or "serum 25(OH)D".) You can order this test directly from an online provider like directlabs.com. Or, if you are getting a routine checkup, insist they include vitamin D in your blood panels. (Unfortunately, it's often not included.)

Depending on whom you consult, you will arrive at somewhat different recommendations for what constitutes a normal or appropriate range for 25(OH)D. Recommendations from assorted vitamin D advocates range between 40-80 ng/mL, with the Vitamin D Council recommending 60 ng/mL for cancer prevention. Nora Gegaudas, CNS, CNT, author of *Primal Body, Primal Mind* and leading functional medicine practitioner in the paleo community, suggests that shooting to land between 60-80 ng/mL is sensible for most people, with greater values recommended for people with autoimmune conditions. These numbers are higher than what a mainstream physician might recommend—generally anything over 30 ng/mL is seen as "fine."

Recently, the "more is better" message has been tempered a bit. While much less likely than a vitamin D deficiency, it's possible to develop problems with excessive vitamin D levels, especially if you are deficient in vitamin A. Furthermore, there is believed to be some variation in opti-mal vitamin D levels based on ethnicity, with those of non-White ances-try able to thrive in lower ranges than light-skinned folks.

Chris Kresser, leading expert on ancestral and paleo health and nutri-tion and author of *Your Personal Paleo Code*, argues that there is no good evidence that levels above 50 ng/mL deliver any health benefits, citing a review of over 1,000 studies conducted by the Institute of Medicine. However, Kresser agrees that levels up to 60 ng/mL are still healthy for most people. Toxicity concerns start to arise if you are in the 100-150 ng/mL range.

There are some important caveats to these general recommendations. If you are of non-White ancestry and have levels of 50 ng/mL, you might be borderline high, based on analyses of non-Caucasian and traditional hunter-gatherer populations. If you are below 30 ng/mL, you should consider aggressive action to get more sunlight and/or supplement. To determine your vitamin D health, you should also consider your levels of other agents such as vitamin A and parathyroid hormone (PTH), which I will explain in the next section.

To optimize vitamin D production, strive to expose the large surface areas of your skin (arms, legs, torso) to direct sunlight *for about half the amount of time it takes to sustain a slight burn*. This is a pretty low-risk endeavor that allows for plenty of individual flexibility for factors like time of day, time of year, skin tone, and reflectiveness of the ground surface. (Water and sand intensify the sun's rays and shorten your timelines for optimal exposure.) Exposing large skin surface areas is the key. If you are worried about wrinkling and cancer risk on the skin areas that are most at risk of overexposure and are most visible and sensitive—face, neck, and hands—go ahead and cover them with clothing or sunscreen routinely. They represent an extremely minimal amount of your vitamin D potential anyway. If you diligently bag enough rays during the summer months, enough to maintain a slight tan, you will store enough vitamin D to sustain you through the winter.

•••••••••• GROK ⚡ TALK ••••••••••

The benefits of sun exposure for overall health are much too numerous to list here, and while vitamin D is certainly a prominent reason to get plenty of sunlight, it is not the only one. Another reason to make sure you are soaking up the sun's rays is that sunlight plays a critical role in entraining (regulating) your circadian rhythm. Exposing yourself to sunlight, especially first thing in the morning, will help you sleep better at night. If that isn't enough, sun exposure boosts serotonin production; low serotonin levels are implicated in Seasonal Affective Disorder and negative mood states. Sunlight is also thought to have a direct positive effect on the immune system and is sometimes recommended to help treat various autoimmune and skin disorders, such as vitiligo, eczema, and psoriasis. Sun exposure also lowers blood pressure, which in turn reduces the risk of heart attack and stroke.

Research suggests that children who spend more time outside in natural light are less likely to develop nearsightedness. What's more, if you are outside getting sunlight, you are enjoying the benefits of

*fresh air (charged with energy-boosting negative ions and counter-
ing the stale, fatiguing indoor air we spent too much time breathing);
you are activating distance vision, giving your eyes a much-needed
balance to excessive focusing on close-up screens; you are potentially
getting the "earthing" benefits from direct connection with natural
ground surfaces (search MarksDailyApple.com for interesting commentary on the topic; there are anti-inflammatory and hormonal
benefits associated with bare feet and ground contact); and you are
generally calming your nervous system to balance the commonly
overstimulating and cramped indoor spaces in which we operate.*

*So, in the name of vitamin D and the many fringe benefits, counter
the momentum of our indoor-dominant lifestyles and conventional
wisdom's irresponsible fearmongering about sun exposure by making
a concerted effort to regularly spend time relaxing outdoors. And if
it's the opportune time of day and year in your area, make sure to
safely expose large skin surface areas to direct sunlight in pursuit of
a slight tan. While it's possible to get some of the health and vitamin
D benefits from tanning beds and UV lamps when used correctly, it's
much better to get the real thing when you can and reap the many
other benefits of being outside in the fresh air and in nature.*

Making the Most Out of Vitamin D—Why More Might Not Be Better

While there is much attention given to the dangers of too little vitamin D, and deservedly so, it is also possible to have excessive levels of vitamin D in your body. Vitamin D toxicity is most likely to result from taking too many supplements over a long period of time. It's impossible to become vitamin D toxic from sun exposure, since the body automatically regulates vitamin D production by tanning the skin (and consequently shutting down further vitamin D production) when you've had enough. Regarding diet, even a deliberately high-vitamin-D diet won't provide nearly enough to put you into the excess zone. The concentrated dose that supplements provide make it necessary to exercise some caution against indiscriminate pill popping. The best idea is to get your levels tested before beginning a supplementation program, and then retest frequently.

Even if you are a diligent tester, it is not enough to simply monitor your vitamin D intake and blood serum levels. Vitamin D works in concert with other compounds in your body and must be balanced with them in order to maintain health. Of utmost importance is the synergistic relationship between vitamin D and vitamin A. Having too little vitamin A increases the risk of vitamin D toxicity at otherwise lower levels. Potassium and vitamin K also work synergistically with vitamin D. If you are making an effort to increase your sun exposure and/or are taking vitamin D supplements, it is imperative that you also take steps to ensure your vitamin A, vitamin K, and potassium levels are adequate.

If you are eating primally with plenty of vegetables, seasonal fruits, and Big Ass salads, you are likely getting enough potassium and vitamin K. However, vitamin A is derived predominantly from animal sources, especially liver. Your body can also derive vitamin A from beta carotene in vegetables, but this process is neither efficient nor sufficient to supply adequate vitamin A.

Evidence from modern hunter-gatherers shows that their diets, which tend to be rich in animal products and organ meats, contain high levels of vitamin A to balance out their frequent sun exposure. The same is not true for most modern humans. This is why many experts now recommend adding cod liver oil to your diet, which is the easiest way to boost vitamin A consumption. (Cod liver oil also contains a nice dose of vitamin D.) The Weston A. Price Foundation website lists recommended brands available in the U.S. and abroad. Adding a teaspoon a day should be enough for most adults. Gedgaudas suggests taking a little more after prolonged periods of sun exposure, since sun actually depletes vitamin A. Kresser recommends also taking a magnesium supplement because magnesium might protect against excess vitamin D and is difficult to get through diet alone.

Nutrition expert Dr. Chris Masterjohn argues that vitamin D levels on the low end of normal are not problematic if you also have low levels of parathyroid hormone (PTH), which can also be determined with a blood test. This is because PTH regulates the conversion of 25(OH)D into a more active form of vitamin D in the body. If PTH is high, above 30 pg/mL according to Dr. Masterjohn, and vitamin D is low, that suggests that there is not enough vitamin D available in the body, and supplementation and sun exposure are recommended. On the other hand, if vitamin D is borderline low (25 to 30 ng/mL), but PTH is also low, that probably reflects a functioning vitamin D regulatory system and is not cause for concern.

Granted, it's starting to get a bit more confusing than "Hey, spend more time in the sun!" What's most important to understand is that insufficient sun exposure is a serious health risk; you should identify your risk factors in this area, expose yourself sensibly to the sun during the times of year and day of peak solar intensity in your area, and test your levels frequently—particularly if you are in a high-risk category. Based on the current evidence, 60 ng/mL is a sensible recommendation for most people. This might be on the high end of normal for dark-skinned individuals but probably does not represent a toxicity risk unless paired with low levels of vitamin A. Lighter-skinned individuals can probably aim a bit higher and still be okay, as long as they are getting their vitamin A. Individuals with autoimmune illnesses should work closely with their doctors to determine their individual needs. They should be especially mindful when considering supplementation, which might alleviate symptoms in the short term but potentially cause imbalances in the long term. And remember, the best way to boost your vitamin D levels is through safe sun exposure. If you do, your body's natural vitamin D regulatory system should ensure that you are getting just the amount you need and never too much.

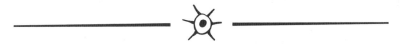

HOW TO SCREEN YOUR OPPONENT

If you do find yourself spending enough time in the sun to encounter a burning risk, you should have a protection plan. Unfortunately, conventional wisdom lets us down again by touting sunscreen as a fail-safe method. Credible research has shown that, historically, most sunscreens have not blocked the UVA rays that can cause melanoma, instead blocking the UVB rays that cause burning. This creates a tremendous problem, of course, because without burning as a deterrent, people spend more time in the sun bagging UVA rays and, hence, increasing their cancer risk. Bad news!

Furthermore, many of the popular agents used in sunblock products may have toxic properties, especially when you consider the standard recommendation to reapply these synthetic chemicals frequently to your porous skin. On sunscreen, Nora Gegaudas says, "The only people genuinely benefitting from sunscreens in this world are those who sell them. Most SPF sunscreens use a base of omega-6 oil (likely rancid), and then tend to be formulated with many toxic and carcinogenic chemicals for the ultimate effect of blocking not only sunlight but vitamin D production as well."

Nevertheless, worries about skin cancer are valid, particularly for those with fair skin, red or blond hair, and light eyes, or those with numerous moles; these folks are six times more likely to develop melanoma than those with darker features.

If you must be out in the sun for extended periods of time, it is far preferable to use clothing, especially technical fabrics designed to provide extra sun protection, to minimize your exposure to harmful UVA rays and to prevent burning. There are numerous apparel brands touting enhanced SPF (sun protection factor) effectiveness available online or in high-quality specialty sports stores. If you are partial to good ol' cotton, realize that it too will offer significant SPF effects.

Examining your skin after a day in the sun will reveal just how well your clothing protects you. As a backup to protection via clothing, use a premium sunscreen that protects against UVA, UVB, and the newly described UVC rays. Check the Environmental Working Group website (ewg.org) for updated ratings on quality sunscreens. Opt for mineral sunscreens that protect against the sun's rays by forming a physical barrier on the skin, preferably one with zinc oxide as its active ingredient; avoid chemical sunscreens (with active ingredients such as oxybenzone or octinoxate) that are absorbed into the skin and can disrupt hormone function and may have other toxic properties.

Beyond exposing yourself sensibly and being careful to always use protection (can you believe I slipped that line past my editors?!), a diet high in antioxidants and free of offensive pro-inflammatory foods like sugars, grains, and chemically altered trans fats and refined high polyunsaturated vegetable/seed oils can go a long, long way toward reducing or eliminating any damage caused by sun exposure. In fact, one of the more common testimonials from people who have adopted a Primal Blueprint eating strategy is, "I can stay out in the sun longer without burning." On the flip side, a bad diet could be an even more profound risk factor than excessive sun exposure for skin cancer. Excess consumption of refined high polyunsaturated vegetable oils has been known to exacerbate the growth of tumors and other inflammation-related health conditions.

My ebook, *The Primal Blueprint Definitive Guide to Sun Exposure and Vitamin D Health* (available at primalblueprint.com/sun-exposure), can help you formulate a customized sun exposure plan. You can also search MarksDailyApple.com for "sun exposure" and "vitamin D" for numerous detailed posts. For now, I want you to second-guess conventional wisdom's knee-jerk, fear-based reaction to skin cancer dangers and the view that the sun is evil.

PRIMAL BLUEPRINT LAW #9: AVOID STUPID MISTAKES

Despite common Fred Flintstone-like depictions, early man was far from a numbskull. Grok was most certainly attuned to his surroundings and was skillful at avoiding mistakes or getting into situations likely to endanger his health. It is a common—but faulty—assumption that our hunter-gatherer ancestors lived "solitary, poor, nasty, brutish, and short" lives. This was the description advanced by 17th-century English philosopher Thomas Hobbes when he argued for the need to have government structure in civilization, instead of living off the land hunter-gatherer style.

Actually, research suggests that Grok and his family were generally healthy (robust is the apropos term), productive, and so appreciative of their lives that they felt the need to express themselves through art. While some hunter-gatherers certainly died young, evidence suggests that many also lived to a ripe old age. In fact, there likely was a selective benefit within tribal units for grandparents, meaning that getting older may have actually had an evolutionary advantage. Clan elders benefited the group by providing services such as babysitting and by transferring important knowledge and history.

But, if they were so robust, and if our genes truly evolved to allow us to live long lives, then why was the average life span relatively short? I had always assumed that it was due to events like death from childbirth, infections, accidental poisoning, or even tribal warfare. But then I got a real-life taste of what might have affected life span more than anything else. Far from nasty and brutish, it was the mundane lapses in judgment, even minor ones, that likely spelled doom for many primal humans.

My unusually bad dive during an Ultimate Frisbee match in September, 2007, resulted in a torn quadriceps muscle, displaced kneecap, ruptured prepatellar bursa, and smashed nerve. An X-ray revealed no other tendon or ligament damage, and my orthopedist said the soft-tissue injury would heal in 8 to 12 weeks. He advised me to use pain as my guide and come back slowly. Because I had no pain at all (smashed nerve, remember?), I felt like I was recovering fairly quickly—to the point of even resuming my beach sprints in early December, followed by a snowboarding trip over Christmas break. But despite wrapping the knee every day and taking it fairly easy (wink, wink—and again no pain), I came home with a very swollen, black-and-blue knee. By the end of the week, I was unable to bend it more than a few degrees.

An MRI revealed a large organized hematoma over the quad and kneecap; it needed to be removed surgically, otherwise I would carry it with me forever. During surgery, my surgeon discovered that the original torn quad muscle had never repaired itself and was leaking blood into the space, causing the hematoma, so she removed the hematoma and stitched the quad back to the patellar tendon.

Here I was, 54 years old, looking forward to living well past 100, but I was effectively incapacitated for more than four months by an injury caused by a random fall. (Truth be told, I had second thoughts as soon as I jumped.) Of course, I had the luxury of modern surgical procedures to repair the damage and eventually recovered fully. Had this happened 10,000 years ago, my inability to run away from a predator might well have spelled the end for me—all because of a momentary lapse of judgment. Even today, a small accident that active younger folks barely sneeze at (e.g., a fall from a ladder while hanging the holiday lights, or turning an ankle on a staircase) can mean something entirely different for someone elderly and sedentary.

I drive way too fast to worry about cholesterol.

—Stephen Wright
Stand-up comedian

The Darwin Awards—Long Live Natural Selection

As society continues to modernize exponentially, we are arguably exhibiting less and less common sense in avoiding stupid mistakes. I believe part of the reason is that deep down, we know we can afford to make them. Our intricate system of safety nets has compromised our capacity to take responsibility for our role in the "accidents" that occur and are chronicled by the news media daily.

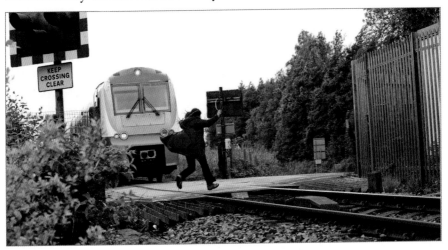

Look no further than YouTube or the Jackass movies and television shows to confirm that we are actively inviting unnecessary struggle and suffering into our lives, all in the name of expressing the youthful sense of adventure that has been stifled by the constraints and predictability of the modern world. The *Darwin Awards* satirical book and website annually bestow special distinction on those who "improve the gene pool by removing themselves from it" with particular brilliance. Here are some of my favorite winners from recent years:

Hot Rod: A Texas motorist spilled a gas can in the back of his car. While searching for the can at night, he flicked on a cigarette lighter to get a better view, igniting the vehicle.

Nacho Libre: A Pennsylvania man was critically injured when, distracted by a plate of nachos on his lap, he crashed his motorcycle into a telephone pole.

CSI—Alternate Ending: A police officer in Illinois was trying to show another patrolman how their fellow officer had accidentally killed himself. While reenacting the shooting incident from the previous week, he forgot to unload his gun and shot himself in the stomach. While driving himself to the hospital to seek treatment, he was killed in an auto accident.

Up, Up, and Away: A Catholic priest in Brazil attached a lawn chair to dozens of helium balloons and launched his homemade craft. Winds picked up and he drifted out to sea. Well prepared for this potential adversity, he fired up his satellite phone to call for help but could not figure out how to operate his GPS unit to provide an accurate location for rescuers. Rescuers were unable to locate him—ever… although bits of balloon were found later on mountains and beaches.

Off the Falls: A man attempted to pilot a rocket-boosted jet ski off the side of Niagara Falls. The idea was for the rocket to launch the jet ski beyond the danger of the falls and then deploy a parachute and float to safety. The damp air caused both the rocket and parachute to fail as he rode off the edge of the falls. Miraculously, he survived the 160-foot drop but drowned because he didn't know how to swim and was not wearing a life jacket.

Each of us must admit that we have brought various levels of misfortune and trauma into our lives from lapses in concentration or critical thinking. As we attempt to reflect on these stupid mistakes, often we default to blaming bad luck instead of reenacting the chain of events with a deep, honest assessment of our accountability. In fact, the concept of taking responsibility seems to have all but disappeared from modern life. If we truly deconstruct those times when we have been the victim of circumstances, it's quite likely we can discover that exact moment when we were distracted, made a poor choice, or ignored the clear warning signs that might have helped us to avoid the entire incident.

Vigilance and Risk Management

Each of us possesses the genetically-hardwired skills of vigilance and risk management. Like any other skills—or muscles—we have to use and develop them or they will atrophy. Unfortunately, the obsessive effort society makes to diffuse all forms of risk and danger suppresses the use of these natural instincts: endless warning signs on roads and in public venues, safety hazard labels on every consumer product, and sensationalized news reports about the dangers of toxic playground bark or pajamas catching fire. Furthermore, continued technological innovations in the name of comfort and convenience collectively push us toward running on autopilot, often to our detriment, through various mundane elements of daily life.

Drive through Europe, and you'll notice very few warnings or safety precautions on the roadways—even high in the Alps they don't bother with guardrails. Take a spin through the canyons near my home, and you will see miles upon miles of safety barriers, guardrails, runaway truck ramps, and diamond-shaped yellow signs with admonitions and icons warning you of assorted dangers that lurk around every corner. Nevertheless, every year tragedy strikes our local community with fatal accidents (typically induced by alcohol and/or speeding) on these obsessively protected roads.

Meanwhile, the traffic fatality rates in France, Germany, Great Britain, Switzerland, and Scandinavia—per capita and per vehicle miles driven—are significantly lower than those of the United States. Interestingly, some progressive traffic engineers, in the U.S. and abroad, are popularizing the concept of *shared space* as a tool to reduce accident rates. The concept relies on human instincts, such as eye contact, in favor of traditional traffic signals and signs. For example, the removal of bike lane striping on a roadway may actually make cycling safer by increasing driver vigilance. This seemingly counterintuitive concept speaks to the power of nurturing our natural instincts to navigate potentially hazardous situations effectively when we are not pacified by excessive safety measures.

As we strive to succeed in modern life, we must be willing to take personal responsibility for our actions instead of defaulting to speed-dialing a personal injury attorney whenever we come to misfortune. If you get hit by a motorist running a red light, it most certainly is his fault, but you may fare better if you remember to fasten your seat belt and look for oncoming traffic despite the color of the traffic light. I can't remember if an errant throw or overly aggressive defensive play was involved in my Ultimate accident, as I prefer to focus on the fact that I hurled myself through the air irresponsibly and then tried to come back into action too quickly afterward. When I take responsibility for my actions, my misfortune becomes a growth experience—an appealing alternative to feeling like a victim or placing any importance on the notion of bad luck.

Similarly, whenever I honk and mumble "asshole" to someone who has just cut me off on the road, I reflect that I might have cause to say it to myself, too—for being in a rush, being too aggressive or impatient, or diverting my focus from the road momentarily. Maybe the motorists who incur my wrath truly do deserve a little choice feedback, but I can honestly reflect and pin some of the blame for the situation on myself almost every time.

This theme also applies to dietary habits. You can blame lousy food options in airports, the limitations of your budget, or your distressing family genetic predisposition to store excess body fat, but you may be better served to accept some personal responsibility when you make poor food choices or find yourself facing a serious diet-related health issue. Take the extra time to pack healthy snacks for your travel. Take a deeper look at your lifestyle priorities, make some compromises, and stretch your food budget a bit to make the best possible choices. View your family history as a catalyst to cultivate vigilance and risk-management skills instead of as a curse. In this way you can turn negatives into positives and create excellent leverage to be the best you can be, regardless of "bad luck" or excuses.

12 WAYS TO AVOID THE BLACK SWAN

Dr. Doug McGuff, a primal-friendly emergency room physician in South Carolina, co-author of *The Primal Prescription*, and expert consultant in high-intensity training and fitness medicine, offers up his advice on the stupid mistakes topic with his list of "12 Ways to Avoid the Black Swan." The list is inspired by his experience treating emergency room patients every day, so it represents some of the most important things you can do to not end up there!

    1. Humm along the road: Drive the biggest vehicle you can afford to drive, or get an old heavy-duty truck if you can't afford a Hummer. (Hummer haters will be pleased to know that car companies are making progress with eco-friendly oversized vehicles.) Your greatest risk of death in daily life comes from a motor vehicle accident, and a larger car always fares better (Force=Mass x Acceleration). Also, if your midlife crisis plans include a motorcycle or sports car, realize that you might resolve your midlife crisis by avoiding old age all together. Oh, and never text while driving. Texting and driving increases your risk of a traffic fatality by a factor of 23.

    2. Quad-riplegic: Never get on a four-wheeler ATV as they have produced more quadriplegics than anything else I have seen.

    3. Stationary bikes rule!: Do not road cycle or jog on public roads/roadsides. To do so is to put your life in the hands of a text-messaging 17-year-old. [*My note:* My cycling friends counter with data showing that routine cycling is statistically pretty safe. Indeed, I think most cycling accidents skew toward rider error/brazenness instead of inherent risk. If you insist on road riding, ride with a rearview mirror mounted to your helmet, and ride single file—save the chit-chat for the coffee shop after.]

4. Stay grounded: Do not fly a plane or helicopter unless you are a full-time professional pilot. If you are a doctor, lawyer, actor, athlete, stockbroker, or other well-to-do professional, do not get a pilot's license. Expertise in one area of life does not transfer to piloting, often with fatal consequences.

5. Run from trouble: If you are walking down a sidewalk and are approaching a group of loud and apparently intoxicated males, cross to the other side of the street immediately. If anyone tries to start a fight with you, the first step should be "choke them with heel dust."

6. Microwave anyone?: If your gas grill won't start... walk away. Never throw gas (or other accelerant) on a fire.

7. Plunge feet first into adventure: Never dive into a pool or body of water (except in a pool diving area marked nine feet or deeper after you have checked it out feet-first).

8. Do it yourself... not: Never get on a ladder to clean your gutters, or on your roof to hang Christmas lights. Do not cut down trees with a chainsaw. I have seen too many middle age males (with a bug up their ass to get something done) die from these activities. In general, any house or lawn work that you can hire for an amount equal to or less than your own hourly wage is money well spent.

9. Stay put: If you are retirement age and plan on moving to a new home... think twice. The stress pushes many seniors over the edge. If you do, buy a fully functional existing house. I have lost count of the number of retirees that have died of heart attacks while going through the stress of custom-building their retirement dream home.

10. Kick and scratch: If anyone tries to force you into your car or car trunk at gunpoint, don't cooperate. Fight and scream all you can even if you risk getting shot in the parking lot. If you get in the car, you will almost certainly die (but after considerable torture and suffering).

11. Cut ties: If you are in any personal or professional relationship that exhausts you or otherwise causes your recurrent distress, then end the relationship immediately.

12. Lotto-notto: Don't play the lottery... you might win. Any unearned wealth, or wealth that is disproportionate to the objective value you provide will destroy you. Lottery winners and sports/movie stars share a common bond of disproportionate rates of depression, addiction, and suicide.

Everybody gets so much information all day long that they lose their common sense.

—Gertrude Stein
American author and art patron (1874-1946)

PRIMAL BLUEPRINT LAW #10:
USE YOUR BRAIN

Art De Vany, Ph.D., author of *The New Evolution Diet*, draws a compelling link between exercising our minds and our genetic nature as free, independent, adventurous human beings. He argues:

> Modern life is cognitively deprived. Imagine the information processing capabilities that were exploited by an ancestor foraging for food alone, or with a small band on open Savanna. Alert to every clue that indicates the presence of game, plants, and predators, aware of self, wind direction, the habits of animals, and with intimate knowledge of the land, trusting and depending on long-evolved instincts and other members of the band, adapting to rapidly changing circumstances, a foraging human in the Paleolithic would appear to us to have extrasensory perception. This is the setting for which your mind is evolved.
>
> Modern life leaves our minds restless and under utilized because we are confined, inactive, and comfortable.

Modern life leaves our minds restless and under utilized because we are confined, inactive, and comfortable.

—Art De Vany, Ph.D.
Author of *The New Evolution Diet*

At first glance, few might agree that our minds are restless and underutilized. Many of end us our days running on fumes, feeling like our minds will explode if we send or receive any more e-mail. But while the modern world features plenty of complex thought and a constant and rapid progression in human innovation—technological and otherwise—our overstimulated lifestyles compromise our ability to use our brains with maximum effectiveness. In the workplace, the mismanagement of information overload from email, text, instant chat, and the like—all available on mobile devices to boot—can stifle creativity and innovation, not to mention diminish our energy levels, motivation, and health. Consequently, many of us operate in a reactive mode, constantly—and often futilely—trying to keep pace with the information with which we are bombarded.

In the book *The Dumbest Generation*, Mark Bauerlein blames digital technology for compromising the intellectual development of young people. "When we were 17 years old, social life stopped at the front door. Now [via Facebook, texting, Snapchat, Instagram, etc.] peer-to-peer contact… has no limitation in space or time," he observes. Hence, time to read, daydream, free-associate, or gain an adequate understanding of current events, history, and other mainstays of cultural sophistication goes by the wayside.

If we back up and examine the true definition of stress as "stimulus," it is clear that we require a certain amount of daily stress to thrive, prosper, and be happy. Yet, in today's world our minds are *over*stressed, but technically underutilized, because we lack the balance that creative intellectual outlets, play, healthy diet, exercise, sleep, and other winning behaviors promote. Eight hours of brainpower is probably a sensible limit to devote to your daily work efforts. However, engaging your mind with things that stimulate your creativity in other ways and for which you have a passion is critical to mental health and overall wellbeing. Here are few suggestions to model Primal Blueprint Law #10—Use Your Brain:

Pursue New Hobbies: Learn a foreign language or musical instrument, take dancing lessons, tackle a jigsaw or crossword puzzle, write a fiction short story—or anything else you can imagine that sounds interesting and challenging.

Discipline Your Brain Use: Pay close attention to balancing your daily intellectual stimulation with time to rest, relax, and mellow out. Integrate behaviors that are truly calming instead of spending your leisure time in front of a screen delivering more stimulation. Instead, spend time in quiet reflection or engaging with nature. Realize that multitasking is a stressful, unproductive mode, and guard against the constant potential for distraction. Instead, focus on a single peak performance task at a time.

Exercise the Muscle: Instead of outsourcing as much brain function as possible to technology, make a habit of challenging your brain during your routine daily endeavors. Replay your favorite song and try to memorize the lyrics, bust out your school yearbook and try to recall the names of your long-lost classmates, or add up numbers in your head instead of always relying on a calculator. Search for Sheppard Software's "Place the States Game" online, and see how close you can come to dropping individual states into their correct spot on a blank U.S.A. map. There are endless opportunities to keep the brain fresh throughout your day.

CHAPTER SUMMARY

1. Get Plenty of Sleep: Despite being a critical component of good health and stress management, sleep is regularly compromised in modern life due to the pull of technology and hectic schedules. Insufficient sleep can lead to numerous health problems and declines in cognitive function. Try to align your sleep habits as closely as possible with the rising and setting of the sun. Pay special attention to minimizing artificial light and digital stimulation after dark. Create a calm, dark, relaxing sleeping environment, observe gradual transitions into and out of sleep, and observe consistent bed and wake times. Naps can produce many health benefits, including recharging creative thinking skills, solidifying emotional memories, reinforcing learning, improving cognitive function, and helping you automatically catch up on the type of nighttime sleep in which you are deficient.

2. Play: The regimented nature of modern life leaves many adults—and even kids—deficient in play. The profound psychological benefits of play are integral to healthy cultures, communities, and individuals, including a direct relationship to work productivity. Engage in some unstructured outdoor physical exertion each day to counter the negative effects of a sedentary, technological existence.

3. Get Plenty of Sunlight: An optimal amount of daily sun exposure (depends upon many personal variables, including skin pigmentation and environmental conditions) can produce numerous health benefits and alleviate many health risks because it enables your body to synthesize optimal levels of vitamin D. The dangers of sun exposure are overdramatized, and many suffer from vitamin D deficiency today due to insufficient sun exposure. Risks of skin cancer are greatly minimized if you avoid sunburns and cover or screen the most vulnerable areas (face, neck, and hands).

Strategically expose the large surface areas of your skin (arms, legs, torso) to direct sunlight for about *half the amount of time it takes to sustain a slight burn.* Dietary sources of vitamin D are vastly inferior to sun exposure. Vitamin D supplements can be useful in the winter months when sunlight is of insufficient intensity to allow for vitamin D production. Make sure you balance vitamin D levels with adequate vitamin A (cod liver oil is the best source), vitamin K, potassium, and magnesium. When you've had enough sun, clothing is the best protection, as sunscreens have some health objections and may be less effective than advertised.

4. Avoid Stupid Mistakes: Avoiding stupid mistakes was a critical survival factor for Grok, because margin for error was much lower in his time. Today, modern life attempts to shield us from all manner of danger, yet—possibly because we are desensitized by all these protection mechanisms—we still seem to find a way to invite trauma and tragedy into our lives by making stupid mistakes. You must practice your hardwired, evolution-perfected skills of vigilance and risk management to navigate successfully through even the mundane elements of daily life. This will prevent unnecessary suffering and promote longevity.

5. Use Your Brain: Technological innovation and overstimulation have compromised our ability to use our brains to maximum effectiveness. You must exert great discipline to leverage technology to your advantage instead of falling victim to it by spacing out, burning out, or otherwise misusing your greatest human gift: complex thought. Pursue new challenges, such as music, language, hobbies, or adventures that stimulate your brain and allow you to depart from your daily routine. Balance peak cognitive tasks with sufficient time for relaxation. Be vigilant against the constant potential for distraction and the perils of multitasking. Instead, focus on a single peak performance task at a time. Beware of outsourcing brain function to technology and keep sharp by throwing little cognitive challenges into your daily routine.

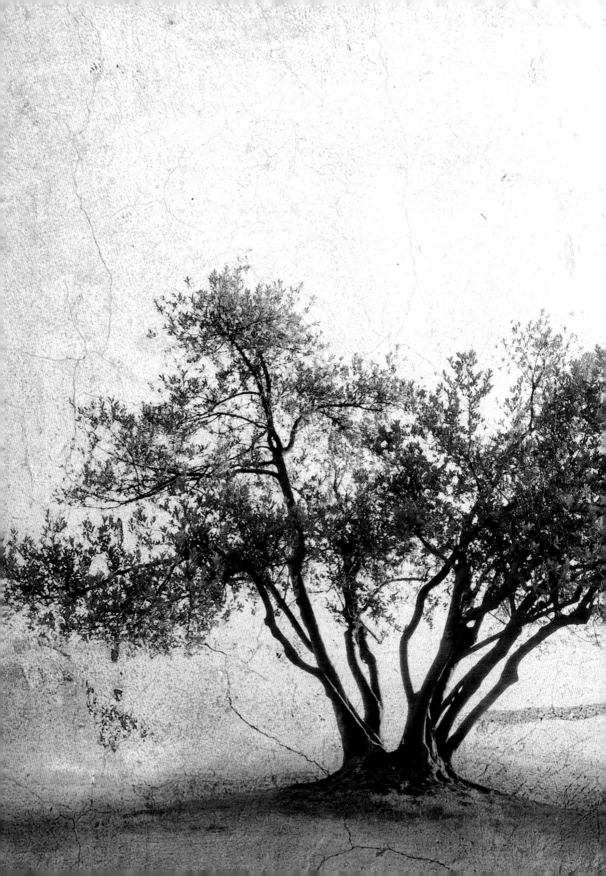

CHAPTER NINE

A PRIMAL APPROACH TO WEIGHT LOSS

Meet Ya at the Sweet Spot!

IN THIS CHAPTER

I provide a step-by-step process for losing an average of one to two pounds (one-half to one kilogram) of body fat per week. You'll learn how to optimize protein, carb, and fat intake in order to ramp up fat metabolism, maintain high dietary satisfaction levels, and avoid the risk of depleting muscle tissue and suffering from the usual rebound-rebellion effect of severe caloric restriction. I discuss how deregulating food intake and fasting intermittently can be effective calorie-restriction tools, and how exercise can accelerate progress toward your body composition goals.

I review two weight-loss case studies (Ken and Kelly Korg, naturally!), calculating their average daily caloric expenditure and optimal daily intake of each macronutrient—Primal Blueprint style—to produce targeted and effective fat loss. We'll examine a sample daily food diary that contains a detailed caloric analysis and macronutrient breakdown for each delicious, nutritious meal, plus a daily total, to demonstrate how easy and satisfying it is to eat healthy, primal fare. The case studies result in a loss of around eight pounds (3.6 kg) for Ken and Kelly in a single month. Finally, I provide troubleshooting tips for possible setbacks and plateaus that arise when trying to lose weight in the real world.

Your health and likely your life span will be determined by the proportion of fat versus sugar you burn over a lifetime.

—Dr. Ron Rosedale, author of *The Rosedale Diet*

T hese are the critical elements of the Primal Blueprint weight-loss approach:

- **Minimize carb intake** to moderate insulin production and enable the body to burn stored body fat for energy.
- **Target protein intake** according to lean body mass and exercise level to maintain or increase muscle mass.
- **Optimize fat intake** to achieve satiety, provide energy, and eliminate hunger.
- **Deregulate meal habits and engage in occasional Intermittent Fasting (I.F.)** to produce caloric deficits that lead to greater fat loss.
- **Exercise primally** to fine-tune fat metabolism and build or tone lean muscle without the drawbacks of chronic cardio.
- **Avoid excessive regimentation or obsessing on results** in favor of appreciating the process and viewing body composition goals with a long-term perspective.
- **Remember that optimal health** is the underlying goal of living primally. LGN (*looking good naked*) is just a pleasant side effect.

By now you understand that the Primal Blueprint is a way of life as opposed to a regimented, gimmicky crash diet. I thought carefully about whether to put the presumptuous claim of "effortless weight loss" on the cover, lest it be misinterpreted as empty blather. However, I believe deeply that if you honor the Primal Blueprint principles at least 80 percent of the time, long-term weight management will happen as a natural byproduct of your enjoyable, stress-balanced lifestyle.

Easier said than done, right? While we have literally thousands of success stories compiled at MarksDailyApple.com, we also communicate occasionally with folks whose progress is not always smooth and steady. I'd like to shift gears in this chapter and get a little more precise about macronutrient intake. By following the steps covered in this chapter, you will be able to reduce excess body fat without the struggling and suffering inherent in any fat-loss program that's based on a carbohydrate-heavy, low-calorie diet.

The idea is to hit the sweet spot where carbs have been reduced just enough so that your body prefers to burn fats and a moderate amount of ketones instead of relying so much on regular ingestion of dietary carbohydrate for its primary energy source. This carbohydrate sweet spot for rapid fat loss is between 50 and 100 grams per day for most people. Where you land in this range depends on your size, age, sex, and metabolism. Consume more carbs than that (up to 150 grams a day), and you'll maintain body composition quite easily without adding fat, but you'll have to work a little harder to burn it off. On the other hand, it's certainly healthy to take in less than 50 grams per day of carbs once in a while (as I've said, you could actually live on zero carbs for quite a long time), but the idea is to stay at a comfortable intake level that doesn't entail suffering or unnecessary deprivation of nutrient-dense foods like vegetables.

In the sweet spot, you will maintain high energy levels (no more insulin crashes), you can exercise (including regular intense sessions) without getting exhausted, and you won't experience any of the unpleasant outcomes of sudden, severely-carb-restrictive diets that put you into ketosis without having prepared your body to effectively use those ketones as fuel. These include the annoying "ketone breath," insufficient vitamin/mineral intake (due to the severe restriction of vegetables and fruits), and poor compliance due to the deprivation and inconvenience involved in trying to bottom out on carb intake.

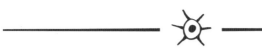

BEING PATIENT GETTING INTO THE SWEET SPOT

If you are coming from a grain-based, high-carbohydrate diet, you may experience some challenges in the first few weeks of primal-style eating. It takes a while for your fat-burning genes to kick into high gear and to become less dependent upon the dietary carbohydrate that has been your go-to energy source for decades. If you experience bouts of low energy, mental fogginess, headaches, or strong carbohydrate cravings, you may need to engage in a gradual reduction of average daily carbohydrate intake until you are ready to operate in the sweet spot and achieve rapid fat loss.

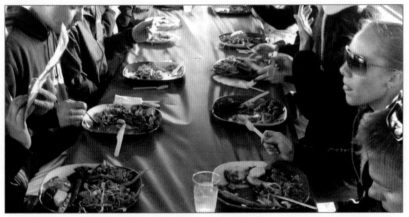

I counsel many new primal enthusiasts not to worry about dropping body fat in the first few weeks of transforming to primal-style eating, but instead to: a) definitely cut out grains, sugars, and refined vegetable oils and eat only healthy fats and high-nutrient-value carbohydrates (e.g., colorful vegetables, sweet potatoes, squash, berries), and b) consume as much fat as necessary to experience high satiety levels at meals and lessen the chance of sugar cravings. If you are "allowed" to chow down on big handfuls of macadamia nuts and hard-boiled eggs any time you have a hankering for a snack, you will avoid carb binge backslides and progress nicely toward fat-adaptation. You may not lose much body fat at first, because you are getting most of your caloric energy from high-fat meals. But once you become fat-adapted, you will notice your appetite and energy levels stabilize, that you require fewer calories to achieve satiety at meals, and finally that you can skip meals (and start burning off excess body fat!) with no strain or struggle.

It's imperative to trust that the process of fat-adaptation will work and not be averse to liberal consumption of healthy dietary fats. Many would-be paleo converts make the mistake of cutting carbs per primal/paleo guidelines but are also averse to liberal fat intake due to a flawed belief system ingrained by conventional wisdom that eating fat is fattening.

Honestly, going to town on fat is essential for your successful transition to primal eating. Another common mistake dieters make is to cut carbs, moderate fat, and default into a high-protein diet. As we learned in Chapter 4, excess protein is toxic to the body. Consuming more protein than is necessary to meet your basic metabolic needs results in the excess being converted into glucose via gluconeogenesis. If you don't burn that glucose right away, it gets converted into fat and stored. A high-protein diet might as well be called a high-carb diet when considering the effect it has on your fat reduction goals.

Once you are fat-adapted from a prolonged period of ditching grains and sugars and moderating carb intake, you can then progress toward a more spontaneous and intuitive eating style where you pay close attention to your hunger and satiety levels, get plenty of sleep to optimize your appetite and fat-storage hormones, and can then create that natural caloric deficit between what you consume and what you burn that is balanced by burning stored body fat. You enjoy rich, satisfying meals, are never hungry or deprived, and you drop excess body fat as a byproduct of fat-adaptation instead of a deprivation/restriction obsession. This is the essence of the Primal Blueprint approach to weight loss and why success lasts for years and years with minimal risk of attrition back to the ranks of carbohydrate dependency.

As you continue to eat in the sweet spot (or dip into the maintenance zone on certain days, no biggie), your eating habits will send signals to your genes to upregulate fat-burning processes and downregulate fat-storage processes. You'll become both fat-adapted and keto-adapted, able to derive energy minute-to-minute from your stored body fat. By eating in the sweet spot, you can expect to drop one to two pounds (one-half to one kilogram) of excess body fat per week, until you reach your personal *set point* (more on this in a minute). This may not seem like much in comparison to the headline on the flyer tacked to the telephone pole, or the flashing Internet banner ad. However, unless you plan to lose water and muscle tissue (and I know you don't), losing one to two pounds of fat per week (your personal maximum rate within this range depends on your existing body weight, metabolic rate, and activity level) means an average daily deficit of 500 to 1,000 calories. You cannot realistically (or safely) lose any more than a pound or two a week of body fat without depleting muscle mass or becoming fatigued.

Before diving in to the details, I want to emphasize that the goal of losing body fat is about being as healthy and vibrant as possible, not as skinny and/or ripped as possible. Humans are meant to have a variety of shapes and sizes—some tall or short, broad-shouldered or narrow, long-legged or long-torsoed, very muscular or lanky, and everything in between. However, we are not meant to be significantly overweight, with tens or even hundreds of extra pounds of fat literally weighing us down. When I talk about losing excess body fat, the idea is not to pigeonhole you into a particular standard of "primal beauty." Rather, it is about you finding your personal ideal body composition.

When I say your personal ideal, I am referring to your "set point," meaning the level of body fat and muscle mass and tone that you are designed to have when you give your genes the input they need and expect. I think (and anthropological and archeological evidence back me up here) that the natural human form is lean and strong. Some people will end up with very low body fat and a ripped physique without even trying; most others can get there if they are willing to put in the work and discipline. I firmly believe that a primal lifestyle is the easiest, lowest-stress path to achieving that. However, just because someone has the capacity to achieve a particular physique does not mean they are obligated to do so. Only you can decide what your personal body composition goals are.

If you have been living primally for a while, and your progress toward your goals is slowing or perhaps even halted, it is up to you to do an honest assessment of where you are vis-à-vis where you would ideally like to be. If you are still carrying a bit of body fat but can honestly say that you have dedicated yourself to living as primally as possible (respecting your real-life responsibilities, like that pesky job that cuts into your hiking time), perhaps you are at your set point. If so, you will have to redouble your efforts if you hope to sculpt a different physique. The closer you are to your natural set point, the harder it will be to change your body. However, if you know you have been loosey-goosey with your food, exercise, and sleeping habits, you more likely have settled into a plateau. Remember, your body strives for homeostasis and will constantly adapt to whatever you are doing. In this case, it is time to buckle down if you want to continue to lose body fat. This is especially true with the most often overlooked variable for successful fat reduction—sleeping habits. Excess artificial light and digital stimulation after dark have a profound effect on your primary hunger hormone ghrelin (making you hungry, particularly for carbs) and your primary satiety/fat-storage hormone leptin (making you more likely to store fat than burn it).

Discussing the realities of familial genetic variation in body composition is not an excuse to be lackadaisical in your commitment to primal principles and then decide, "Well, I guess I'm just genetically programmed to be a little softer through the middle." It is simply a reminder that we do not all have to look alike. For many people, there is probably a tipping point at which the effort and dedication required to push through to the next level in terms of losing fat or building muscle mass would be sufficiently burdensome, stressful, or time consuming that they must decide whether it is worth it. If you are motivated to continue your fat-loss efforts, this chapter provides the tools to do so.

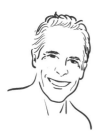

MARK TALK ──────────────────────
Feeling Good About Looking Good

Physical appearance has probably always been important for humans, as it is for many species— just ask the peacock. There is nothing wrong with wanting to look good. Just make sure that you are mindful of where your standards for "looking good" come from. We all know that the images of celebrities with which we are bombarded are airbrushed and filtered false perfection, and moreover that they represent only one possible idea of beauty. And yet, it can be incredibly difficult not to hold ourselves to these standards, which for most of us are simply unrealistic (unless we, too, are being paid handsomely to present a certain image and can hire chefs, personal trainers, and a "glam squad" to keep up the façade).

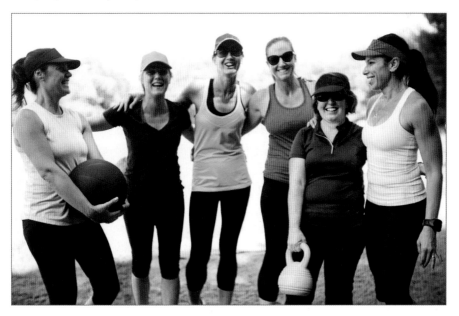

Olympic distance runner and popular blogger Lauren Fleshman (asklaurenfleshman.com) did the world a service with a revealing 2013 blog article called "Keeping It Real." Her discussion about distorted standards of beauty was accompanied by a stunning photo of her on the runway modeling fitness attire—six-pack in full glistening glory—followed by photos taken later that same week of her exercising in similar attire. Some memorable comments accompanied the pics: "This is what I looked like with my belly not turbo-flexed and sucked in," and in conclusion:

"Everyone has thigh cheese. It's part of life. No one is perfect."

Remember, your self-worth is not measured by biceps circumference or the number on the scale (which I don't mind if you throw away, by the way). I want you to want to be healthy, fit, and able to do everything you enjoy for a long, long time; that is the essence of primal living. If aesthetic goals are part of the package for you, I fully support that with the caveat that you must pursue them in the right spirit. We are almost always more disparaging toward ourselves than toward anyone else. Instead of falling into the trap of negative self-talk and self-criticism, focus on the positive steps you are making toward your health and wellbeing, and let the aesthetic changes happen naturally.

WEIGHT-LOSS MACRONUTRIENT PLAN

The plan is as follows: obtain a calculable level of protein sufficient to preserve lean muscle mass, strictly limit carbs to an average of 50 to 100 grams per day, and use fat as the main variable you adjust in order to obtain the satisfaction you need from your diet each day so that you aren't stressed or anxious about your weight-loss journey. To ensure your success and comfort during the fat-reduction period, please make an extra effort to have primal-approved snacks available at all times. These include vegetables and certain fruits like fresh berries, and nutritious high-fat foods like hard-boiled eggs, natural jerkies, nuts and seeds, olives, avocados, sardines, and high-cacao dark chocolate. If you're feeling deprived during your primal journey, or have cravings for some of your old grain-based standbys, have a few celery sticks smothered in almond butter, a hard-boiled egg, a couple squares of 85-percent dark chocolate, then call me!

It's difficult to habitually under-consume protein. Your appetite will guide you to increase protein with intense cravings!

Protein

As you learned already, you only need a maximum of around 0.7 grams of protein per pound (1.54 grams per kilo) of lean body weight per to effectively repair, build, and/or maintain lean muscle mass and to adequately support numerous other metabolic functions that depend upon dietary protein. This means a person with 100 pounds (45 kg) of lean body mass needs only 70 grams/280 calories of protein per day (one gram of protein contains four calories). For a person with 150 pounds (67.5 kg) of lean body mass, this amounts to only 100 grams/400 calories of protein per day.

I'm not asking you to undergo an expensive DEXA scan test to pinpoint your lean body mass and then track every bite to ensure that you nail your exact protein requirements every day. Your appetite will guide you effectively to meet your protein requirements. That said, if you experience low energy or a perceived reduction in muscle mass, you may want to delve further into just what you are eating to be sure the levels are in proper range. Jot down everything you eat for a few days, and then use an 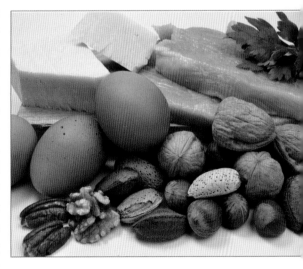 online food calculator such as Fitday.com to determine how many grams of the various macronutrients you are consuming. I've provided some suggested meals with detailed nutrient breakdowns later in this chapter to give you a feel for how healthy and satisfying the Primal Blueprint weight-loss plan can be.

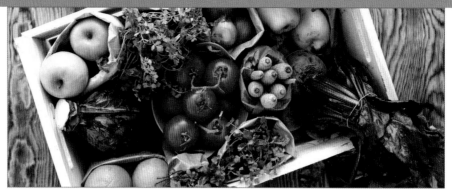

Carbohydrate

Limiting your average carb intake to 50 to 100 grams per day will effectively moderate your insulin production and optimize your fat-burning system. At this level of carbohydrate intake, your body will be stimulated to burn more stored fats and manufacture a little extra glucose in the liver through gluconeogenesis in order to meet its energy needs. I've discussed the gluconeogenesis process as a bad thing in the context of the fight or flight response triggered by chronic cardio (or, in rare cases, a protein-deficient extreme diet), but it can just as easily be a wonderful, adaptive, energy-balancing mechanism when you eat primally. In this case, dietary protein will provide the raw material for gluconeogenesis instead of your precious muscle tissue.

> *You can enjoy abundant servings of vegetables and some well-chosen fruit and still lose excess body fat—provided you ditch sugars, grains, and legumes.*

As an added benefit of this process, your liver will generate a moderate amount of ketones that will help spare muscle tissue and provide added fuel for cells that might otherwise require glucose. Hence, limiting your carbs to well under 100 grams per day will put you in a very mild (and desirable, because you'll be burning fat like crazy) state of ketosis. You probably won't even notice it, but for the appreciable increase in steady-state energy now available. If your carb intake drifts above 100, your increasing blood glucose levels will start to redirect energy pathways more toward glucose burning.

I'm not asking you to split your carrot sticks down the middle or to skimp on salad portions to stay under 100 grams. As you can see from this chapter's examples, you can still enjoy abundant servings of vegetables and ample servings of other nutritious carbs like seasonal fruit and still land in the optimum carb intake range for insulin moderation and weight loss. The key is to virtually eliminate all forms of sugars, sweetened beverages, and grains from your diet. Accomplish this and you can expect a steady reduction in excess body fat. If you struggle to drop fat at the rate you desire, you can get a little stricter and ditch legumes, sweet potatoes, and possibly even fruit for a stretch. Journal your food intake and generate reports from Fitday.com to see where you might be slipping on your carb intake goals.

REALLY, IT'S ALL ABOUT THE CARBOHYDRATE CURVE

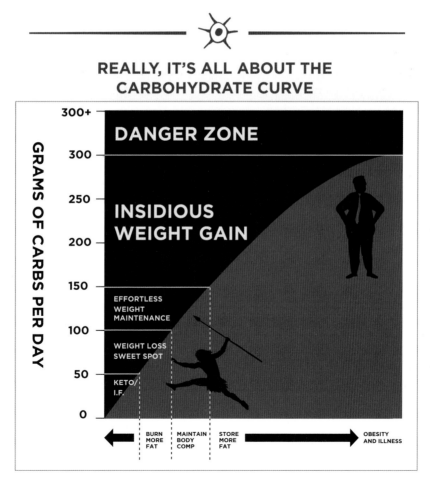

Your body composition *success* is overwhelmingly dependent on controlling your carbohydrate intake and, consequently, your insulin output. Exercising sensibly, getting sufficient everyday movement, managing your stress levels, and accounting for genetics are lesser factors in the equation. Your *failure* to maintain desirable body composition may have assorted contributing factors—unlucky genetics, overly stressful exercise, insufficient sleep, emotional eating issues, and more—but an excess body fat condition *almost always includes excessive carbohydrate intake.*

Eat in the 100- to 150-gram maintenance zone, and you won't gain fat (unless you have an extremely severe overeating problem... but even then it will be hard!). Eat in the 50- to 100-gram sweet spot, and you will lose excess body fat, no matter who you are and how hard it's been to drop weight in the past.

Fat

When you eat only as much protein as your body requires (respecting the updated Primal Blueprint guidelines of only .5 grams per pound of lean mass), and strictly limit carbohydrates to 50 to 100 grams per day during the fat-loss phase, it's easy to see how you can reduce body fat at an accelerated rate. Even an active male will be consuming less than 1,000 calories per day before considering fat intake. Hence, the variable you will adjust in order to meet your energy and total calorie consumption needs ends up being fat. If you are committed to success, you will

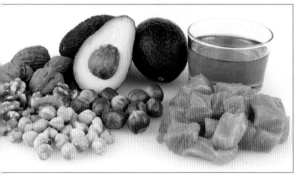

make a concerted effort to eat only what you need (in fat and in total calories) to feel satisfied and energized. Since fat has such a high satiety factor, a little will go a long way. Even something like a small handful of nuts can sustain you for hours when you skip meals or need a quick snack to keep you going. With the right meal choices and healthy snacks around, your weight-loss experience will not involve the typical struggling and suffering of a "diet." After you reduce the amount of body fat you desire, you can consume even more liberal amounts of fat without worrying about gaining weight.

Reject carbohydrate dependency caused by the Standard American Diet and reclaim your Homo sapiens genetic factory setting as a fat–burning beast!

While the "eating fat is okay for weight loss" idea might seem contradictory at first glance, it is scientifically valid; without insulin, eating fat will not make you fat! If you don't produce insulin, your body has no way to store the excess calories as body fat. Note, however, that if I give you an inch and you take a mile—pounding high-fat foods all day "as directed by Mark Sisson"—you will not succeed in losing fat either. If you slam macadamia nuts all day, you will obtain your energy requirements from ingested fat, rather than the storage depots on your body. This is not a big deal, but as you become more fat-adapted, you'll notice it's no trouble to skip a meal and smoothly maintain your energy, mood, and cognitive focus by tapping into internal sources of caloric energy. Furthermore, your appetite will self-regulate to a point at which you eat when you are hungry and become comfortable eating only as much as you need to feel satisfied. Proceed with your dietary transition at a pace most comfortable to you, and realize that this is the essence of primal living: rejecting a dependence on dietary carbs that is the hallmark of the Standard American Diet and reclaiming your *Homo sapiens* genetic factory setting as a fat-burning beast!

KEN KORG: SUGGESTED EATING FOR PRIMAL WEIGHT LOSS

Let's look at a case study of our old friend Ken Korg, a 44-year-old, 5'11" (177.5 cm), 197-pound (89 kg), moderately active male with 25-percent body fat (metric equivalent: 25 percent; sorry, still too much!) who wants to lose weight aggressively (near the maximum suggested rate of two pounds per week) following the Primal Blueprint. We'll calculate Ken's estimated daily caloric expenditure and suggested macronutrient intake based on Primal Blueprint guidelines. Then, I'll present a list of suggested meals and snacks with accompanying macronutrient analysis. This will show how Ken can enjoy sensible, satisfying meals and snacks and still achieve a dramatic improvement in body composition by meeting the average macronutrient guidelines for a single month.

Throughout these examples, remember to focus on the concept of averages. While it's instructive to examine a detailed daily example of both expenditure and intake to understand how we can properly achieve caloric deficits, in reality you will have days when you exceed your carb limit, go above or below your ideal protein intake, and exercise more or less than the averages in our calculations. Ultimately, this isn't about counting and tracking every calorie in and calorie out but about developing an intuitive sense of what works best for you on a bigger scale, over several days, a week, or even a month, as you make primal lifestyle choices.

Caloric Expenditure

The basal metabolic rate (BMR) estimates were derived using a BMR calculator. (bmi-calculator.net is one of many online resources.) BMR factors in your age and weight to estimate the number of calories your body burns if you simply stay in bed all day. An Activity Factor adding additional calories to the daily estimate is derived using the Harris Benedict Formula (also available at bmi-calculator.net), which takes into account typical levels of activity. You can input your personal variables and generate similar estimates for total daily caloric expenditure.

1. **Basal Metabolic Rate:** Number of daily calories Ken burns to support basal metabolic functions (at his age and body composition) = 1,923

2. **Activity Factor:** Harris Benedict Formula for additional calories burned when "moderately active": BMR × 0.55 = 1,057

3. **Total Average Daily Calorie Expenditure:** BMR (1,923) + Activity Factor (1,057) = 2,980

Macronutrient Calculations

- Ken wants to lose eight pounds (3.6 kg) of body fat. Each pound requires a caloric deficit of 3,500 calories. 3,500 calories per pound × 8 pounds ÷ 30 days = 933 calorie deficit per day
- Desired average caloric intake per day = 2,047 (2,980 average caloric expenditure less 933 deficit)
- Minimum daily protein intake = 0.5 grams per pound (1.1 gram) of lean body mass (as discussed in Chapter 4)
- 197 pounds at 25-percent body fat = 148 pounds (67 kg) of lean body mass
- Average daily protein intake = 148 pounds × 0.5 grams per pound = 74 grams (296 calories)
- Desired carb intake = 75 grams (300 calories) to get into the sweet spot on the Carb Curve
- Desired fat intake = 161 grams (1,449 calories) to get back to the 2,047 daily calorie total

. You can see right away that the suggestions will not be difficult for Ken to follow. That amount of fat calories will provide ample energy and satiety at each meal, while the hitting the minimum amount of protein will ensure that his body recovers from exercise stress and maintains healthy metabolic function so that he continues to burn an average of 2,980 calories per day. It's likely that Ken will bump up to 0.7 grams of protein over the long term when he consumes more dietary calories instead of being in fat loss-caloric deficit mode with the calculations here. In his past dieting efforts, Ken tried to cut back on calories in general. He made a little extra effort to cut back on fatty foods in particular but was not nearly diligent enough with carbs to stimulate fat reduction.

Each time he tried to lose weight in the past by cutting back on fat rather than carbs, Ken's energy and exercise level declined slightly. Meanwhile the carbs prevalent in his diet led to insulin production, driving the calories he consumed into fat cells. Hence, his body fat percentage has stayed pegged at 25 percent for years despite repeated efforts at dieting. Let's see how the results can differ when eating Primal Blueprint style.

Ken Korg Food Journal

BREAKFAST

Primal Omelet

Eggs (three medium) with cream
  (1 ounce) and shredded cheddar
  cheese (1 tablespoon)
Chopped mushrooms, red onions,
  and red peppers (3/4 cup total)
Topped with sliced avocado
  (2 ounces) and fresh salsa
  (2 tablespoons)
Fresh blueberries (1/4 cup)
Cup of black coffee

FitDay.com Analysis

Total Calories: 477
Protein: 23 grams, 92 calories
  (19 percent of meal's total)
Carbs: 22 grams, 88 calories
  (18 percent)
Fat: 33 grams, 297 calories
  (63 percent)

LUNCH

Primal Salad

Mixed salad greens (2 cups)
Chopped onions, carrots, jicama,
  red peppers, and cherry
  tomatoes (2 ounces each)
Chopped or shredded chicken
  (3 ounces)
Sesame seeds (1/3 ounce)
Chopped walnuts
  (1/2 ounce or 7 halves)
Oil-based dressing (2 tablespoons)

FitDay.com Analysis

Total Calories: 586
Protein: 31 grams, 124 calories
  (21 percent)
Carbs: 30 grams, 120 calories
  (21 percent)
Fat: 38 grams, 342 calories
  (58 percent)

DINNER

Salmon and Vegetables

Broiled wild salmon (6 ounces)
Steamed asparagus and zucchini
(6 ounces each) with butter
  (1 tablespoon)
Red wine (5-ounce glass)

FitDay.com Analysis

Total Calories: 566
Protein: 39 grams, 156 calories
(28 percent)
Carbs: 16 grams, 64 calories
  (11 percent)
Fat: 26 grams, 234 calories
  (41 percent)
Alcohol: 16 grams, 112 calories
  (20 percent)

SNACKS

Snacks

Hard-boiled egg
Macadamia nuts
 (1-1/2 ounces or 17 nuts)
Venison jerky (one 4-inch strip)

FitDay.com Analysis

Total Calories: 457
Protein: 14 grams, 56 calories
 (12 percent)
Carbs: 8 grams, 32 calories
 (7 percent)
Fat: 41 grams, 369 calories
 (81 percent)

DAILY TOTALS

Calories: 2,086
Protein: 107 grams, 428 calories
 (21 percent)
Carbs: 76 grams, 304 calories
 (15 percent)
Fat: 138 grams, 1,242 calories
 (60 percent)
Alcohol: 16 grams, 112 calories
 (5 percent)

Ken Korg

Caloric deficit from average
daily expenditure (2,980) = 894*
Projected net fat loss over
30-day period: **8 pounds**

* To make up for the caloric intake deficit, Ken will derive his additional 935 daily calories from stored body fat, which becomes his primary energy mechanism to fuel a busy day. Quite an improvement from his previous roller coaster of carbs, caffeine, insulin and blood glucose spikes and crashes, and fatigue.

YOU WON'T BELIEVE WHAT'S PRIMAL!

The diary entries for Ken and Kelly illustrate the concept that Primal Blueprint weight loss does not have to be a spartan exercise of weighing and measuring bland food, choking down powdered "replacements" for real food, relying on pre-packaged and heavily processed "diet" meals, or otherwise engaging in repetitive, restrictive eating habits. While the rules of Primal Blueprint macronutrient intake are clear-cut, there is tremendous opportunity for flexibility within these guidelines.

Primal Blueprint eating offers tremendous flexibility for personal preference, allowing you to actually enjoy the process of transitioning to primal eating.

At MarksDailyApple.com, we have hundreds of recipes, shopping tips, and detailed meal-planning strategies that will help you actually enjoy the process of eating healthfully, perhaps to an even greater extent than you enjoyed your pre-primal dietary habits. You can also check out *The Primal Blueprint Cookbook,* the *Primal Blueprint Quick & Easy Meals,* and the many other primal/paleo cookbooks available today. Take a glance at this list of recipes that are posted on MarksDailyApple.com—yep, they're all primal-approved!

- Arugula Endive Salad with White Wine Vinaigrette
- Spicy Thai Coconut Soup
- Broiled Halibut with Garlic Aioli and Steamed Broccoli
- Crustless Quiche with Spinach and Scallions
- Baked Mahi Mahi with Pesto and Tomatoes
- Grilled Flank Steak with Sautéed Beet Greens and
- Creamy Horseradish Beets
- Smoked Salmon with Asparagus and Poached Egg
- Spicy Korean Seaweed Salad with Shrimp
- Sautéed Broccoli Rabe with Sundried Tomatoes and Pine Nuts

KELLY KORG: SUGGESTED EATING FOR PRIMAL WEIGHT LOSS

Now let's evaluate Kelly Korg, our 40-year-old, 5'4" (162 cm), 148-pound (67 kg), very active female with 27-percent body fat. While her goal of losing nearly eight pounds of body fat (3.6 kg) in a single month is ambitious for a female, she is fit enough to tolerate intense exercise and create substantial caloric deficits with sensible Primal Blueprint meals. She will actually reduce her total weekly exercise time and corresponding calories burned in favor of a more sensible program with slower-paced cardio, more rest, and shorter, more intense workouts.

Caloric Expenditure

1. **Basal Metabolic Rate:** 1,411

2. **Activity Factor:** Harris Benedict Formula for additional calories burned when "very active": BMR × 0.725 = 1,023

3. **Total Average Daily Calorie Expenditure:** BMR (1,411) + Activity Factor (1,023) = 2,433

Macronutrient Calculations

- Goal of losing eight pounds of body fat per month = 933 per day average caloric deficit
- Desired average caloric intake per day = 1,500 (2,433 average caloric expenditure less 933 deficit)
- Minimum daily protein intake = .5 grams per pound (1.1 grams per kg) lean body mass
- 148 pounds at 27-percent body fat = 108 pounds of lean body mass (49 kg)
- Average daily protein intake = 108 pounds × .5 grams per pound = 54 grams (216 calories)
- Desired carb grams = 75 (300 calories) to get into the sweet spot on the Carb Curve
- Desired fat grams = 109 (984 calories) to get back into the 1,500 daily calorie total

You can see right away that the primal eating plan will be much more pleasant for Kelly to follow than her previous efforts to severely restrict calories, interspersed with inevitable carb binges. The fat calories will provide satiety at each meal (missing from her last diet, which featured heavily processed, high-carb liquid shakes). Hitting her protein minimum will ensure that her body recovers from exercise stress, and maintains her lean muscle tissue daily metabolic rate at 2,433 calories.

Kelly Korg Food Journal

BREAKFAST

Steak and Fruit
Flank steak (4 ounces)
Blueberries (1/2 cup)
Peach (1/2 of whole)
Green tea (1 cup)

FitDay.com Analysis
Total Calories: 245
Protein: 25 grams, 100 calories
(41 percent)
Carbs: 16 grams, 64 calories
(26 percent)
Fat: 9 grams, 81 calories
(33 percent)

LUNCH

Chicken Club Lettuce Wrap
Lettuce (3 large leaves)
Diced cooked chicken (4 ounces)
Sliced red pepper (1/2 cup)
Plum tomato (1 medium)
Avocado (1/2 of whole)
Mayonnaise (1 teaspoon)

FitDay.com Analysis
Total Calories: 371
Protein: 37 grams, 148 calories
(40 percent)
Carbs: 13 grams, 52 calories
(14 percent)
Fat: 19 grams, 171 calories
(46 percent)

DINNER

Beef Stir Fry
Sliced beef steak (4 ounces)
Olive oil (1.5 tablespoons)
Sliced zucchini (1 medium)
Sliced mushrooms (1 cup)
Spinach (1 cup)
Sliced bamboo shoots (1/2 cup)
Sesame seeds (1/4 ounce)

FitDay.com Analysis
Total Calories: 624
Protein: 38 grams, 152 calories
  (24 percent)
Carbs: 10 grams, 40 calories
  (6 percent)
Fat: 48 grams, 432 calories
  (69 percent)

SNACKS

Hard-boiled egg (1 large)
Apple (1 medium)
Almond butter (1 tablespoon,
  spread on apple)

FitDay.com Analysis
Total Calories: 291
Protein: 10 grams, 40 calories
  (14 percent)
Carbs: 29 grams, 116 calories
  (40 percent)
Fat: 15 grams, 135 calories
  (46 percent)

DAILY TOTALS

Calories: 1,531
Protein: 110 grams,
  440 calories (29 percent)
Carbs: 68 grams, 272 calories
  (18 percent)
Fat: 91 grams, 819 calories
  (53 percent)

Kelly Korg
Caloric deficit from average
daily expenditure (2,433) = 902
Projected net fat loss over
30-day period:
8 pounds

WEIGHT-LOSS EXERCISE PLAN

While my view that 80 percent of your body composition success is determined by how you eat is difficult to prove scientifically, the anecdotal evidence is overwhelming. Go to the starting line of a major marathon or Ironman triathlon and take note of the surprising level of excess body fat sported by many of these highly trained athletes. The same goes for the droves of gym rats and aerobics devotees with physiques that belie their tremendous devotion to fitness. There's no better proof that regardless of how many calories you burn, consuming excessive processed carbohydrates ultimately inhibits your ability to access and burn stored body fat efficiently around the clock. Instead, when you are locked in a sugar-burning state, all that arduous training results in an increased appetite, combined with insulin-driven sugar cravings, leading to more poor food choices. Unless you are a genetically gifted, extremely devoted endurance athlete (i.e., racing at the front of the pack with a motorcycle escort), it's a vicious cycle that you cannot escape no matter how hard you exercise.

While it's true that exercise moderates the insulin response (a sugary energy gel consumed during a tough workout will be burned quickly and will not prompt an insulin release like it would if you sucked it down at your desk), burning lots of calories (particularly with overly stressful chronic cardio) and eating lots of carbs throughout the day will simply make you carb-dependent for energy. Invariably, left to its own devices, your body will want to overcompensate by tempting you to eat slightly more than you need to refill the tank, as if it's actually thinking, "What if this clown decides to do this again tomorrow? I'd better be ready!" This is how so many people have programmed their genes over the years, protecting them against depletion by stimulating an appetite increase in response to hard exercise.

Beyond the appetite increase, chronic exercise patterns have been scientifically shown to make you lazier throughout the day. Seriously—it's known as the *compensation theory*. Some of this compensatory behavior is conscious ("Sure, why not take the elevator? I already ran five miles this morning."), but there is also a subconscious component. The compensation theory asserts that you generally move less energetically throughout the day and are more liberal with your appetite and caloric intake. Buoyed by a deep down sense of accomplishment from your chronic workouts, you essentially grant yourself free license to veg out and pig out!

The bottom line is that you will not lose fat effectively with exercise-driven weight-loss efforts unless you moderate insulin production.

The bottom line is that you will not lose fat effectively with exercise-driven weight-loss efforts unless you moderate insulin production. Of course, a sensible exercise program will improve your health, sense of wellbeing, and muscle tone, and will somewhat minimize the negative effects of a high-carb diet by making you more insulin sensitive, but it won't get rid of that spare tire. On the flip side, since evolving to a Primal-Blueprint-style eating pattern, I have been able to maintain my ideal body composition effortlessly while working out literally one-tenth as much as I did in the past. During my recovery from knee surgery in 2007, I was able to maintain my exact weight and eight-percent body fat on zero exercise for a month and very limited exercise for a few more months after that.

Of course, we all have genetic differences that account for the reality that "results may vary." Regardless, focus on the concept of triggering the ideal expression of *your* own genetic potential through the combination of Primal Blueprint diet and exercise behaviors. Consider an age when you were pleased with your fitness level and physique. It *is* possible to approximate your appearance and energy levels at age 18 or 21, reversing years or even decades of suboptimal diet and exercise practices.

Be content with long-term improvement in your body composition and a wholehearted enjoyment of the process. If you can focus on the intrinsic value of your choices—to pursue better health, invest in your longevity, take control of your eating behavior—you will be much better off than if your satisfaction depends on the scale. Concentrate on how great you feel, and your motivation and compliance levels will be strong even years down the line.

By the way, you are welcome to pursue the program with more enthusiasm and discipline to produce accelerated results by dialing in your carb intake and fine-tuning your workouts, but you must align your efforts with your fitness level. A serious athlete who has added a few pounds in the off-season can ramp up training easily and return to his or her ideal weight relatively quickly. An old-time pro triathlete I coached was once asked how long it took after he resumed his training program to drop the seven pounds he'd typically gain during the off-season: "A couple long rides," he deadpanned. On the other hand, a novice unaccustomed to regular exercise must follow a more patient approach to avoid burning out. Following are some primal exercise recommendations to turbocharge your weight-loss efforts.

Be not afraid of growing slowly,
be afraid only of standing still.

—Chinese Proverb

Increase General Everyday Movement

When you conduct cardiovascular workouts at "180 minus age" heart rate or below, you enjoy assorted health benefits with little risk of fatigue or burnout. Couple your aerobic sessions with a major effort to increase general everyday movement in every possible way—walking or cycling instead of driving for nearby errands, taking the stairs, parking at the edge of the lot, strolling the neighborhood after dinner, and enjoying leisurely hikes on the weekends. One friend of mine makes business calls while walking briskly on a treadmill (a great icebreaker, by the way: "Hey, what's that hum in the background?").

Make Your Hard Workouts Harder

Your strength and sprint workouts must be brief and intense in order to elicit the desired hormonal response that leads to accelerated fat loss. Be sure that you are well rested before these sessions or skip them if you don't feel 100 percent. Make sure these workouts are not too lengthy—just 4-6 short sprints and strength workouts lasting 10-30 minutes—no longer. Doing prolonged, overly stressful high-intensity sessions promotes carbohydrate dependency and burnout.

Chill Out and Break Through

I cannot emphasize strongly enough how important it is for you to reject the conventional wisdom toward weight loss that obsesses on daily calories burned, strictly controlled portion sizes, and other restrictive nonsense. If you are hungry, eat (the right stuff). If you are motivated, exercise (the right way). And if you are tired, rest! When you are dragging, your energy is needed to rebuild broken-down muscles and your body's systems. Pushing a fatigued body through exercise will only lead to depletion, burnout, and undesirable sugar cravings.

If you are hungry, eat (the right stuff).
If you are motivated, exercise (the right way).
And if you are tired, rest!

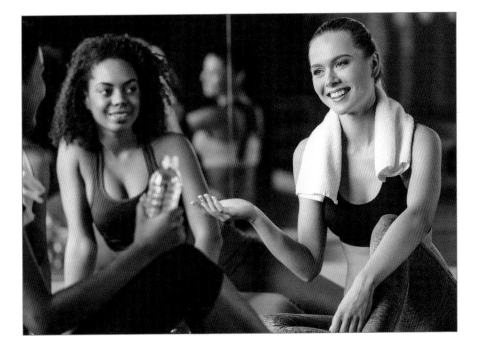

The key to exercise and weight loss is to wisely balance periods of stress and rest. It will be easier for you to reach your peak efforts when you allow adequate time for recovery and rebuilding. With the athletes I advise, I call these peak efforts *breakthrough workouts*—sessions that are difficult and challenging enough to help you "break through" to a higher fitness level (or, in our context here, stimulate a reduction in body fat).

Whether you want to reduce your 10k time or drop ten pounds, it comes down to directing optimal gene expression, primarily through diet, and secondarily through an effective workout plan with occasional breakthrough sessions. From a genetic/survival perspective, it's clear that taking fat off is more difficult than packing it on. Only by harnessing your energy with careful attention to stress management and the occasional bouts of brief, very intense, good old-fashioned hard work can you expect something different than the "same old same old": scale numbers, clothing sizes, race times, and so forth.

SHHH! SISSON'S SIX-PACK SECRETS

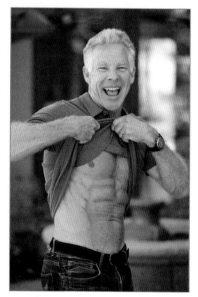

"Washboard Abs on a High-Fat Diet, No Ab Workouts and No Cardio" was the title of one of my most popular MarksDailyApple.com posts. A "six-pack" is widely considered the hallmark of a lean, fit, well-toned physique. Consequently, fitness enthusiasts spend countless hours performing crunches and sit-ups and burning zillions of calories on the treadmill, coupled with obsessively limiting the number of calories they take in, in pursuit of this "gold standard" that is often unrealistic, especially for females. Let's discuss the primal way to develop strong, functional abs without having to exhaust yourself in the gym or starve and dehydrate yourself.

First, moderating carb intake and insulin production is by far the most effective way to improve muscle definition and toning, not only in your abdominal area but everywhere else. That's right, laying off the Cap'n Crunch is better than doing 300 crunches. With your diet optimized, the best way to exercise your abs is to involve them in all manner of movement, both in workouts and in daily life. When you do pushups, tighten your abs (pressing the navel toward the spine); the same is recommended during pull-ups, squats, lunges, curls, and other complete body exercises. Raking leaves, carrying your toddler, reloading the bottom drawer of the copy machine, lugging groceries out of the trunk and onto the kitchen counter, and infinite other daily activities—including simply sitting at your desk or in your car—can all be considered opportunities for a mini ab workout.

When you are engaged in basic movement, sitting or walking, you should tighten your belly as if you are going to be punched in the gut while blowing out the candles on your birthday cake. Hold it for 10, 20, or more seconds a few times every hour. Now do it while slightly tilted to one side. Repeat for the other side. For even better results and a stronger core, you can also simultaneously contract your buttock muscles. After a while, it will become second nature to squeeze your abs spontaneously. Engage your abs, eat right, that's all there is to it!

Suggested Weekly Exercise Schedule

Walk, walk, walk. Hike, hike, hike. Move, move, move. This might seem like strange advice to help you get lean and toned. However, by now you should have a clear understanding of why ill-advised frequent moderate-to-high-intensity workouts simply burn glucose and increase appetite, and that your exercise program on the whole is only dealing with

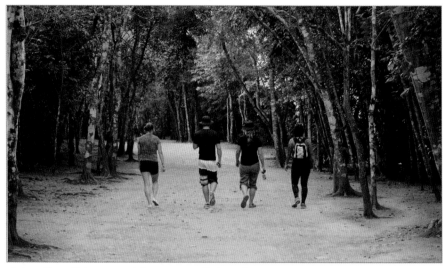

PrimalCon Tulum participants stroll thru the Mexican jungle, touring the 9th century settlement of Coba.

the 20-percent slice of the weight-loss pie. After all, walking around the block or hiking up to the water tower doesn't burn enough calories to contribute notably to weight loss. However, increasing your daily movement will build you from the inside out—toning muscles and strengthening joints and connective tissue so that you can thrive on the high-intensity workouts that strongly influence body composition.

Coupled with Primal Blueprint eating habits, your active lifestyle will refine your fat-burning skills so that you become an efficient fat-burning machine around the clock and easily reach your ideal weight in a matter of weeks or months, as seen with the Korgs' case studies. Best of all, as you scan the suggested daily meal plan (earlier in this chapter) and the weekly exercise plan (next), you'll see that it's easy to eat and exercise in a primal manner for the rest of your life. Here's a sample of what Kelly and Ken did to "go primal" with their workouts:

Sunday: Two-hour hike at low intensity. (The Korgs can do this together and get quality time as well.)

Monday: Easy 45-minute spin on stationary bike and 15-minute walk after dinner.

Tuesday: Fifteen- to 30-minute intense strength-training session. Go for an effort of 8 to 10 on a 10-point scale. Try the Primal Essential Movements (pull-ups, pushups, squats, and planks). Further details are available at MarksDailyApple.com in the free downloadable ebook *Primal Blueprint Fitness*, as well as *The Primal Blueprint 21-Day Total Body Transformation* and a series of instructional videos available on YouTube. (Search "Mark Sisson Primal Essential Movements.") Fifteen-minute walk after dinner.

Wednesday: Rest.

Thursday: Easy 45-minute stationary bike ride or hike.

Friday: Sprint session at grass field, school track, or even the beach. You can also sprint indoors on an elliptical machine or stationary bicycle. Duration, including warmup and cooldown, is about 20 minutes. Choose from the recommended sessions based on ability level in the Bonus Material at the end of this book.

Saturday: Ten-minute intense strength-training session. Go for an effort of 6 to 7 on a 10-point scale.

Exercise Analysis
Total Duration: Around five hours—most of it comfortable cardio.

Total Calories Burned: Who cares! Enough to accelerate fat reduction and get in shape without suffering.

Muscle Groups Exercised: Arms, legs, core, and everything in between or attached.

Total Scenery Enjoyed: A ton more than someone on a treadmill or an elliptical or in a spin class.

Total Fun Had: Lots!

What a far cry from Kelly Korg's exhausting regimen of predawn high-intensity workouts, nutrient-devoid shakes replacing real meals, and the resulting fatigue, energy-level swings, and sugar cravings! Kelly, on the Primal Blueprint plan, could wake up leisurely with the rest of the family and enjoy herself with comfortable exercise sessions (possibly including some of her less-than-optimally-active family members?). Instead of suffering several mornings a week—and sacrificing hours of sleep that are crucial for her health, not to mention her fat-loss efforts—she could pick a few key opportunities to engage in high-intensity breakthrough workouts that leave her exhilarated and accelerate her fat reduction. In six months' time, she'll have shed some 24 pounds of body fat and likely have added a few pounds of well placed, lean, toned muscle tissue. She'll be happier and more energetic, and she'll look better than she has in decades, with less effort and less struggle than before.

Meanwhile, Kelly's neighbor Wendy (remember her, the peppy network marketing enthusiast who dropped eight pounds in two weeks?) will almost assuredly weigh the same or more than she did when she started her cleansing diet six months prior. Furthermore, because 99 percent of network marketing participants lose money (from a survey of the largest and most reputed network marketing operations, after considering all expenses and inventory purchased from the company for resale), she'll probably have a lot of cleansing diet kits gathering dust on the garage shelves.

I.F. YOU WANT TO LOSE *EVEN MORE FAT*, TRY IT!

As we reflect on the tidy examples of Ken and Kelly Korg nailing their daily caloric deficits with delicious, fulfilling meals, I must stress once again the concept of averages and expanding your timeline out from a day or week to at least a month-by-month view for measured progress. The meal diaries for Ken and Kelly obviously represent a good—make that perfect—day. In real life, your ability to optimize your meal choices and caloric intake will be more difficult than the examples (based on some of my own favorite meals) printed here. I realize there will be days, and even longer periods, when you slip away from the ideal.

However, you can get back on track and even make up ground easily because of the metabolic leverage you create with Primal Blueprint eating habits. When your insulin production is moderated and your fat metabolism is optimized, you have a greatly reduced need to snack or even eat regular meals. As you'll see from my 72-hour personal journal (sidebar in the next chapter), my own day-to-day caloric intake varies wildly due to my whims and schedule variations.

When your body has reprogrammed gene expression to be able to get energy from fat whenever it wants, hunger tends to subside, and blood sugar and energy levels stabilize. Why not tap into this new "skill" and take full advantage? You can easily make up lost ground when you slip a little, and you can also accelerate the process of fat reduction to virtually whatever speed you want (up to the maximum mentioned previously) by engaging in a classic primal strategy called Intermittent Fasting (I.F.).

You choose just when and how to practice I.F. Your decisions should fit with your personality, lifestyle, schedule, and unique habits and preferences. I recommend starting by simply waiting until you experience hunger to eat your first meal of the day. Since you are already fasted for some eight hours when you awaken, this represents a great way to track your progress with becoming fat-adapted. If you are hungry right away, go ahead and break your fast with breakfast. Over time, you should find yourself easily being able to last until lunchtime with good energy and no food. Teaching your body to operate for 16 hours without calories improves your insulin sensitivity, turbo-charges your fat metabolism, and promotes longevity by slowing cell division in favor of improved cell repair. Personally, a compressed eating window is my standard practice—I generally eat only between the hours of noon and 8:00 p.m. daily.

Another intuitive way to engage in I.F. is to skip a meal when you don't feel hungry. Numerous studies show that I.F. offers a multitude of benefits, including loss of body fat (obviously), lowered blood pressure, improved insulin sensitivity and glucose uptake, a decrease in inflammation and oxidative damage, and improved longevity by virtue of slowing cell division in favor of improved cell repair. I fast when I feel a disturbance in immune function, such as a sore throat or stuffy head, and believe that my recovery is quicker as a result.

These benefits are achieved when certain genes are "turned on" to repair specific tissues that would not otherwise be repaired in times of caloric surplus. The idea is that this genetic adaptation allows certain cells to live longer (as repaired cells) during famine because it's energetically less expensive to repair a cell than to divide and create a new one. That might help explain some of the phenomenal longevity results produced by studies on animals eating restricted-calorie diets; with mice, longevity continues to improve as calories are restricted by 10 percent, 20 percent, and even 50 percent of normal.

Animal studies have shown that I.F. reduces spontaneous cancers, which could be due to a decrease in oxidative damage and/or an increase in immune response. Pockets of research around the globe strongly suggest that deregulated meal timing and generally moderated caloric intake produce many health benefits (particularly for those who are overweight) and promote longevity with virtually no negative side effects.

It's important to note, however, that some studies and plenty of anecdotal evidence suggests that males and females respond differently to I.F. For some women, especially pre-menopausal women, I.F. can potentially disrupt normal hormone production and lead to dysregulated menstrual cycles, fertility, appetite, and so on. This makes sense if you consider that pre-menopausal women's bodies need to be especially attuned to signs of starvation in order to protect themselves and their fetuses and offspring during pregnancy and breastfeeding. Thus for everyone, but for women especially, it is important to be very intuitive when you begin incorporating I.F. Start small and build up to longer and/or more frequent fasts as long as they seem to be producing desirable effects, but scale back or stop if you perceive that your body is overly stressed. Many women enjoy I.F. as long as they pursue it mindfully and adjust their approach as needed. A simple rule of thumb to follow is eat when you are hungry! That's right, I.F. is not about suffering; it's about fine-tuning your fat-burning genes by not eating if you aren't hungry!

Whatever method of fasting/caloric restriction you engage in, the net effect is to send signals to your genes to upregulate fat burning, downregulate glucose burning, and even manufacture more energy producing mitochondria in your cells. If you ever notice yourself "hangry" when you miss a meal, that is a sign that you are still somewhat carbohydrate dependent. No problem, just eat some food (make sure it's primal-aligned with emphasis on high-satiety fat—resist dosing with sugar when you're hangry) and carry on with your patient efforts to become more fat-adapted.

To be clear, I.F. is a strategy best employed after a sustained period of eating primally, especially if you are coming from a SAD eating pattern, so that your body becomes proficient at burning fat. Fasting is easier to handle when you control insulin production with Primal Blueprint-aligned foods and much harder when you are entrenched in a typical American diet with lots of carbs and the resulting insulin (and energy) highs and lows.

Regular meals are overrated!

If you have tried fasting or skipping meals in the past but (as with Kelly Korg) concurrently ate a diet that is moderate to high in carbs, you can likely relate to becoming irritable and exhausted when you miss even a single meal. In my days as an endurance athlete, I burned so many calories and relied so heavily on carbohydrates to refill the glycogen stores that I drained daily, I'd feel like I was on the verge of a hypoglycemic coma if I did so much as skip breakfast. Now I marvel at how often I forget to eat—and the fact that doing so has no impact on my energy levels. That's the true power of shifting from sugar burning to becoming an efficient fat burner.

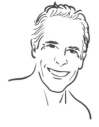

MARK TALK

Crazy as it may seem after a lifetime of cultural programming about the importance of eating regular meals (especially breakfast!), there are many health benefits to waiting until you are hungry to eat. However, this is true if and only if you are fat-adapted and able to access internal sources for energy. If you are carb-dependent and you force yourself to fast, skip meals, or try a restrictive calorie diet, your body will shift into starvation mode. Surely you've heard this refrain before: skip a meal and your metabolic rate slows down, and what calories you do eat are more likely to be stored as fat.

Yep, carbohydrate dependency is no fun. The only way to break free is to moderate insulin production in your diet, thereby reprogramming your genes to burn stored body fat. Once fat-adapted, you can drop excess body fat through strategic fasting and calorie restriction, without the risks that arise when you are carb-dependent. It takes about three weeks of devoted dietary modification to downregulate sugar-burning genes and upregulate fat-burning genes, so stick with it at first! When you can wake up and last a few or more hours before needing breakfast, it's a good indication you are fat-adapted. Then, you are on you way to effortless lifelong weight management.

Freeing yourself from an addiction to regular doses of energy from ingested calories is the essence of "going primal." Experiencing these primal "symptoms" yourself ("Hey, I'm actually not hungry!") will recalibrate your entire belief system about food and meals.

If you take a moment to reflect on the principles of evolution and homeostasis, it's clear how messed up our modern eating culture is. It should not be hard for humans to sustain daily energy levels and optimal body composition but we make it hard by constantly filling our bodies with foods that we are not adapted to eat. Eat strictly primal-aligned foods for twenty-one days or more to allow your genes to upregulate fat-burning mechanisms and to moderate insulin levels, before playing around with Intermittent Fasting. I promise that you will experience this epiphany: that you are eating the way evolution designed us (perhaps for the first time since infancy), that it is easy and fun, leading to breakthroughs in your fat loss and long-term weight management.

WEIGHT-LOSS TROUBLESHOOTING

If you are making a sincere effort to drop body fat with the Primal Blueprint and are not satisfied with your results, here are some issues that might be tripping you up, along with some suggestions to alter your routine.

Get into the Sweet Spot and Stay There!

If the fat is not coming off quickly enough after a month or two of Primal Blueprint efforts, the best remedy is to restrict carbohydrate intake further and stay in the sweet spot of 50 to 100 grams per day (on average) for several weeks, or even trying to go ketogenic for short stretches. Once you reach your body composition goals, you'll be able to relax your carbohydrate restrictions, land in the maintenance zone of 100 to 150 grams per day, and maintain your existing body composition indefinitely.

While you might experience difficulty adjusting to the severe reduction of dietary "staples" (e.g., grains and pleasure foods, including sweetened beverages and snacks), your body will quickly adapt to an eating style that is aligned with your genes. Yes, I know, getting your carbs down to 50 to 100 grams per day is easier said than done. That is why many people get stuck in the mode of "trying" to cut back instead of making a firm commitment to modify their habitual intake of certain foods by replacing them with ample servings of foods that are more nutritious and technically more satisfying to their bodies than their favorite carb treats.

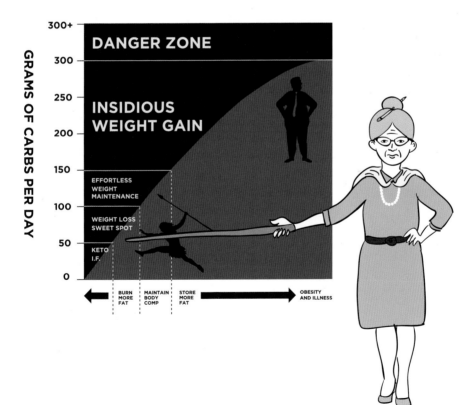

It will require great discipline to maintain an average of 50 to 100 grams (remember, most of us are accustomed to throwing down 300 grams or more per day), but you only have to do it for a short time—say a month or two—depending on your starting point and how ambitious your goals are. By "great discipline," I'm not talking about suffering with a cloud of anguish and guilt hanging over your head. I'm simply recommending you eat plenty of eggs, meat, chicken, fish, nuts, and seeds, plus all the vegetables you want and fruits (with a little bit of restraint and selectivity), and stay away from grains, sugars, and processed foods.

I strongly recommend using an online food calculator to know exactly where you stand instead of guessing. I find the mere act of having to write down everything I eat for one or two days increases my awareness of dietary habits and provides an effective check and balance against idle grazing or overeating when awareness is low. Chart everything you eat for a few days and then enter the results at FitDay.com to get a truly accurate accounting of your carb intake. Even today, with what I consider a pretty decent knowledge of the macronutrient content of many foods, I continue to be surprised at some of the results that the online calculators spit out.

Moderate Stress Levels

Body fat reduction simply doesn't work well when you are skimping on sleep, working too hard, or experiencing high levels of emotional and psychological stress. To successfully change your body composition for the long term, you must have the time, energy, and patience to devote attention and care to the topic. Rushing through meals or reaching for sweet foods when you are stressed is not aligned with the simple lifestyle of the Primal Blueprint.

It's time to start walking your talk, rather than burning the candle at both ends. Allow your genes to express themselves optimally by making healthier choices. Perhaps you can relate to Ken Korg's constant, moderate-to-high workplace stress, plus the financial strain of maintaining his suburban lifestyle with a little bit of keepin' up with the Joneses thrown in. Such chronic stress wreaks havoc on your sympathetic nervous system, causing hormone imbalances, sugar cravings, sleep distur-

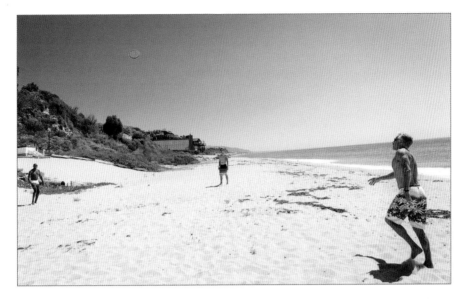

bances, flagging energy levels, and trouble losing weight. Nor do those choices lead to a happy, fulfilled life.

You simply must take a hard look at the sources of stress in your life and start making positive changes toward reducing (ideally, eliminating) chronic stressors. This is also where those Primal Blueprint lifestyle laws come into play. Getting enough sleep (including naps, to optimize appetite and the release of metabolic hormones), sunshine (vitamin D enhances all cellular function, including fat metabolism), and play, relaxing, and using your brain will assist your weight-loss goals on many levels. While the insulin control and intense sprint sessions might be the sexier elements of the Primal Blueprint weight-loss plan, you should not discount the importance of the supporting lifestyle elements that can make or break your success.

Sleep More

When you skimp on sleep, you disturb key appetite and metabolic hormones that can sabotage your otherwise devoted weight-loss efforts. Lack of sleep spikes ghrelin, a key appetite-stimulating hormone, and dysregulates leptin, a key hormone that controls whether you burn or store fat. Blasting your eyeballs with artificial light and digital stimulation after dark suppresses melatonin (the hormone that causes you to

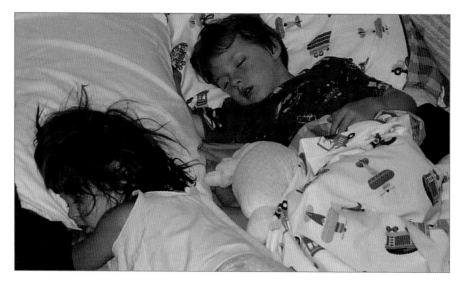

feel sleepy) and spikes the stress hormone cortisol, which leads to sugar cravings. Suppressed melatonin also disturbs the function of glucagon, the hormone that liberates stored body fat and glycogen to be burned for energy. The list goes on, but you get the point: your delicate hormone system, which influences fat metabolism among many other things, is integrally tied to your sleep patterns.

To lose excess body fat, you must avoid excess artificial light and digital stimulation after dark. You also must strive to receive adequate sleep every night (at least eight hours for most people, perhaps more for some individuals and during winter months). If your weight-loss efforts are stalled, especially if you have been conscientiously eating in the sweet spot, do an honest assessment of your sleep habits. If you are not receiving sufficient high-quality sleep most nights, observing regular bed and natural wake times, and avoiding artificial light at night, this is the next thing you must get in order.

Adopt a Positive Mindset

The subject of body composition is too often laden with a sense of failure, deprivation, restriction, self-limiting beliefs ("I have the fat gene"), and superficial judgment from society. Yet I believe there is a bigger picture that involves optimism, positive thoughts, and enjoyment of the process that you can choose to adopt when you pursue body composition changes. When working toward any goal, psychological research suggests that you will enjoy greater happiness and perceived wellbeing, and perhaps be more successful, if you approach the goal with the mindset that you are working toward mastery. This can include taking control of your weight, learning how to optimize your health, or overcoming a long-term health issue. When the rewards you experience are intrinsic – such as feeling more vibrant and energetic, appreciating the investment you are making in yourself, modeling healthy behaviors for loved ones- rather than extrinsic (for example, the numbers on a scale), you are likely to experience more success and to enjoy the process. Focusing on the process rather than the outcome can also be beneficial because it allows you to observe and appreciate even incremental steps in the right direction, and it rewards commitment to the goal even when progress is slow.

It is critical to approach the subject of fat loss with a positive attitude and an appreciation for the journey. Your primary motivation must be to enjoy a higher quality of life and better health. This sense of purpose will far overshadow any disappointment related to not losing body fat as quickly as you might want. A change in body composition is not something to obsess about, measure, and judge as a success or failure each day or each week. Instead, it should be an effortless byproduct of primal living, a consequence of lifestyle changes driven by ideals higher than wanting to look good in a bikini for your summer vacation in Hawaii (although there is nothing wrong with that goal if it's within a healthy, big picture context).

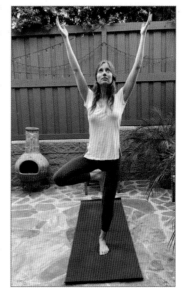

The great thing about mindset is that it is something you can control. It may take effort, but you can actively work on quieting negative self-talk by consciously shifting your attention to the positive changes you have made, and the milestones you have reached. Pick a favorite inspirational quote or mantra to use when negative feelings start bubbling up. Like anything else, it gets easier the more you do it, so start practicing today.

---★---

HOW TO LOSE LIKE A WINNER

The sensible limit on the rate of losing body fat is evident when you consider that one pound of fat contains 3,500 calories, and adults only burn between 1,500 and 3,000 total calories per day, much of which comes from food. What about the "Biggest Losers" glorified on the television program, or in before-and-after magazine contests, who alter their body composition dramatically in a short time? These results are achieved with a combination of incredibly grueling exercise coupled with severe caloric restriction, an approach that is simply untenable in the real world and impossible to follow long term. Generally, any extreme weight-loss effort results in a significant reduction in water retention and lean muscle mass, and just a bit of fat loss.

A crash weight-loss program (or any other form of extreme stress, such as a family crisis) prompts a prolonged fight or flight response in your body. Buzzed on stress hormones, you can triumphantly complete your six-, eight-, or twelve-week program—particularly when the bright lights of television and monetary incentives are there to motivate you. Afterward, you are likely to collapse in exhaustion when the fight or flight response wears off, and your body's energy reserves are depleted. In this post-traumatic-stress state, many become sedentary (or much less active, in any case) and tend to overeat—a genetically programmed reaction to an ordeal perceived as a starvation threat.

Lo and behold, the "before and after" success story typically becomes a "before and after and back to before ... and a little more" reality check! There is absolutely no reason to struggle or suffer to achieve your body composition and health goals. In fact, if you are, I can guarantee that your approach is flawed and destined for long-term failure.

When you embrace the Primal Blueprint as a lifelong transition away from conventional wisdom's flawed grain-based diet into something aligned with your genetic requirements for health, you'll realize there is no hurry here—and that you'll have complete control over your physique for the rest of your life. Fine-tune your eating habits or workout patterns for a few weeks, and you can drop fat and add or tone muscle as simply as turning a number on a dial.

P.S. Do you know how some of those amazing before/after contest winners haul in the big bucks with their mind-blowing transformations over short time periods? Rumor has it that certain opportunistic super-fit hardbodies will cease training and commence a crash course in chowing junk food and spending lots of time on the couch. After a few weeks of devoted sloth and gluttony, they will snap a "before" photo—with the requisite sad face, poor lighting, and likely bloated with an extra gallon of water in the tank. Once the money shot is secured, they will plunge back into intense training and return to their sculpted ways in a matter of weeks. Leading up to the "after" money shot, they'll stop eating for a day and dehydrate themselves in a sauna until the veins start popping like the Los Angeles Area Freeway System map.

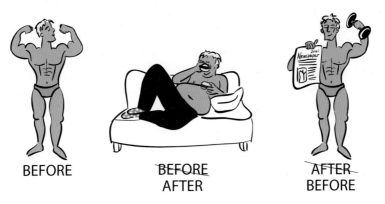

BEFORE   ~~BEFORE~~
              AFTER

              ~~AFTER~~
              BEFORE

In essence, they become "Before (ripped)-After (sloth and gluttony)-(and back to) Before" success stories—the opposite of the poor schlubs who are trying to play by the rules and get into shape too quickly!

Accept Your Plateaus, Then Carry On—Primally

When I say you can "average a pound or two a week" of fat loss, I'd like you to consider this statement with the perspective of a four-month or six-month timeline. I know we are conditioned to a "what have you done for me lately" mentality, but we are dealing with lifestyle change here, not journal entries of happy faces or frowns each day based on your scale numbers or food calculator graphs and charts.

> *Your genetically ideal weight is where you are healthy, energetic, and comfortable.*

I guarantee that making some elementary primal changes (eliminating grains and excess sugar from your diet to regulate your carb intake to a below-100-grams-per-day average; adjusting your exercise program to refrain from chronic cardio, and adding some brief, intense sessions to the mix) will result in a certain amount of effortless weight loss. However, there is a range of possible outcomes based upon individual factors such as your compliance rate as discussed in the Troubleshooting section, your stress levels, and how long or severely you have diverged from Primal Blueprint laws before embarking on this journey.

After a sustained period of fat loss, it's not uncommon to see results level off and hit a plateau—even if you are still carefully restricting your carb intake. For example, a female might effortlessly go from 185 pounds to 152 pounds in six months, at which point she might long to drop into the 140s and find the process a bit more difficult. This is a natural and expected homeostatic drive kicking into action in response to fat reduction. Fat is essential to survival, so your genes might downregulate insulin receptors or trigger an elevation of hunger hormones in the interest of survival. In many cases, your plateau is where your body feels comfortable, healthy, and energetic, and hence it will rebel against further fat-reduction efforts. Knowing this, you might decide that it's not really worth the additional effort and focus to go beyond your "healthy, energetic, comfortable weight" to a tenuous lower weight. Accept that plateaus are going to happen, for a valid genetic reason, and see if you can practice some acceptance.

If It Were Easy...

One of my favorite sayings—whether it has to do with business, fitness, or balancing the varied demands and responsibilities of daily life—is: "If it were easy, everyone would be doing it." There is a reason you don't see 80 percent of American adults sporting single-digit body fat or dozens of joggers flying by in the park at a pace of six minutes per mile. If you are unsatisfied with your results after months of devoted effort, I recommend focusing on two things to help stimulate a breakthrough. First, be more diligent about restricting average daily carb intake. Second, introduce some high-intensity sprints (preferably weight bearing) into your fitness routine.

In the first case, many people unwittingly eat too many carbs—this is where journaling can be helpful. With sprinting, the shock of

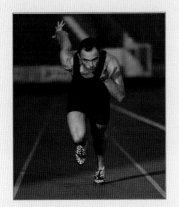

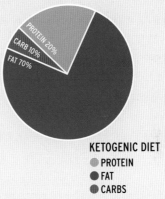

KETOGENIC DIET
- PROTEIN
- FAT
- CARBS

asking your body to perform at 30 MET (Metabolic Equivalent of Task—an all-out sprint requires metabolic function 30 times higher than when you are at rest) can accelerate fat reduction in a way that hours of additional cardio simply cannot.

CHAPTER SUMMARY

1. Primal Blueprint Fat Loss: You can lose an average one to two pounds of body fat per week (one-half to one kilogram) by taking in targeted, optimal levels of each macronutrient daily, fasting intermittently, doing Primal Blueprint-style workouts, and approaching the challenge with a positive, process-oriented, big picture attitude. Don't stress about results or apply an overly regimented approach. Instead, cultivate an intuitive approach where you honor natural appetite and focus on the enjoyment of eating delicious, satisfying foods.

2. Macronutrients: Adequate protein intake (0.7 grams per pound, or 1.54 grams per kg, of lean body mass) will preserve muscle tissue (and metabolism) during calorie-restriction efforts, avoiding the "crash-and-burn" effect of most diets. Maintaining the "sweet spot" intake of 50 to 100 grams of carbohydrates per day will moderate insulin production and allow stored body fat to be utilized as a primary energy source. Fat intake will be the main variable to ensure you are satisfied and nourished at each meal, making your weight-loss efforts effective, realistic, and even enjoyable.

3. Korgs' Weight Loss: Ken and Kelly Korg can achieve their ambitious fat-reduction goals by eating delicious, nutritious Primal Blueprint-style meals. When the carb intake sweet spot is observed, and protein requirements are met, ample amounts of fat will provide a high satiety factor at meals but will not result in excess fat storage thanks to low insulin levels.

4. Exercise: Increase low-level activity, both from structured aerobic sessions at a heart rate of "180 minus age" or below and increased general everyday movement. Conduct brief, high-intensity sessions to stimulate adaptive hormones in the bloodstream and accelerate fat reduction. Take care to avoid chronic exercise patterns (both from aerobic workouts at excessive heart rates and high-intensity workouts that are too long in duration). These stimulate appetite and result in diminished everyday activity per the compensation theory. Relax any preoccupation with burning calories for weight management. Focus instead on balancing stress and rest and making intuitive workout decisions.

5. Intermittent Fasting: Whether deliberate or as a natural outcome of fluctuating mealtimes (now that stored body fat instead of ingested carbs is your preferred energy source), I.F. will create natural caloric deficits that lead to fat reduction and effortless long-term maintenance of ideal body composition. A great way to start with I.F. is to simply wait until you are hungry to eat your first meal of the day. You can track your progress with fat-adaptation accordingly.

6. Troubleshooting: If your progress slows, try being more diligent in hitting the carb intake sweet spot (using an online nutrient calculator to know exactly where you stand), moderating your stress levels (by utilizing the Primal Blueprint lifestyle laws), sleeping in accordance with your natural circadian rhythm, and adopting a positive mindset.

7. Plateaus: Expect that your progress may stall after some good results, due to natural homeostatic forces trying to keep you at your set point. Practice some acceptance that your "comfortable, healthy, energetic" weight may be different than an arbitrary lower goal weight that is tenuous to reach and maintain.

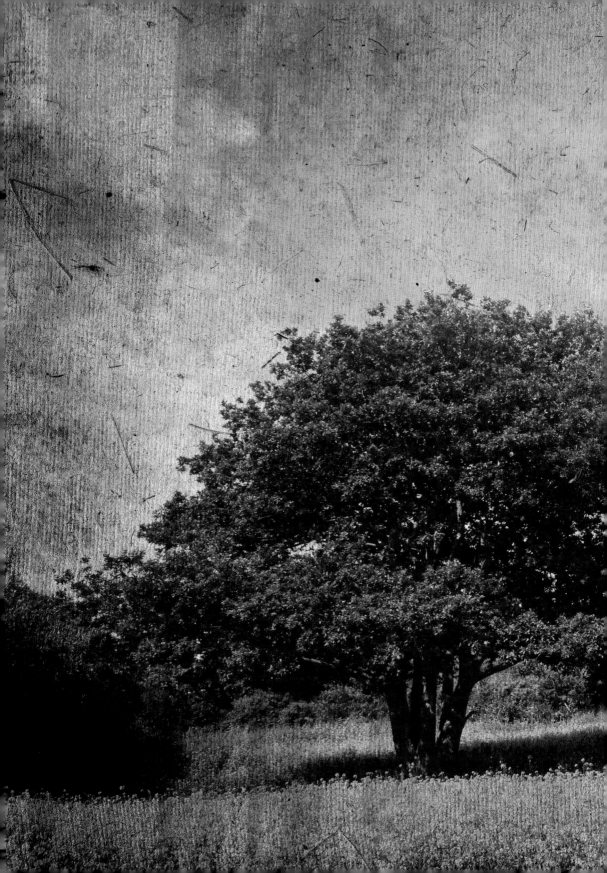

CHAPTER TEN

CONCLUSION

Time to Party Like a Grok Star!

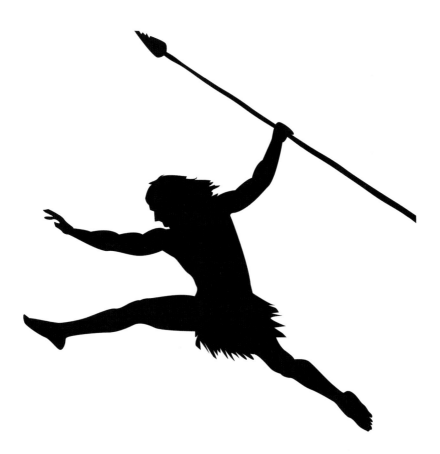

A s we near the end of the book, I want to call attention to the special place in my heart that Chapter 2, "Grok and Korg," occupies. I've been fascinated by the primal concept for nearly three decades. (I self-published my *Training and Racing Duathlons* book using the name Primal Urge Press in 1988!)

As an athlete and a coach, I've reflected on the primal theme constantly—inspiring athletes to balance the unnatural act of endurance training with proper recovery and lifestyle support and to temper our primal competitive human instincts with common sense to avoid burnout.

My work in the fields of nutrition and personal training, and my immersion into the health community on the Internet, have enlightened me about the realities of everyday modern life for the masses. While we are making progress in some ways, I am increasingly disturbed by the seemingly inexorable drift farther and farther away from natural, healthy, evolved behavior in the technological world.

As my staff and I worked through the stages of Chapter 2—conceptual, research, first draft, editing, soliciting external feedback, and revisions—I finally had the chance to print a fresh copy, sit on a lounge chair in my yard, and truly "read" the material for the first time. I have to admit I was downright horrified. I questioned whether people would think the commentary was sensational or unrealistic and be turned off accordingly. I returned to my computer, reviewed all the references, conducted more research, and generally made darn sure this was an accurate and realistic picture of modern life.

Unfortunately, the draft withstood my own devil's advocate scrutiny as well as that of numerous health, medical, nutrition, psychology, and sociology experts. Family and career men in their 40s and 50s take prescriptions left and right, families frequently feel that life is too hectic and stressful to align with the broad definition of health, and teenagers often feel overpressured and disconnected from parents. Today's kids have too much body fat and too little physical fitness. We eat too much beige stuff and not enough green stuff. We avoid exercise and sit at desks all day staring at a screen in the name of increased productivity. We go home at night and stare at a bigger screen in the name of relaxation. We stay up too late and then awaken to the stressful screech of an alarm clock. We are stressed by bills, traffic, noise pollution, digital pollution, the past, the future, and all kinds of anxiety we manufacture in our restless minds. Our first line of defense when our genes react to these lifestyle habits as they are programmed to do is prescription drugs, which treat symptoms quickly but, over time, weaken our natural ability to maintain health.

As we bombard our genes with these lifestyle risk factors, they respond the only way they know how in an often futile attempt to maintain homeostasis and a desperate effort to keep us alive in the short term—with inflammation, early cell death, insulin resistance, atrophy, and so on. If you consider the dietary habits, activity level, and body composition of your family above-average, you can congratulate yourself while remembering that "average" is actually borderline obese. (Sixty-four percent of American adults are classified as overweight, of which about half are classified as obese.)

In California, 40 percent of 10-year-old schoolchildren fail to attain a bare minimum aerobic conditioning performance standard known as the *Healthy Fitness Zone* (established by the Cooper Aerobics Institute), meaning that hundreds of thousands of "average" kids in California are technically classified "at risk" to develop serious health problems related to inactivity because they can't complete a mile run at a slow jog. *Forty percent!* Take a zero off that figure and I think you'd approximate the relevant statistic during the time of my youth. And this is in what might be considered a progressive, fair-weather state, with a rate of overweight and obese children that is lower than the national average. (According to the Kaiser Family Foundation in 2011, 30.4 percent of Californian children aged 10 to 17 were overweight or obese, compared to 31.3 percent nationwide. What's incredibly troubling is the state performing the "best"—Utah—still measured 22.1 percent of children being classified as overweight/obese.)

As we reflect on how far we have drifted from Grok's simple lifestyle and ponder how we can better honor and reprogram our genes by following the Primal Blueprint, it is critical to proceed with a clean slate and a deep conviction that you are doing the right thing. This is not an easy task. Numerous elements of the Primal Blueprint flat out oppose the mainstream dogma that government espouses or that Big Agra and Big Pharma promote with billions of advertising and marketing dollars.

One must also wonder how society has strayed so egregiously far from the healthy living that Grok enjoyed and devolved to the carb-overdosed, pill-popping, overfed, overweight, overstressed Ken Korg. How can the conventional wisdom that you have believed for years and decades be wrong and even dangerous? The truth is, human nature is to blame. Just like Grok, programmed into our genes is a desire to manipulate and rule our environment for our benefit, to pursue a more advanced, more comfortable life. Our indomitable human spirit has accomplished many great things but has also created tremendous fallout from our constant quest for "progress."

Humans have conquered the world. As a species, we are the fat cat. Yet now, peak physical and intellectual performance and self-discipline are no longer requirements for survival. Humans have become self-indulgent and driven by short-term gratification. Like the miners who stripped and poisoned the land and waterways during the California gold rush, we have done similar damage to our bodies in the name of making life easier, more convenient, and more productive.

In Eric Schlosser's *Fast Food Nation*, he reveals how the fast-food phenomenon exploded in popularity in the 1950s because fast food made life easier: no more cooking or lengthy waits for expensive meals. Families across all socioeconomic levels were suddenly able to live the good life by dining out on delicious food. Unfortunately, the fare served up was disastrous not only to the human body but also to the human spirit—destroying a centerpiece of family fabric that was the shared home-cooked meal of fresh, nutritious foods.

When there is interest and demand to make life easier, profit seekers often swarm in and exploit this element of the human spirit. Nowhere is this more evident than in the field of health. While I am all in favor of capitalism and making a profit, it seems that where health is concerned, today we must question the approach, motives, and trustworthiness of many of the traditional pillars of health, human compassion, and expert knowledge. We must admit that doctors, despite their extensive knowledge, training, and loyalty to the Hippocratic Oath, are focused on treatment rather than prevention. The sad reality is that most of their business comes from dealing with symptoms—not causes—of easily preventable conditions. As with drugs, it's wonderful to have extensively trained and prepared doctors standing ready when we need them, but it seems the preferred solution to all medical issues today is to throw money at the problem (as evidenced by the remarkable comment from a solo family practice doc I know who lamented that his "business was down" due to the 2008 economic recession!), hoping for a quick fix instead of making the necessary lifestyle changes to get to the root of the problem. The fact that doctors receive little or no training in nutrition is nothing short of abysmal.

Our government's laws, subsidies, and diet-education efforts are seemingly driven more by lobbyists for the beef, grain, and dairy industries than by unbiased scientific evaluation and concern for human health. In the media, the historical checks and balances provided by honorable and unbiased investigative journalists have been deemphasized and devalued by giant ratings-driven corporations. Salacious "click-bait" stories that elicit fear, anger, or other strong emotions are what sell, regardless of their legitimacy. Even our scholarly community is subject to free-market influences that potentially bias the objectivity and even the premise of many studies.

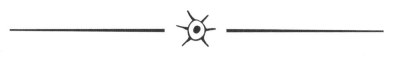

THE KORG KOMEBACK!

Let me reiterate my distaste for a perfectionist mentality toward diet, physical appearance, lifestyle change, and even school, career, and competitive athletics. Respecting the broad definition of health and the legacy of the simple lifestyle that our ancestors lived, we need to reject the measuring and judging forces of society and pursue fun and peace of mind in conjunction with health and fitness goals.

Admittedly, your efforts to go primal will possibly require some serious adjustments to your comfortable modern existence. If you feel overwhelmed or take occasional exception to my strong positions, keep in mind my 80 Percent Rule as well as the suggestion to take one step at a time.

While the Korgs seem quite far down a disastrous road, they can also quite easily turn things around, step by step, with minimal pain, suffering, negativity, or disruption of the things they love to do in life. If Ken modifies his late-night activities by snacking on macadamia nuts instead of cheesecake, watching less television in favor of reading or a quick stroll around the block with the dog, and turning the lights out at 10:30 P.M. instead of midnight, he'll fall asleep more easily and wake up refreshed the next morning, without having to rely on Ambien. This means more quality time with the kids, including *walking* young Cindy to school.

If Ken brings the macadamias, some carrot sticks, and a couple hard-boiled eggs for snacks at work and chooses lunch wisely at the supermarket deli (one-third pound of sliced tri tip stuffed inside a red bell pepper costs less than Chinese buffet), he'll better maintain energy and concentration during the workday, increase his productivity, and better handle workplace stress. Ken will leave the office at 6 P.M. feeling ready to enjoy and appreciate the leisure and family time options that await.

If Kelly reduces the stress of her exercise program and eats delicious, satisfying Primal Blueprint meals, she will get her blood sugar and energy levels under control and tap into her stored body fat for a steady, reliable source of energy. With Kenny, a few sensible and consistently enforced limits on digital entertainment and bedtimes will help him reconnect with the family, focus better in school, and consider the option to eliminate his medication.

Talk about little things making a big difference! There is no better example to illustrate this maxim than the momentum (particularly the unbridled increase in physical energy) created by healthy lifestyle changes begetting further healthy lifestyle changes.

ON YOUR OWN

It is sobering, to say the least, opening our eyes to the direction the bullet train carrying modern society is heading. In my opinion, the heaviest realization of all is that you are *on your own*. The imagined safety net of government, modern medicine, or the food or pharmaceutical industries looking after your health is a facade. Oh sure, you'll be cared for very, very well if something catastrophic happens (that is, if you have good medical insurance), whether it's a high-risk childbirth, serious injuries from a car accident, or one of the small fraction of cancers that are not lifestyle related. But when it comes to eating healthy, getting in shape, avoiding stupid mistakes—even building a career and a nest egg—the world can lead you astray and separate you from your cash (and other assets, such as health, emotional wellbeing, etc.) in the blink of an eye.

The Elitist Race

I read with amusement the occasional critiques of the Primal Blueprint eating style as being "elitist"—too expensive (eschewing inexpensive grains and switching from conventionally grown animals and produce to the pasture-raised or organic variety) and impractical for the average person to follow. Furthermore, astute observers point out that there are not enough local, pasture-raised animal products or produce to sustain the entire population. I acknowledge this observation and how it opens up a can of worms and big picture questions about global overpopulation (made possible by the cultivation of grains to feed the expanding masses) and the sustainability of life on our planet in general. Indeed, in this context, making healthy choices is elitist and also puts you into a competitive situation for scarce resources. That said, basic economic theory confirms that if more people demand local, pasture-raised animal products, they will become more affordable and more plentiful; if more people take a stand against industrial food or manufacturers peddling poison, there will be less availability and advertising of these products. Also, when you say healthy eating is expensive, you might want to compare the cost of quality food to the long-term costs of medical care for lifestyle-related health conditions. The cost of a single major surgery outweighs decades of making "elite" food choices over conventional ones!

When it comes to eating right and exercising, there is no 'I'll start tomorrow.' Tomorrow is disease.
—V. L. Allineare

Over the past century of rapid technological progress, we've figured out how to manufacture and package food and mass-produce animals, producing huge profits without regard to the health, humane, or ecological consequences. Stepping back for a moment to grab a wide-angle view of the wide angles in the buffet line at a Vegas casino, it's evident how ridiculously out of control this situation has become. No offense, but America looks like one giant yard of fattened cattle ready for slaughter.

In comparison, being elitist doesn't seem bad at all. Right now, the race is on and you are welcome to participate. So take a deep breath and spring for the pasture-raised animal products and organic leafy greens at the farmers' market, especially if you are pregnant or have a two-year-old in his most crucial brain development stage. Come to think of it, make that especially if you are age 20, 30, 50, or 70 and have an interest in enjoying a long, healthy, happy life.

I put a dollar in one of those change machines. Nothing changed.
—George Carlin

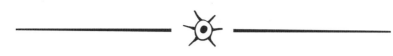

MARK-ING TIME FOR 72 HOURS

I'm often asked to reveal the details of my dietary habits and daily routine to interested MarksDailyApple.com readers and seminar guests. The truth is, I'm short on secrets but big on guidelines and practical tips that will help you successfully navigate the particulars of your daily life, including the innumerable challenges to being primal that we all face in the modern world. That said, I hope my real-life experiences give you some perspective that I'm a regular guy trying to run a business, enjoy a family, be as healthy and fit as possible while also aging with grace and acceptance, and generally enjoy the heck out of my awesome life.

I first completed a 72-hour journal of food intake and general daily activities back in January of 2009 for publication in the original *Primal Blueprint.* Reviewing this passage, titled, "To Dallas and back in 72 hours," was a fun reflection into my old eating and work routines. So much has changed since then, so I realized it was time for an updated journal. Back in 2009, with the primal movement still in its infancy, I was schlepping to Dallas every two weeks to appear on cable television programs to help promote my vitamin products. I was drinking more red wine, eating more carbs, and consuming more total calories than I do today. The Internet was still a minimal player in marketing/promotions for my business, my kids were still in the house, and we had five employees in my company instead of the 25 we have today.

By many measures, you could consider my life less stressful back then, but I wouldn't trade the excitement of my life today for anything. My business now extends beyond vitamins into publishing books and educational products, creating healthy kitchen products like mayonnaise, salad dressings, and energy foods, launching a primal-themed fast-casual dining restaurant chain, and serving as an investor and advisor to several startup companies associated with the primal/paleo movement. The entrepreneurial nature of my endeavors allows me to pursue the highest expression of my talents—which is to lay down a vision, chart the course, invest my heart, soul, and savings into the ventures, and then empower top-quality people around me to shine to the highest expression of their talents.

As you will see from the journal entries, I follow the Primal Blueprint lifestyle laws naturally, thanks to family and friends; a lifelong appreciation of the outdoors and physical fitness; a dynamic, challenging and constantly stimulating career; and a positive attitude—one that I've worked hard to cultivate over the years.

The exercise of keeping an accurate journal for 72 hours helps me realize that it's not about the often-mentioned "consistency" when it comes to winning diet, exercise, and lifestyle practices, nor is it about the assortment of questionable "hacks" (a word that straight up annoys me every time I hear it) that seem to be so popular today. Instead, I argue that following your passions, being flexible, and choosing to settle for nothing less than awesome every day are the real recipes for health and happiness. I admit that it's probably easier for me to engage in healthy lifestyle habits than for others, thanks to my athletic background, flexible work schedule, and health-oriented career path. However, whoever you are, you have the potential and the right to pursue happiness and health. Don't let nobody tell you different! Find a way to choose fresh, nutritious foods instead of defaulting to the junk that surrounds us. If your sleeping habits are insufficient, turn off your screens at night and make sleep the number one time-investment priority that it should be. When life gets hectic and stressful, do the best you can and realize that your body is really, really good at managing stress and dealing with inconsistent lifestyle patterns if you create a healthy foundation represented by the 10 Primal Blueprint laws.

Here, then, are my journal entries for a three-day stretch in May of 2016, featuring my standing Sunday routine of an intense, two-hour Ultimate Frisbee match and a lot of R&R to balance it out, a basic day at work in Malibu, and then off on another airplane trip to the annual Paleo f(x) convention in Austin, TX.

SUNDAY

7:00 A.M.: Wake up and drink large cup of strong coffee with a bit of cream and sugar. Tackle *LA Times* Sunday crossword puzzle in 23 minutes (PB Law #10, Use Your Brain).

10:30 A.M.: Head out to battle royale Ultimate Frisbee game in Malibu. Intense two-hour competition (counts toward both Law #7, Play and Law #5, Sprint Once in a While) with an assortment of young-uns that keep me young (or sometimes wishing I was young...).

1:00 P.M.: Prepare world-famous Primal Salad (search YouTube for "2 minute salad") with tons of greens, chopped veggies, walnuts, tuna salad made with Primal Kitchen mayo, and drenched in Primal Kitchen avocado-oil-based dressing.

Afternoon: Nurse aches and pains with light stretching while enjoying some Netflix offerings with Carrie. 20-minute nap in the sun (Laws #6, Get Plenty of Sleep and #8, Get Plenty of Sunlight).

4:00 P.M.: Handful of macadamia nuts and two heaping spoonfuls of Nikki's Coconut Butter, Honey Pecan Pie flavor.

5:00 P.M.: A bit of office work and Skype session with Primal Blueprint General Manager Aaron Fox in Australia. (Yep, it's his Monday, so I oblige!)

7:30 P.M.: Grass-fed steak (10 ounces), two cups of steamed broccoli and Brussels sprouts, dripping in butter.

8:00 P.M.: Several squares of 85-percent organic dark chocolate bar.

Evening: Short walk with Carrie and dog Shanti around neighborhood (Law #3, Move Frequently), binge-watch three Netflix episodes of *Silicon Valley*. Take a cold plunge (a few minutes moving around in mid-60s pool water), followed by a few minutes of rewarming in spa.

10:00 P.M.: Retire to bed for some pleasure reading. Lights out, and out like a light, by 10:30 P.M. (Ultimately, feeling my age after that Ultimate game.)

MONDAY

6:45 A.M.: Wake up. Enjoy some coffee with a bit of cream and sugar. Head to desk to hit email, phone calls, and record a podcast.

10:00 A.M.: Head to Malibu Gym for an easy 30-minute stationary bike session (heart rate 100-120 bpm), helping legs recover from Frisbee. Return home, shower, more office time.

1:00 P.M.: Entering my "compressed eating window" for first meal in 17 hours. Primal salad with leftover steak and the usual fixin's.

2:00 P.M.: Drive to Oxnard for meetings at company headquarters. Try some homemade baked sweet potato discs wrapped in bacon offered in the break room—some extra carbs today to recover from Sunday.

4:00 P.M.: Try new cashew collagen flavor of Primal Kitchen bar. Delicious!

5:00 P.M.: Decompress on drive home by stopping at the beach for 20 minutes of disconnected time. Think of a cool idea for my presentation at Paleo f(x).

7:30 P.M.: Sushi restaurant. Sashimi plate, miso soup, seaweed salad, and some cold white rice for a dose of prebiotics. (Cooked and cooled white rice is digested as resistant starch, not carbohydrate as it would be in a warm/hot state.)

9:00 P.M.: Couple of shows on Netflix, followed by a cold plunge/spa warming.

10:00 P.M.: Retire to bed for some pleasure reading. Lights out by 10:30 P.M.

TUESDAY

6:45 A.M.: Coffee with a bit of cream and sugar. A bit of time in office and then pack for afternoon flight to Austin, TX, for Paleo f(x) convention.

9:00 A.M.: Quick trip to Malibu Gym for five sets of 10 wide-grip pull-ups, followed by Maximum Sustained Power (MSP—detailed in the book *Primal Endurance*) deadlift session with sets of 5, 5, 4, 2, 2, 2 = twenty reps of 250 pounds. (Let's see if I can get to 300 pounds by next book reprinting!) Total workout duration 18 minutes.

11:30 A.M.: Primal omelet with four pasture-raised eggs, assorted chopped veggies, melted cheese, bacon, and avocado.

12:15 P.M.: Head to airport, fly to Austin. Big handful of raw almonds on airplane.

8:00 p.m.: Dinner in Austin, BBQ ribs with sauerkraut and creamy tomato soup.

11:00 p.m.: Lights out, ready for a busy conference."

Mark's Diet: 3-Day Macronutrient Analysis

SUNDAY

- Coffee and salad: 20g carb, 31g protein, 38g fat
- Macadamia nuts: 4g carbs, 2g protein, 22g fat
- Coconut butter: 7g carbs, 2g protein, 18g fat
- Dinner: 26g carbs, 66g protein, 38g fat
- Dark chocolate: 10g carbs, 3g protein, 15g fat

TOTALS: 67 grams carb = 268 calories, 14%

104 grams protein = 416 calories, 22%

131 grams fat = 1,179 calories, 63%

Total = 1,863 calories

MONDAY

- Coffee and salad: 20g carb, 31g protein, 38g fat
- Sweet potato with bacon: 12g carb, 5g protein, 4g fat
- Primal Kitchen Cashew Collagen Bar: 14g carb, 15g protein, 15g fat
- Sashimi, miso soup, seaweed salad, cold white rice (again, resistant starch, not carbs): 9g carb, 73g protein, 26g fat

TOTALS: 55 grams carb = 220 calories, 15%

124 grams protein = 496 calories, 34%

83 grams fat = 747 calories, 51%

Total = 1,463 calories

TUESDAY

- Coffee and omelet: 12g carb, 30g protein, 44g fat
- Almonds: 6g carbs, 6g protein, 14g fat
- Dinner: 24g carb, 37g protein, 26g fat

TOTALS: 42g carb = 168 calories, 14%

73g protein = 292 calories, 24%

84g fat = 756 calories, 62%

Total = 1,216 calories

3-DAY TOTALS
164 grams carbs = 656 calories, 14%
301 grams protein = 1,204 calories, 27%
298 grams fat = 2,682 calories, 59%
Total = 4,542 calories

3-DAY AVERAGES
54 grams carbs = 218 calories, 14%
100 grams protein = 400 calories, 26%
99 grams fat = 894 calories, 59%
Total = 1,512 calories

I obtained some interesting insights from this exercise. First, my total caloric intake is pretty low for a guy of my lean muscle mass and activity level. It's lower than it was seven years ago when I did this exercise for the first *Primal Blueprint* printing and generated an average daily intake of 1,842 calories (including a high day of 2,676 calories, which I assuredly never eat close to today). Sure, I might be burning fewer calories at 63 than I did at 55, but I doubt that's the reason. Instead, I believe I have continued to refine my fat-adaptation and caloric efficiency to the extent that I require fewer calories to sustain energy, health, concentration, and of course total dietary satisfaction at every meal.

Second, astute observers will notice that I don't eat that many calories, and fall well short of long-standing expert recommendations for active exercisers to consume an average of one gram of protein per pound (2.2 grams per kilo) of lean mass per day. For me, that would be 153 grams of protein. (I weigh 170 pounds at ~10 percent body fat, so lean mass = 153 pounds.) As discussed in Chapter 4, I am now on board with the latest science that suggests we need less protein than previously believed, and that a pattern of excess protein intake can accelerate aging and increase cancer risk.

RETHINKING YOUR GOALS

Consider for a moment the possibility that setting and pursuing specific, tangible goals is screwing you up more than helping you succeed. Do you strain, struggle, and suffer to obtain predetermined times, paces, and distances in your workouts—following a set workout regimen or training plan and tracking everything with a Fitbit and training log—thinking that a robotic approach to fitness will bring success? Do you buy in, at some level, to the superficial elements of modern culture, where everything we do is measured and judged (and weighed), and success (and often happiness) is defined by what we accomplish and accumulate?

I know I once did, big time. My fervent desire to achieve my athletic goals—run in the Olympic marathon trials, average 100-mile weeks, beat my training partners—ruined my physical health and ended my running career. When I returned to competition as a triathlete, I had a more easygoing, light-hearted attitude. I enjoyed the challenge of a new sport and pushing the limits of human endurance, just for the heck of it. Gun-shy from my injury history, I adopted a more relaxed approach. I listened to the signals from my body and backed off when my energy levels declined or aches and pains crept up. I enjoyed longer, slower bike rides into the mountains, connecting with nature and enjoying a sense of adventure in exploring new routes. I built my fitness in a comfortable manner and felt refreshed, energized, and inspired about my training—a far cry from the out-and-out suffering I endured from recurring intense running sessions with a fit pack of training partners.

Lo and behold, with my casual approach I became the fourth fastest Hawaii Ironman triathlete in the world one year, avoided injuries, and had a great time. After retiring from professional racing and pursuing a "real" career, I continued competing just for kicks on the amateur level well into my late 30s. I had no goals, structured training program, or training log. I was just having fun, inspiring and being inspired by my personal training clients, and mixing with the professional athletes that I coached at the time. At the same time, I enjoyed, by my standards, excellent results... with less effort. Often I would see the "game faces" worn by other amateurs (as I now was, mind you)—tense, anxious, snapping at their loved ones, looking like they weren't having much fun or experiencing much personal growth.

It's simply no fun to predicate your happiness on whether you reach your goals. Failing to reach your goals will lead to disappointment and dwindling motivation levels. Even reaching your goals can lead to a dead end and a flawed mentality. Many "winners"—in sports or other competitive arenas, such as business—develop a distorted sense of self-worth, leaving them vulnerable to up-and-coming opponents or negligent about behaving themselves in ordinary society because of our twisted hero-worship of winners and the wealthy.

There is a phenomenon in endurance sports known as the *post-marathon blues* (or post-Ironman blues for triathletes)—so common that it's been discussed in psychological journals. It seems that on the occasion of the glorious achievement for which they've trained diligently for months or even years, many athletes get that "now what?" feeling that leads to a profound sense of letdown. Ideally, we would use our physical accomplishments as catalysts for continued growth (including moving on to less extreme fitness pursuits perhaps!), exploration, and challenge, not an excuse to get depressed and pig out on jellybeans in the weeks after the big event.

We must take a close look at the goal-setting process to avoid these common pitfalls and bring a relaxed, fun-first approach to our diet, fitness, body composition, career, and other lifestyle pursuits. The primary reason for switching to a Primal Blueprint eating style should be enjoyment—eat foods that taste great, stabilize your energy levels, optimize the function of all the systems in your body, provide long-lasting satisfaction, and alleviate the psychological stress of regimentation and deprivation that accompany many diets. Yes, you will look better, become stronger, have more energy, avoid illness, disease, and obesity, and enjoy other quantifiable results, but these motivators pale in comparison to the instant gratification you get at every single meal from eating the foods that your body was meant to eat.

If you have any psychological stress about your diet, reject it flat out and start eating foods and meals that make you happy, drawing upon the long list of foods that fit the minimally-restrictive Primal Blueprint eating style. Do whatever you need to do to enjoy your life, including indulging once in a while with a clear conscience and a big smile. If you are not having fun with your current workout regimen, junk it and figure out other endeavors that turn you on. Instead of struggling and suffering to keep pace with your peppy group exercise instructor or your training partners, adopt the Primal Blueprint suggestions to make your sustained workouts comfortable and energizing so they become fun again. Throw in some exhilarating fast activities occasionally to get you excited about pushing your physical limits, and enjoy tangible breakthroughs including weight loss, more energy, and peak performance. Play once in a while. Forget the notion of consistency in this context, and align your exercise program with your energy level, mood, and life responsibilities. Push yourself when you are rested and motivated, and rest when you are tired.

Once you discard unnecessary goals that are mentally and emotionally stressful, you can focus your attention on process-oriented goals. Goals such as having fun, aligning workout choices with energy levels, and tackling new endeavors should define your exercise mentality. That said, great champions have an esteemed ability to blend a process-oriented approach with a strong competitive drive to achieve measurable results. It's certainly okay to aspire to specific results (e.g., losing 10 pounds or completing a 10k, marathon, or triathlon), but you must never lose sight of the concept that the rewards come from the chase, not from reaching the finish line.

You can lose 10 pounds very quickly via any number of ill-advised methods. The true joy from changing your physique comes not from a surgeon's knife or a brutal calorie-restriction diet coupled with an exhaustive workout routine. The most lasting rewards come from the positive, fun lifestyle changes you implement to make it happen.

It is time for you to accept the grand purpose of the Primal Blueprint and reject other motivators that are confusing, petty, or contradictory to your health and wellbeing. To get more connected with the ideal represented by Grok, we have to pare down, not accumulate. The power and the magic are in the simplicity—a refreshing break from the complexity of modern life, the sordid influence of ego on your endeavors and emotional state, and the pop culture messages that can easily make you feel like a loser if you aren't as tight as the beautiful person on the magazine cover.

Grok did not traffic in any of this nonsense. Granted, he was preoccupied with survival, and we surely don't need to regress to that point to enlighten our mentalities. What we can do is leverage the Primal Blueprint laws in our daily lives to become healthier, fitter, happier, and more connected with our basic nature as human beings. Make it your goal to honor your genes and your destiny to make the most of your life on earth, without attachment to any outcome.

What are you waiting for? Let's get primal!!

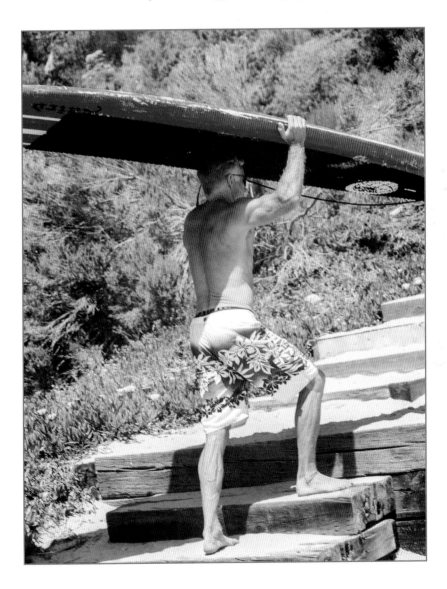

PRIMAL APPROVED—AT A GLANCE

DIET

Baking Ingredients: Coconut, almond, or other nut flours, tapioca starch, arrowroot powder (for occasional use in paleo/primal-approved baking recipes).

Beverages: Water (according to thirst), unsweetened teas, full-fat coconut milk or unsweetened almond milk (great smoothie bases).

Coconut Products: Butter, flakes, flour, milk, and oil offer healthful medium-chain fats; great substitute for dairy, refined vegetable/seed oils, and wheat flour.

Coffee: Enjoy in moderation (cream and minimal sweetener okay); don't use as energy crutch.

Condiments: Yellow mustard; mayonnaise and salad dressings made with avocado oil or olive oil and without excess or artificial sweeteners.

Dairy: Raw, fermented, high-fat, and organic products are preferred (cheese, cottage cheese, cream cheese, kefir, whole milk, yogurt); consume in moderation.

Dark Chocolate: Primal-approved snack/treat. Cacao content: at least 75 percent, ideally 85 percent.

Eggs: Local, pasture-raised, or certified organic for high omega-3 content.

Energy Bars: Primal Kitchen bars and other low-sugar bars (rare finds; even the most natural and nutritious bars offer a significant carbohydrate load).

Fats & Oils: Avocado and domestic extra virgin olive oil for eating. Coconut oil, grass-fed butter, and animal fats (bacon grease, chicken fat, lard, tallow) for cooking.

Fish: Wild-caught from remote, pollution-free waters. Small, oily, cold-water fish are best. Salmon, mackerel, anchovies, sardines, herring = SMASH hits! Certain farmed fish are approved (domestic Coho salmon, trout, and some shellfish—not shrimp). Check seafoodwatch.org for up-to-date recommendations.

Fruit: Locally grown (or wild), organic, in-season preferred. Berries are premier choice. Go strictly organic with soft, edible skin fruits. Moderate intake of higher glycemic/lower antioxidant fruits. Wash thoroughly.

Herbs and Spices: High-antioxidant, anti-inflammatory, immune-supporting, flavor-enhancing.

Meat & Fowl: Local, pasture-raised, or UDSA-certified organic critical. If you must eat conventional meat, choose the leanest possible cuts and trim excess fat to minimize toxin exposure.

Nutritious Carbs: Optimize carb intake for body composition, recovery, and hormonal balance goal. Opt for abundant vegetables, extra fruit, nuts and seeds, dark chocolate, sweet potatoes, yams and other starchy tubers, quinoa, and wild rice.

Nuts, Seeds, & Their Derivative Butters: Nutritious, satisfying snack. Try nut butters on dark chocolate. Raw almond milk is a great substitute for dairy milk.

Prebiotics: Cooked and cooled white rice and white potatoes, green bananas, raw potato starch.

Probiotics: Fermented foods like kefir, kombucha, pickles, sauerkraut, and yogurt, and even dark chocolate!

Snacks: Berries, canned tuna or sardines, celery with cream cheese or nut butter, cottage cheese with nut or fruit topping, dark chocolate, hard-boiled eggs, jerky, nuts, olives, seeds, trail mix, and other high-fat and/or high-protein, low-carb primal foods.

Supplements: Daily multivitamin/mineral/antioxidant formula, omega-3 fish oil capsules, prebiotics, probiotics, protein powder, and vitamin D complement healthy eating nicely.

Vegetables: Locally grown, organic, in-season preferred. Go strictly organic for large surface area (leafy greens) and soft, edible skins. Wash thoroughly.

EXERCISE

Complementary Flexibility/Mobility Practices: Practices like yoga and Pilates develop mobility and flexibility, with the added benefit of strengthening a variety of muscles, notably the core. Mobility exercises target tendons, ligaments, and fascia that support the entire musculoskeletal system. Hold positions for two minutes (or even longer).

Move Frequently: Blend increased everyday movement (short walking breaks, evening strolls, etc.) with structured cardio workouts at 180-age heart rate.

Schedule: Vary workout type, frequency, intensity, and duration, always aligned with energy levels. Be spontaneous, intuitive, and playful!

Shoes: Gradually introduce some barefoot time for low-risk activities to strengthen feet and simulate natural range of motion. Choose shoes with minimalist design (Vibram FiveFingers, Nike Free) to prevent cuts and other injuries. Ease into it!

Sprinting: All-out efforts lasting 8 to 20 seconds every 7 to 10 days when fully energized. Regular, less strenuous "wind sprint" sessions for conditioning.

Strength Training: Brief, intense sessions of 10 to 30 minutes. Full-body, functional exercises that promote broad athletic competency.

Stretching: Minimal, full-body, functional stretches to transition from active to inactive; Grok Hang and Grok Squat.

LIFESTYLE/MEDICAL CARE

Medical: Rx drugs ideally would be reserved for acute conditions. Try making lifestyle modifications now to avoid prescription drugs later! Check with your doctor about ordering additional blood tests (CRP, Lp2A, A1C, fasting blood insulin) to assess disease risks.

Play: Change attitude—it's not just for kids! Enjoy daily, outdoor physical fun! Enhances work productivity and stress management.

Sleep: Minimize artificial light and digital stimulation after dark; consistent bed and wake times; calm transitions into and out of sleep. Awaken naturally without alarm. Nap when necessary and possible.

Stupid Mistakes: Become vigilant to modern dangers (e.g., texting and driving) to manage risks. Avoid multitasking and overly stressful or regimented lifestyle practices. Focus on peak performance!

Sunlight: Fear not the mighty orb! Expose large skin surface areas often (protecting sensitive areas that tend to be exposed too much such as your face and hands) and in short increments that do not allow burning.

Use Your Brain: Engage in fun, creative intellectual pursuits to stay sharp and enthusiastic for all of life's challenges.

PRIMAL AVOID—AT A GLANCE

DIET

Baking Ingredients: Corn products (meal, starch, syrup and HFCS), other starches and syrups, grain-based flours, powders (gluten, maltodextrin, milk), sugars and sweeteners (dextrose, fructose, lactose, malitol, xylitol, agave, artificial sweeteners, brown sugar, cane sugar, evaporated cane juice, honey, molasses, powdered sugar, raw sugar, table sugar).

Beverages: Bottled, fresh-squeezed, or refrigerated juices (Odwalla, OJ, Ocean Spray, etc.); "energy drinks" (Red Bull, Rock Star, Monster, etc.); soy milk, rice milk, and other non-dairy milks that are sweetened (e.g., almond, coconut—although these are great in raw/unsweetened forms); other flavored powdered drink mixes (chai, coffee, or hot chocolate flavored); soft drinks and diet soft drinks; sports performance drinks (Gatorade, Vitamin Water); sweetened cocktails (daiquiri, eggnog, margarita); sweetened teas (Snapple, Arizona).

Coffee: Avoid excessive use or as energy crutch in place of adequate sleep and healthy lifestyle habits.

Condiments/Cooking Items: All products made with sugary sweeteners and/or refined high polyunsaturated vegetable oils: honey mustard; jams and jellies; ketchup; mayonnaise, spreads, and salad dressings made with canola, safflower, sunflower, or other refined vegetable oils; low-fat dressings and spreads.

Dairy: Conventional and GMO milk products with hormone, pesticide, antibiotic, allergenic, and immune-suppressing agents; ice cream; nonfat/low-fat milk; processed (e.g., American) cheese and cheese spreads; sweetened nonfat/low-fat yogurt and frozen yogurt.

Eggs: Limit mass-produced eggs (fed with grains, hormones, pesticides, and antibiotics). Find local, pastured eggs at farmers' markets!

Fast Food: French fries, onion rings, deep-fried foods, burgers, hot dogs, chimichangas, chalupas, chorizos, and the rest of the industrialized fare we are inundated with daily; it's chemically treated, deep-fried, insulin-stimulating, and devoid of nutritional value.

Fats & Oils: Partially hydrogenated; refined high polyunsaturated vegetable/seed oils (canola, etc.); interesterified fats; buttery spreads and sprays; margarine; vegetable shortening; deep-fried foods.

Fish: Most farmed fish, all Asian imports (polluted waters, lax chemical regulation), Atlantic salmon (farmed in dirty conditions), shrimp (farmed in dirty conditions), endangered/objectionable catch method fish, top of food chain fish (shark, sword, etc.—concentrated contaminants).

Fruit: Limit or avoid GMO, remotely grown, or conventionally grown, especially those with soft, edible skins.

Grains: Corn, rice, and wheat; bread and flour products (baguettes, crackers, croissants, danishes, donuts, graham crackers, muffins, pizza, rolls, saltine crackers, swirls, tortillas, Triscuits, Wheat Thins); breakfast foods (Cream of Wheat, dried cereal, French toast, granola, grits, oatmeal, pancakes, waffles); chips (corn, potato, tortilla); cooking grains (amaranth, barley, bulgur, couscous, millet, rye); pasta, noodles; pretzels; puffed snacks (Cheetos, Goldfish, Pirates Booty, popcorn, rice cakes); and all other baked or processed high-carb foods. Even avoid whole grains due to higher levels of objectionable phytates, lectins, and gluten.

Legumes: Alfalfa, beans, peanuts, peanut butter, peas, lentils, soybeans, and tofu. Less objectionable than grains, but still contain anti-nutrients. Unnecessary and possibly counterproductive to health and weight management.

Meat & Fowl: Commercially grown, grain-fed ranch or CAFO animals (with concentrated hormones, pesticides, and antibiotics); pre-packaged processed products (breakfast sausage, dinner roasts, lunch meats); smoked, cured, or nitrate- or nitrite-treated meats (bologna, ham, hot dogs, jerky, pepperoni, salami).

Processed Foods: Energy bars; fruit bars and rolls; granola bars; protein bars; frozen breakfast, dinner, and dessert products; and packaged, grain/sugar-laden snack products. If it's in a box, package, or wrapper, think twice—or find the rare exceptions to high-sugar-content products.

Sweets: Brownies; candy; candy bars; cake; chocolate syrup; cookies; donuts; ice cream; milk chocolate; milk chocolate chips; pie; sugar-/chocolate-coated nuts and trails mixes; popsicles and other frozen desserts; syrups; and other packaged/processed sweets and treats. The less you consume, the less you'll want!

Supplements: Cheap, bulk-produced supplements with additives, fillers, binders, lubricants, extruding agents, and other synthetic chemicals.

Vegetables: GMO, remotely grown, or conventionally grown, especially those with large surface areas or edible skins (leafy greens, peppers).

EXERCISE

Chronic Cardio: Avoid a consistent schedule of sustained cardio workouts at medium-to-difficult intensity (exceeding heart rate of "180 minus age" in beats per minute).

Schedule: Avoid consistent application of stress with insufficient rest (compromises health, energy, and motivation levels). Consistency is *not* key when it comes to fitness!

Stretching: Avoid static, isolated muscle group stretches of "cold" muscles in favor of simple, dynamic stretches.

MEDICAL/LIFESTYLE

Medical: Strive to avoid or wean off prescription medication for lifestyle-related health problems. Reframe "fix it" mentality into a "prevention" mentality.

Sleep: Avoid excessive artificial light and digital stimulation after dark, morning alarms after insufficient sleep, or fighting off a much-needed nap with caffeine.

Stupid Mistakes: Avoid multitasking (e.g., texting and driving), zoning out, or trusting that the world will keep you safe. Don't blame others for your stupid mistakes.

BONUS MATERIAL

PRIMAL BLUEPRINT COMMON STUMBLING BLOCKS AND QUICK TIPS

We've analyzed hundreds of threads and thousands of posts on the MarksDailyApple.com forum and have come up with this list of the most common challenges. Next to each concept is a quick tip that might help your effort and prompt you to refer to the book over time for additional guidance.

Breakfast ideas: Omelet or other egg dish, green smoothie with fat and protein content (coconut milk, Primal Fuel powder, avocado). Let go of the idea that there are "breakfast," "lunch," and "dinner" foods and embrace more flexibility to eat intuitively. Or simply skip a meal when your fat-burning genes are fine-tuned and you're not hungry.

Handling budget issue: Look at the big picture and prioritize expenses. The impact on your budget might actually be offset by getting rid of processed carbs and sweetened beverages and hitting your local farmers' market.

Dealing with non-primals (spouses, kids, etc.): Set an example through your results and energetic disposition, rather than by lecturing. Avoid preaching to resistant folks and focus on those ready to receive your guidance.

Dining out: Be assertive and request menu flexibility to piece together suitable meals centered around animal protein. You can stay primal-aligned at most any restaurant by making some careful choices and requests.

Eliminating chronic cardio: Balancing stress and rest is the key to fitness progress! Adopt an intuitive approach to exercise instead of compulsively logging miles or reps in the name of "consistency." Strictly monitor heart rate during cardio workouts to stay at or below "180 minus age." This will likely involve getting your training partners on board or simply opting to do more of your cardio exercise solo so you can moderate your pace.

Finding good snacks: Review the list of my favorites on pages 225-226. Discover your own favorites from the extremely broad list of primal-aligned options.

Getting enough fat: Inadequate fat intake is likely influenced by decades of cultural programming to minimize intake of all fats, despite the health benefits of many types. Eat as much fat as you desire to enjoy meals, achieve satiety, and eliminate carbohydrate temptations. Just make sure you choose from the list of healthy, approved fats.

Getting enough sleep: Implement the sleeping tips detailed in Chapter 8 and in the Primal Blueprint quick tips that follow, paying particular attention to creating a calm, quiet, dimmed environment the final two hours before bedtime.

Giving up diet soda: Artificial sweeteners confuse your appetite hormones, triggering sugar cravings and even insulin surges. Try flavoring carbonated water (mineral or soda water, not tonic water!) with a generous squeeze of lemon and a bit of salt to get your carbonation fix. There are also several brands of unsweetened, naturally flavored carbonated water on the market now.

Giving up grains: Face it—grains are bland-tasting. It's the stuff you put on grains that makes them taste good! Reframe your perspective about what you really need and reject rigid SAD traditions. Eggs for dinner? Steak for breakfast? Knock yourself out!

Engaging in Intermittent Fasting: The best bet for novices is to eat dinner, then delay breakfast the following morning until hunger sensations are compelling. See how long you can comfortably last without food, then enjoy a delicious primal-approved meal. Check your progress each month, as your ability to regulate energy without ingested calories provides a good indication of how well your genes have been programmed to make you a fat-burning beast.

Finding quick/easy food: Advanced planning is important, since the modern world will not provide very well for your primal needs on the go. Create a stash of temperature stable, easily transportable primal snacks (jerky, apples, nuts, trail mix, Primal Kitchen bars) so you can always have ready-to-go options available.

Learning to cook: Start with simple recipes, build your confidence, and get ever more creative over time. Check out *Primal Blueprint Quick & Easy Meals* or *Paleo Primer* for simple, fun, non-intimidating recipes. Keep your kitchen well-stocked to make things easy.

Listening to your body: Cultivate an intuitive approach to eating, exercise, sleep, and other primal behaviors. This means you must reject external influences (superficial cultural messages, peer pressure, judgmental family and friends) and answer to yourself first and foremost.

Listening to hunger signals: Eat when you're hungry, finish when you're satisfied. Give yourself permission to eat whatever you want, whenever you want, as much as you want (within primal guidelines of course) to achieve dietary satisfaction and promote health. Slow down your eating pace to really tune in!

Managing expectations: Focus on the intrinsic value of living primally, and don't attach your happiness or self-esteem to the results. Take what your body gives you each day (energy, motivation, health, etc.) and never force results on an unnatural time schedule. Stop holding yourself to perfectionistic standards, and let go of the notion that there is some ideal you can and should attain. Trust that the immediate sensations you experience from promoting optimal gene expression (more energy and regulated appetite, hormone, and immune function) will translate into long-term results with body composition and other peak performance goals. Judge your "success" by how good you feel.

Managing stress: Minimize insulin production, eliminate chronic exercise, and align sleep habits with the circadian rhythm. Build momentum with these three big ones, and let further lifestyle refinements fall into place.

Overthinking things: Some passionate primal folks actually go overboard and become inflexible and anxious about their adherence to primal guidelines. This type of mentality, however well-intentioned, can compromise mental and even physical health. Accept that there is a range of potential outcomes—from magazine cover model to ordinary but extremely healthy. Don't get bogged down with external results instead of honoring the most important big picture goal of primal living: long-term health.

Packing lunch/preparing meals: Cook large portions ahead of time, then refrigerate or freeze for quick meals on the go. Chop and store veggies to facilitate quick salad preparation. Portion out barbecue or crock pot meat dishes for quick reheating.

Playing more: Schedule grand outings and involve others. Get involved with kids—the world's foremost experts on play. If you're really out of practice, start small with a five-minute break from work or a quick stop at the park on the way home.

Reading food labels: Should you really be eating food with labels on it?! Emphasize fresh plant and animal foods and minimize consumption of wrapped, packaged, canned, and frozen foods. That said, read labels to avoid refined vegetable oils and sugars. Look at the carbohydrate count—this can clue you in to hidden sugars with sneaky names.

Resisting temptations: Why resist? Reject the struggle-and-suffer mentality and enjoy life! An occasional well-chosen treat is absolutely primal-approved. Honor the 80 Percent Rule and don't stress about perfection or obsess about resisting temptations. Go with the flow and calmly return to your center if you happen to get thrown off track.

Scheduling meals: What for?! You will enjoy more flexibility with your schedule, shopping, and planning as you become more fat-adapted. The need to fuel with unfavorable options just because your body needs some calories will quickly diminish as you become adept at burning stored body fat.

Sourcing primal ingredients: Try backyard gardening (or renting an urban plot), farmers' markets, co-ops, specialty grocers, or the Internet (if you live in a primal-challenged area).

Supplements: The best categories to supplement a healthy diet are: multivitamin/antioxidant, omega-3 fish oil, prebiotics, probiotics, high-protein meal replacement, and vitamin D for the sunlight challenged.

Satisfying sweet tooth: High-cacao-content dark chocolate (75 percent or above; ideally 85 percent) is a primal-approved treat that will satisfy your sweet tooth and provide an antioxidant boost.

Varying your diet: The primal guidelines afford tremendous variety in food choices. However, there is no rule that says you must eat a variety of foods. Personally, I'm a creature of habit and enjoy repeating my favorite primal-approved meals frequently. If you're inclined to experiment and shake things up, go ahead and enjoy yourself!

Working out consistently: Striving for consistency is overrated! Consistency increases risk of injury from chronic exercise patterns and burnout. Focus on intuitively balancing stress and rest. Take what your body has to give you each day instead of blindly following a regimented workout pattern. Don't feel guilty for skipping a workout if you don't feel like it.

Motivating to exercise: People who can't get or stay motivated to exercise generally view it as painful and overly stressful. Do workouts that are fun and make you happy. Head out the door for a hike, haul off a few PEM exercises on a whim, or rest if that is what your body requires. Don't worry about burning a certain number of calories or moving at a certain pace; build momentum naturally with workouts that are fun and enjoyable.

PRIMAL BLUEPRINT LAWS AT A GLANCE

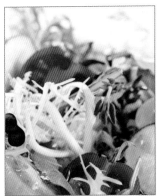

Law #1: Eat Plants and Animals: Transforming your dietary habits is not easy, even for the most disciplined among us. The pull of comfort foods, cultural forces misaligned with health and balance, and our innate resistance to change must be skillfully negotiated. Find primal breakfast, lunch, and dinner meals and convenient snacks that you really love, and use these as a foundation for going primal. There are probably a dozen distinct omelet variations you can create from the starting point of cracking eggs into a mixing bowl.

While my eating habits vary wildly from day to day (see pages 470-475 for a 72-hour journal), I'd say my entire diet revolves around a midday Big Ass Salad that I make on many days of the week. Some days I'll hit it around noon, after skipping breakfast or having a quick morning shake. Other days I'll enjoy it in the late afternoon, providing me enough satisfaction and nourishment that dinner essentially becomes optional.

If you're fond of nuts, prepare some individual servings for your desk, briefcase, car, and home, and make them your go-to afternoon snack. Building productive and easy-to-implement habits such as centerpiece meals or primal snack stashes should mitigate the chances of backsliding into quick-energy sweetened beverages or high-sugar energy bars when your hunger does strike.

Summary

Make primal eating simple and convenient by establishing some go-to breakfast, lunch, and dinner meals, and favorite snacks. Cycle through your five favorites as you build momentum going primal. Keep primal-approved snacks around.

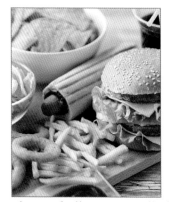

Law #2: Avoid Poisonous Things: Out of sight, out of mind. What better plan to implement here than to simply avoid exposing yourself to health-compromising foods? This is particularly true when it comes to the struggle to wean children away from cultural traditions into a somewhat primal eating pattern. Establish firm guidelines for what is allowed in your home and don't deviate from it. If the tee-ball team wins the championship and all are compelled to celebrate with hot fudge sundaes, your kid should go ahead and enjoy life to the fullest. This is different from stocking caramel sauce, chocolate syrup, and vanilla ice cream in your home for daily doses.

If you find yourself in the midst of tempting foods and are compelled to indulge, do so with a clear conscience and a total focus on the enjoyment that your treat provides. Often, when you reject the silly mind games of guilt and rebellion, you'll discover that those few moments of gustatory pleasure experienced when the treat hits your taste buds are simply not worth the long-term negative consequences of digestive distress or acting in a manner incongruent with your big picture life goals.

Summary
1. Keep offensive foods out of your home, and stay away from junk-food establishments.
2. If you must indulge, do so with a clear conscience and total focus on the pleasure and satisfaction it provides. With taboos eliminated, you may realize that it's not really worth it, and that primal-approved substitutes can provide similar satisfaction.

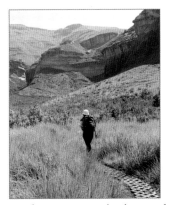

Law #3: Move Frequently: Own this idea about aerobic exercise: it's not about the calories burned, *it's about the frequency of movement.* If you are a cardio enthusiast, slowing down the pace of your workouts will promote fitness more than a chronic pattern of overly-strenuous workouts that compromises hormone, immune, and metabolic function. Apply your impressive levels of discipline and motivation not only to getting out the door and putting in the hours, but to backing off when your intuition suggests. You won't get fat and lose fitness if you include more rest days and recovery sessions in your schedule, I promise! Remember, 80 percent of your body composition success is influenced by diet, and 100 percent of your fitness progress is influenced by common sense.

Focus on taking incremental measures to accumulate more total movement in everyday life, especially if you aren't already very active. Contrary to what certain fitness pundits might spout, those 30-second hops up three flights of stairs, 5-minute walks around your corporate campus, and 15-minute strolls through the neighborhood with the dog definitely add up. You really can become aerobically fit without having a gym membership or a fancy spandex outfit. Just get out and move!

So many people get stuck because we've been conditioned to believe that there is no intermediate category between couch potato and die-hard gym fixture. Tomorrow, examine your daily routine and identify five ways that you can replace mechanized or sedentary habits with physical movement.

Once in a while, go for an extended outing such as a hike that is paced comfortably enough that you'll actually enjoy it and look forward to doing it again. If you're nature-averse, make your hike of the urban variety. You can even walk or bike to a fun destination such as the farmers' market, arranging ahead to get a ride back home. Make an effort to integrate flexibility/mobility activities into your "move frequently" efforts—things like yoga, Pilates, tai chi, basic stretching, and even self-myofascial release (foam rollers, etc.).

a series of progression exercises that are easier than the baseline essential movement. For example, chair-assisted pull-ups or wall pushups will allow a novice or someone with injuries or physical limitations to simulate the resistance and muscle recruitment of the PEM while doing an appropriate number of repetitions to build full-body strength.

Strive to complete one full-length PEM session and one abbreviated PEM session each week on days when energy, motivation, and immune function are strong. A full-length session involves two or more sets of maximum repetitions of each of the four PEMs. An abbreviated PEM workout involves a single set of maximum repetitions in each exercise. Start with two to five minutes of an easy cardiovascular workout before commencing your PEM exercises. After each exercise, take a 30- to 60-second break to get your breathing rate back to near normal. A full-length PEM circuit should take less than 30 minutes to complete, while an abbreviated PEM circuit should take less than 15 minutes.

Summary
1. Keep it simple with the PEMs: pushups, pull-ups, squats, and planks.
2. Use the progression exercises appropriate for your fitness level to achieve an appropriate number of reps.
3. Strive to conduct one full-length PEM circuit (two to three sets of max reps for each PEM) and one abbreviated PEM circuit (one set of max reps for each PEM) per week.

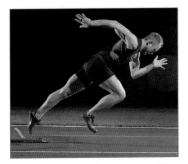

Law #5: Sprint Once in a While: If you are a fitness novice or otherwise intimidated about sprinting, try a few preparatory sessions where you simulate a sprint workout at 80 to 90 percent of maximum intensity. Known as "strides" or "wind sprints" in running parlance, you complete a series of efforts that are shorter and less intense than a maximum effort sprint. You can also do technique drills (high knees, heel kicks, mini-lunges—other movements that exaggerate running range of motion and help reinforce correct technique) to help prepare your muscles and nervous system for eventual workouts at maximum effort.

Almost everyone can eventually enjoy the optimal gene expression benefits of all-out sprinting when you conduct prep sessions at incremental intensities and eventually take it up to 100 percent. Utilize low- or no-impact exercises if running carries a high injury risk for you.

Summary

1. Sprint once every 7 to 10 days and only when you are 100 percent rested and motivated.
2. To prepare for the strenuous nature of sprinting, conduct lower intensity "strides" or "wind sprints" and choose low- or no-impact options if appropriate.
3. Refer to the forthcoming Sprint Workout Suggestions for details.

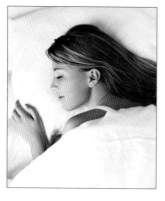

Law #6: Get Plenty of Sleep: Melatonin production has been triggered by darkness for all of human history. When you keep your evening environment unnaturally bright with artificial light or blast your eyeballs with digital stimulation from Netflix or YouTube, cortisol levels spike and carbohydrate cravings can occur, leading to sleep deprivation and excess body fat storage. As soon as it gets dark, minimize artificial light in your home. If you don't want to use candles, try installing orange light bulbs (available at home supply stores) in commonly used lamps, especially in the bedroom. Or you can don glasses with yellow or orange lenses to block the disruptive "blue light" emitted from white bulbs. The tinted bulbs and lenses allow plenty of light in but do not disrupt the production of the sleep hormone melatonin in the manner that white light bulbs and digital screens do.

Mellow things out after dark by choosing relaxing endeavors such as reading, strolling, talking, and board games instead of digital entertainment. Create an ideal bedtime environment: simple, quiet, as dark as possible, clutter-free, cool (65°F seems to be the preferred sleeping temp), and keep it exclusively for sleeping. When you implement calm, relaxing evenings, you set yourself up for success on the other end: waking up naturally, without an alarm, feeling refreshed and energized. Even if you're convinced that you're not a morning person, exposing yourself to direct sunlight as soon as possible after awakening will help elevate serotonin and suppress melatonin, kicking your body into high-energy mode for a busy day.

Summary
1. Minimize artificial light after dark: Use minimal indoor lighting and orange bulbs or lenses.
2. Get your digital technology into night mode: Visit getflux.com and download a free program called f.lux for your computer. f.lux automatically alters the "color temperature" of your computer screen to align with ambient light—easier on the eyes after dark. If your cell phone or tablet offers a nighttime mode, always activate it if you must use your devices after dark.
3. Minimize digital stimulation: Especially in the final two hours before bedtime, choose reading, conversation, board games, or neighborhood strolls instead of going straight from screen to bed.
4. Bedroom: Get rid of all clutter and maintain a simple, stress-free environment. Try blackout curtains and keep the temperature around 65°F.
5. Sleep mask: A handy resource for napping and eliminating potential light distractions during your evening sleep.
6. Napping: Whenever you fall behind on sleep, a 20- to 30-minute nap during the day can help rejuvenate energy and brain function.
7. Morning: Awaken naturally, close to sunrise, and expose yourself to direct sunlight ASAP.

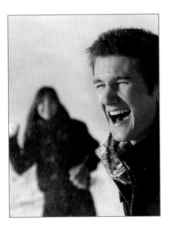

Law #7: Play: Take a few mini-play breaks throughout the day lasting 5 to 15 minutes, and schedule grand play outings once in a while that involve exciting new adventures with family and friends. There are few rules or restrictions to mini play breaks, except to let go of inhibitions and cultural pressure that discourage anything out of the ordinary. Don't be afraid to get strange looks from co-workers when you start playing wastebasket hoops or attempt to juggle some tennis balls in the office courtyard. Don't let the hectic pace of modern life stand in your way here—start modestly if you must with a five-minute endeavor. Once you become comfortable departing from your daily routine, you may experience bursts of creativity. When in doubt, hang around kids, and you'll be playing in no time.

For your grand outing, take a few moments to jot down a wish list of adventures you and your loved ones might like to try. Rank them in order of priority, being realistic with your time and budget. Then, take a couple of initial steps today toward making it happen—schedule your rock climbing lessons, grab a hiking map from the state park website and plot out a route, or rent or purchase necessary gear. Plan the big day and stay accountable by involving others and getting a firm handle on logistics so the adventure is not too daunting when the time comes.

Summary

1. Make mini play-breaks lasting 5 to 15 minutes a regular part of your daily routine. Don't overthink this; just take some time out for amusement.

2. Occasionally step it up with grand outings and adventures. Check things off your bucket list, and spend quality time with friends and loved ones while you're at it. Start now by deciding what your next adventure will be, and take a concrete step or two toward making it happen.

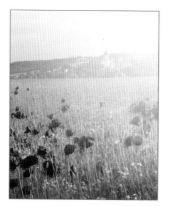

Law #8: Get Plenty of Sunlight: For maximum vitamin D production, expose large surface areas of your skin (arms, legs, torso) to direct sun for about *half the amount of time you think it takes to get slightly burned*. This is a highly individual estimate based on time of year and day, skin pigmentation, latitude, reflectiveness of the ground surface, and other variables. Nevertheless, guesstimating the halfway mark is a pretty low-risk endeavor, so make a strong effort to expose as much skin as possible to direct sunlight during the months of the year when the sun's rays are sufficient to manufacture vitamin D (year-round in the tropics; around eight months in the continental U.S.A.). If your climate/geography, skin color, or lifestyle make it difficult to obtain adequate sunlight during the summertime, definitely get your levels tested. If you are below 30 ng/mL, consider taking vitamin D supplements during the winter months, particularly. Even a sincere effort to obtain sufficient vitamin D from diet will fall well short. Get some sun!

To mitigate skin cancer concerns or reduce the cosmetic appearance of aging, cover frequently exposed, sensitive skin areas (face, neck, hands) with clothing or sunscreen—they contribute minimally to vitamin D production anyway.

Summary
1. Expose large skin surface areas to direct sunlight for half of "burning time" (or half the time it would take for skin to get pink) whenever possible, especially during times of day/year when sunlight is strong.
2. Routinely cover face, neck, and hands to prevent long-term overexposure.
3. Get tested if you have a sun-challenged lifestyle, and consider supplementing with vitamin D during winter months if necessary.
4. Make sure you are getting sufficient vitamin A, vitamin K, potassium, and magnesium through your diet, or supplement if necessary, since these work synergistically with vitamin D in the body.

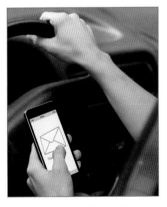

Law #9: Avoid Stupid Mistakes: Reject the concept of humans as good multi-taskers. The human brain is literally incapable of multitasking. Instead, we divert our attention quickly back and forth between stimuli, making us more stressed, less focused, and more likely to make mistakes. Obviously texting and driving is foolish, but when you cut other corners while juggling a hectic daily schedule, bad things can happen. Is talking on a hands-free cell phone while driving cool? Many don't think twice about this, but your brain is significantly less focused on driving while talking on the phone.

Be vigilant and manage risk intelligently by taking nothing for granted—not even a quick ride through town to the supermarket. Your own and other's lives are in your hands each time you get behind the wheel; do you *really* need to have a phone conversation at the same time? Focusing on one task at a time throughout your day—even those that are mundane—will give you the discipline and resolve to stay focused when the stakes escalate, such as every time you turn the key and hit the road.

Summary
1. Multitasking is literally impossible for the human brain. Concentrate on a single task at a time to increase productivity and reduce stress.
2. Be vigilant and manage risk intelligently by taking nothing for granted. Respect the importance of even mundane tasks and hone your ability to focus.

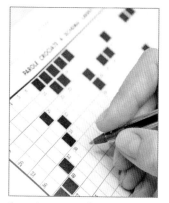

Law #10: Use Your Brain: Engage in creative, intellectual pursuits that counter the grind of daily responsibilities. Give yourself permission to have fun, knowing that tapping into your creative side will enhance your performance in your core areas of responsibility and economic contribution. Get the most out of your brain by strictly filtering and editing the excessive amount of stimulation you are exposed to in daily life and taking frequent breaks away from tasks of intent focus to refresh brain function.

Summary
1. Find creative, intellectual pursuits to balance the daily grind: music, language, crosswords, Sudoku, model airplanes, fantasy sports leagues, or whatever interests you.
2. Find ways to stimulate and challenge your brain throughout the day, such as adding up numbers in your head or recalling names of acquaintances.
3. Treat your brain kindly: take frequent breaks to refresh focus and avoid burnout.

PRIMAL ESSENTIAL MOVEMENTS

Strength training can be simple, convenient, and safe for everyone with the Primal Essential Movements (PEM). Pushups, pull-ups, squats, and planks collectively work all the major muscle groups of the body in a functional manner, providing benefits that are directly applicable to all types of everyday fitness, work, and play activities. You don't have to feel intimidated venturing into a gym, nor assume the inherent risks of loading your body with external sources (meaning gym equipment) for resistance exercises. The PEMs are a great choice for novices and old hands alike because they use *bodyweight* for resistance, comprise simple movements that are easy to learn (and very difficult to screw up and get injured from), and have a series of easier progression exercises that approximate the familiar baseline movement. Even hard-core strength athletes can make the PEMs challenging enough to stimulate fitness breakthroughs.

Begin your strength-training sessions with a two- to five-minute warmup of low-intensity cardiovascular exercise (walking, jogging, stationary cycling, or other cardio machine at a heart rate of "180 minus age" or below). You should break a light sweat, indicating elevated body temperature, and be breathing at a comfortable rate. Conclude each workout with a two- to five-minute cooldown to allow sufficient time to return your breathing rate to normal. Be certain that you have medical clearance before attempting any strenuous workout, including those described in this book.

Next to each exercise listed are levels of "mastery" for males and females. The mastery levels represent your target performance in one set of maximum effort. Your first PEM workout should be an assessment session to determine, by trial and error, your maximum effort level for each essential movement. If you can't complete the mastery number of reps for a particular Essential Movement, drop down to the appropriate progression exercise to enable you to complete a sufficient number of repetitions in your workout. As you improve your performance with your progression exercise, bump up to the next progression exercise or the baseline movement. Advanced strength trainers can integrate numerous adaptations to increase the degree of difficulty beyond the baseline Essential Movements, including donning a weighted vest for the entire PEM session.

Males – Primal Essential Movement mastery
50 pushups
12 pull-ups (overhand grip)
50 squats (thighs, just below parallel to ground)
Plank: 2 minutes holding the Forearm/Feet Plank position
Females – Primal Essential Movement mastery
20 pushups
5 pull-ups (overhand grip)
50 squats (thighs, just below parallel to ground)
Plank: 2 minutes holding forearm/feet plank position

Pushups (lats, pecs, triceps). Mastery = Male 50, Female 20. Assume pushup plank position (arms extended below you, hands forward, body straight). Lower to ground—chest touching first! Keep body dead straight, core and glutes tight, head and neck neutral to torso. Elbows bend backward at 45-degree angle as you lower.

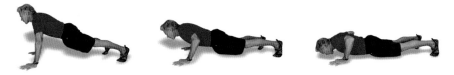

Easiest Progression: Wall Pushups (M50, F30). Do standing push-ups with your arms extended and hands resting against a wall. Maintain plank position as you lower to the wall and re-extend your arms to starting position.

Next Progression: Bench Pushups (M50, F25). Do pushups with hands resting on a bench or other object elevated from ground. Maintain plank position as you raise and lower.

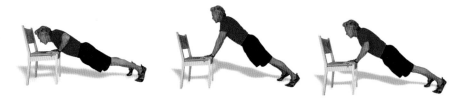

Pull-Ups (back, lats, pecs, biceps). Mastery = Male 12, Female 5. Grasp bar at shoulder width with overhanded grip. Elbows tight, chin tucked, shoulder blades retracted to protect spine. Lead with chest up, keeping lower body quiet. Raise your chin over the bar and gradually lower all the way until your arms are straight (or just before straight if you have joint issues).

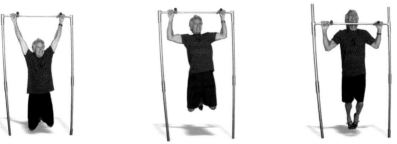

Easiest Progression: Chair-Assisted Pull-Up (M20, F15). Start with your leg loosely positioned on a support chair underneath the bar. Engage your upper body muscles and raise yourself up to the bar. Use just enough leg force to assist getting your chin over the bar. You probably only need to use one leg, but can use two if necessary. Yes, *everyone* can do pull-ups!

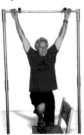
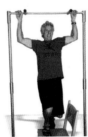
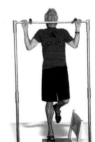

Next Progression: Chin-Up (M7, F4). Many find the chin-up to be slightly easier than a pull-up, particularly if you have wrist, elbow, or shoulder issues. Simply invert your grip on the bar so your palms face you, and raise yourself until your chin is over the bar.

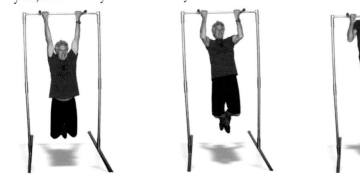

Squats (lower body). Mastery = Male 50, Female 50. Feet shoulder-width or slightly wider apart. Feet face directly forward, or if you must, point them slightly outward. Lower yourself by extending your butt out and bringing thighs to just below parallel to the ground. Envision screwing your feet outward into the ground—left foot counterclockwise, right foot clockwise—tracking your knees over your midfoot as you lower down. Strictly refrain from allowing the knees to cave inward. Maintain a straight spine (it will travel from a 90-degree to a 45-degree angle), but resist the urge to lean forward—chest up! Use your quads and buttocks to absorb the load both sitting and standing. Go down in a smooth and steady movement until your thighs are a bit past parallel to the floor. If you are flexible enough to lower all the way down ("ass to grass") go for it (and work toward it!). Return…Return to a standing position without locking your knees, again making sure your knees track in line with your feet.

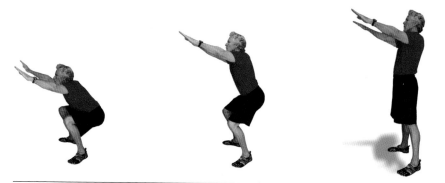

Easiest Progression: Assisted Squat (M50, F50). Hold pole or other support object while lowering into and raising up from squat position. Use support object as little as possible.

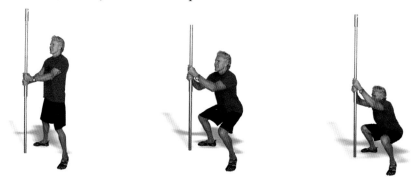

Planks (core and lower back, as well as shoulders, triceps, hip flexors). Mastery = Male 2 minutes, Female 2 minutes. Hold pushup plank position while resting your elbows on the ground. Maintain position until you can no longer maintain straight body position or your arms/shoulders fatigue. An optional movement to stimulate the oblique abs is to lean on one extended arm and rotate body into sideways plank position, preserving a straight line from your head to toe. Hold until failure, and then repeat on other side.

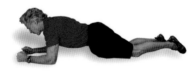

Easiest Progression: Forearm/Knee Plank (M 2 minutes, F 2 minutes). Assume plank position with forearms and knees resting on ground. Engage core muscles and glutes during exercise.

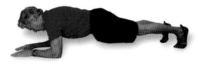

Next Progression: Hand/Feet Plank (M 2 minutes, F 2 minutes). Assume plank position a la pushup starting point, with arms extended and hands and feet on ground.

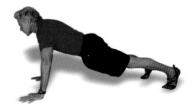

PEM Isolation: For a unique challenge, set an ambitious numerical goal for a single PEM and make that your entire workout one day. Perform reps until failure, then rest as needed and tackle additional reps, counting your accumulated total to reach your goal. For example, some mornings I'll aspire to do 200 decline pushups. These might accumulate in sets as follows: 60, 50, 30, 25, 25, and 15. I might do half the sets in 10 minutes, then get sidetracked for 20 minutes before I finish off the last several sets.

PEM Sprint Workout: This is a fun session that's over with quickly and integrates strength training and sprinting. It's a great challenge to all of your muscle groups and your cardiovascular system.

- One set maximum effort pushups, then immediately sprint 80 meters. Rest 30-60 seconds until breathing returns to normal.
- One set maximum effort plank, then bunny hop 40 meters. Rest 30-60 seconds.
- One set maximum effort pull-ups, then sprint 80 meters. Rest 30-60 seconds.
- One set maximum effort squats, then bunny hop 40 meters. (Wow!)

SPRINT WORKOUT SUGGESTIONS

Begin each workout with a five-minute warmup of low-intensity walking or jogging (heart rate of "180 minus age" or less) followed by light stretching. Conclude each workout with a five-minute cooldown identical to the warmup. Be certain that you have medical clearance before attempting any strenuous workout, including those described in this book.

Novice Sprint Workout – Strides and 85-Percent Sprints

After proper warm up, conduct six warmup strides of 5 to 8 seconds each, with a 20-second rest period between strides. Focus on maintaining good running form and don't worry about your speed. These are just warm ups for your main sprint efforts. After your warmup strides, do six sprints lasting 8 to 20 seconds each at an estimated 90 percent of maximum effort. Take a one-minute rest period between sprints or otherwise enough to be fully recovered and achieve normal respiration before beginning your next sprint.

After two to three sessions over a few weeks' time, increase your sprint efforts to nearly full speed. Use a moving start (jog up to starting line and then begin sprinting) instead of a static start, to minimize injury risk. Where you fall in the range of 8 to 20 seconds is personal preference. Naturally, shorter sprints will be at faster speeds. I like to include both shorter and longer duration sprint sessions into my schedule. Pay attention to the difference between leg fatigue and pain. If you experience any acute pain or tightness, particularly in your hamstrings, wrap up the workout immediately with an easy cooldown and refrain from further intense exercise until your condition completely clears.

Sprint Workout #1 – Strides and Full Sprints

Strides and sprint workout as described for novice workout, except build to maximum (controlled) effort on the sprints. Remember to deliver a consistent quality of effort on each sprint, and stop the workout if your time or perceived effort is unsatisfactory.

Sprint Workout #2 – Hill Repeats

Six to eight times hill sprints lasting 8 to 20 seconds at 90 percent effort. Recover by walking or trotting down the hill. Return to normal breathing before beginning next effort.

Sprint Workout #3 – Accelerations

Six to eight times 30-second sprints with the first 10 seconds at medium effort, second 10 seconds at hard effort, and third 10 seconds at full sprint. One to two minutes recovery between efforts. You can use a running track and do 150-meter repeats accelerating every 50 meters (start at turn apex, accelerate at straightaway, accelerate again at middle of straightaway, finish at traditional finish line) or any other course you can mark with one-third distance intervals.

Sprint Workout #4 – Technique Drills

- **Strides:** Four times eight-second strides at 90 percent effort. Ten-second rest between efforts. One-minute rest before next exercise.
- **Skipping:** Two to four times 50 meters. Drive knee as high as you

can (try to hit your chest), taking off and landing on opposite leg. Then launch off and land with opposite leg, driving other knee high into chest—like an exaggerated skip. Strive for maximum height instead of length. Fifteen-second rest between efforts. One-minute rest before next exercise.

- **Bounding:** Two to four times 50 meters. Take as long a stride as possible, focusing on keeping your balance rather than speed. Thirty-second rest between efforts. One-minute rest before next exercise.

- **Bunny Hopping:** Two to four times 50 meters. Take off on both legs and jump up and forward. Focus on achieving a good balance between height and length. Swing arms to assist effort and ensure a balanced landing. One-minute rest between efforts (you'll need it, trust me). Two-minute rest before next exercise.

- **Full Sprint:** Two to four times 50-meter full sprint. One-minute rest between efforts.

Sprint Workout #5 – Stair Drills

Conduct this workout on stadium or building stairs. Your flight of stairs should take 8 to 20 seconds to ascend. Take 30 seconds rest between each exercise, or more or less as needed to feel refreshed and get your breathing under control.

- Four times warmup stair climbs at 75-percent effort. When you reach the top, return immediately down the stairs at a comfortable pace, then ascend again.

- Two times single stairs. Ascend one stair at a time with rapid leg turnover. Descend comfortably and repeat effort.

- Two times bounding stairs. Ascend by skipping as many steps as you can. Focus on keeping your balance rather than speed. Drive arms for balance and leverage. Descend comfortably and repeat effort.

- Four times full speed stairs. Skip desired number of stairs with each stride to get to the top as fast as possible. Descend comfortably and recover completely between efforts.

Sprint Workout #6 – "Grokball"

This workout, inspired by MarksDailyApple.com regular Grant Peterson, is a refreshing example of the simplicity of fitness in a culture that habitually tries to make things more complex than they need to be. In the amount of time it takes to get through the basic set-up instructions of your heart rate monitor owner's manual, you can capture the essence of Grok with this primal effort.

Take a 5- to 10-pound medicine ball (depending on your own bodyweight and strength level) to an ample-sized athletic field. After a 5-minute light jog, grab the ball and throw it down the field. Sprint after it, pick it up and throw it again, completing repeat trips up and down the field. Discover numerous variations on the throw—overhead like a soccer throw-in, underhand like an old school free-throw, sideways one-armed like a discus thrower, sideways two-armed like a hammer thrower, roll like a bowling ball (one- or two-handed), or face backward and throw over your head two-handed. (Watch out for little kids at soccer practice with the latter.)

Be extremely careful to keep your spine and neck in a neutral position every time you throw. Your legs and core muscle groups will provide the most leverage and receive the most training effect from the throws. Your spine and neck should always be in a straight line (angle to the ground might vary from perpendicular to 45 degrees depending on your throwing style)—don't curve your back or neck fore-aft or side-to-side. Make sure that the force of your effort is absorbed by your legs and core muscles.

Begin with gentle throws that will give you a form check. As you fatigue after a few lengths of the field, you will have to be especially diligent about maintaining proper body position for your throws. When you notice that your ability to maintain correct form becomes compromised due to fatigue, it is time to stop the workout; the same goes if you experience any acute pain in your muscles or joints. Finish your session with five minutes of easy jogging.

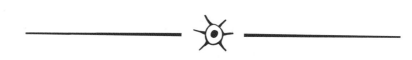

SPRINTING AWAY FROM MALIBU

While I'm aware of the need to address Primal Blueprint enthusiasts living in varied climates with varied options for exercise venues, I obviously have difficulty suppressing my enthusiasm for one of my favorite workouts: beach sprints. (Check out a session on video at MarksDailyApple.com.) As MarksDailyApple.com reader Robert McLeod commented, "Hey Mark, not everyone lives at the beach. What about sprint workout suggestions for winter?" A stationary bike will work just fine, as will any building staircase for the "stadium" workout.

If you don't have a suitable indoor venue, or you are feeling adventurous, try doing sprints on cross country skis, snowshoes, or ice skates. On my visits to the mountains, I've enjoyed doing sprints on snowshoes up a very steep hill in deep powder. It's a fascinating athletic juxtaposition to compare the sensations of moving quickly on packed sand with barely moving up a steep hill at high altitude, while using the same motion and same effort level.

Cycling Sprint Workout #1 – Interval Ladder

Cycling sprints should only be done on a stationary bike due to the high degree of technical difficulty and automobile danger associated with sprinting on a bike outdoors. Take a five-minute warmup on the bike at easy-to-moderate effort. For the main set, sprint 10 seconds, rest 10 seconds. Then a 20-second sprint with a 20-second rest. Then 30-second sprint, 30-second rest. Then another 30-second sprint, 30-second rest. Then a 20-second sprint, 20 second rest. Then a 10-second sprint, 10-second rest to complete the ladder workout. Five minutes easy pedaling cooldown.

Cycling Sprint Workout #2 – "Thirty-Twos"

Six to eight times 30-seconds all-out with two-minute recovery between efforts. The extended recovery time in this workout helps improve power—the number of watts you can produce at maximum intensity. The interval workouts (cycling workouts #1 and #3) are more focused on developing oxygen-carrying capacity, since recovery intervals are shorter in relation to work efforts. *Note*: Thirty seconds is longer than the maximum recommended running sprint of 20 seconds, because cycling is less strenuous than running.

Cycling Sprint Workout #3 – Tabata Intervals

Tabata is a workout system where you achieve a desired number of minutes of intense effort in sprinting, weightlifting, or any other maximum effort exercise, using the consistent work/rest ratio of 20-seconds sprint, 10-seconds rest, 20-seconds sprint, 10-seconds rest—repeated for usually four minutes by Tabata enthusiasts. Going for just four minutes is a great workout, but some people like to pedal slowly for a few minutes and then commence another one or two four-minute Tabata sessions.

A FEW WORDS ABOUT DIETS AND DIETING
Recapping the Primal Argument
Against Conventional Wisdom

While it's encouraging to see the increasing mainstream acceptance of the primal/paleo/ancestral health eating style, we are still swimming upstream against the massive forces that have entrenched a grain-based diet into Western culture. If you are struggling in your mind about who is "right," I believe any confusion can be alleviated when you consider a larger context and the different paradigm the Standard American Diet operates in.

Proponents of the SAD try to convince us that humans need to center our diet around carbohydrates, especially grains. Furthermore, they want us to believe that the many diet-related health problems with which so many people struggle are due to factors other than carbohydrate consumption. And yes, eating fat while eating excessive amounts of processed carbohydrates (especially in comparison with our ancestors) can contribute to excess body fat due to the high insulin production.

When you reject the flawed starting point of a grain-based, high-carbohydrate diet, you begin to see the rationale of the Primal Blueprint in its proper perspective. Carbohydrates are not required to survive. Our evolutionary history and any scientist will confirm this. If you eat primally, your fat-burning genes will upregulate (or turn on) and you won't need regular meals to get through the day. If insulin and glucose are not running rampant in your bloodstream (thanks to cutting back on carbohydrates), then your risk of systemic inflammation and cellular damage is greatly minimized. At this point, eating fat—lots of *the right kinds* of fat—will support health and long-lasting energy.

If you are still conflicted, try ditching grains and sugars for 21 days and see how your body reacts. Or, if you have been struggling with weight management, check out the Success Stories link at MarksDailyApple.com to get a sense of the physical transformation people are experiencing when they go primal—on the heels of years of frustration from trying conventional diets.

Beyond the glaring distinction between primal eating and a grain-based, high-carb diet there are certain other points to consider. Vegetarians will have objections to my emphasis on meat, but these objections are almost entirely countered (saving the philosophical ones, which involve a personal belief system and not a dietary quality debate) by emphasizing local, pasture-raised animal products and consuming high-antioxidant vegetables and fruits along with your meat.

If you've seen research suggesting that meats and high-fat diets are unhealthy, this conclusion is likely heavily influenced by eating overcooked or heavily processed meat laden with nitrites and other toxins; consuming high-fat foods in conjunction with moderate-to-high-carb diets (because insulin drives the fat into storage and promotes systemic inflammation that allows ingested cholesterol and saturated fat to cause trouble in your arteries); consuming partially hydrogenated trans fats and refined high polyunsaturated vegetable/seed oils (troublemakers who get the whole class of "fat" blamed for their bad behavior); and obtaining insufficient high-antioxidant foods such as fresh organic produce.

Some dieticians argue that the avoidance of whole grains and legumes compromises nutrient intake, since these foods have long occupied a prominent position in the diet recommended by conventional wisdom.

We already know that grains and legumes stress the insulin response system and are inferior sources of vitamins and minerals—particularly on a per calorie "bang for your buck" basis—compared to other plants and animals. Furthermore, a grain-based diet results in excessive fiber consumption and health risks associated with the aforementioned anti-nutrients (lectins, glutens, and phytates) on a noticeable allergic level and a more insidious subclinical level.

Those in the low-fat camp might shudder at all the fat that primal enthusiasts enjoy from animal meats, fish, fowl, eggs, avocados and avocado oil, nuts and seeds, coconut products, butter, olives and olive oil, and dark chocolate. However, we know that heart disease is related more to excessive insulin production and the inflammatory elements of your diet than it is to fat intake. The continued popularity of the sentiment that too much fat is bad for you simply blows my mind. It's time to separate once and for all good fats from bad. Fortunately, the health dangers of partially hydrogenated trans fats are now well accepted, and the backlash against toxic refined vegetable oils is building. Meanwhile, the health benefits of consuming omega-3 and monounsatured fats are being widely embraced.

We're getting there, but we need to also recognize that saturated fat is not evil either—unless you wolf down too many carbs in conjunction with them or rely exclusively on feedlot animals, overly cook them, or fail to consume high-antioxidant plant foods.

Dr. Ron Rosedale, author of *The Rosedale Diet* and acclaimed for reversing type 2 diabetes, obesity, and heart disease through diet, says, "A high-complex-carbohydrate, low-saturated-fat diet is an absolute oxymoron. A high-complex-carbohydrate diet is nothing but a high-glucose diet, or a high-sugar diet. Your body is just going to store it as saturated fat (since we have very limited glycogen stores in muscle and liver), and the body makes it into saturated fat quite readily."

The Biggest Losers

"Who will be the biggest loser this week?"—goes the tag line of the popular boot camp weight-loss competition on television. The answer is definitely the public. You simply can't lose 10 or 20 pounds of body fat in 10 or 20 days—period. It's a parlor trick. Most of the weight lost is from reduced water retention (four grams of water bond with every gram of stored glycogen in the body). Some of the weight lost is precious muscle, leaving only a small fraction of the impressive total as actual body fat. What's more, contestants follow extremely low-calorie diets that are still carbohydrate-heavy and feature plenty of processed, low-fat, artificial-sugar-laden frankenfoods. At the "finish line" of extreme, unsustainable crash diet/workout efforts, big losers are left depleted, exhausted, and prone to a rebound effect of overeating and under-exercising. This is the human organism's survival instinct kicking in and trying to restore, replenish, and recover from the hormonal and metabolic disregulation caused by the extreme experience of a crash diet.

You may have heard the oft-reported government survey figure that 97 percent of dieters gain the weight back within five years. Also troubling is a recent study from Dr. Traci Mann, a UCLA psychology professor who tracked the long-term success rate of participants in 31 popular diets. The study reported that 41 percent of participants gained back more weight than they lost within one year. While Mann admitted the number seemed "depressing," she also revealed that "we have strong reasons to feel that this number *under-represents* the true number of participants who gained back more weight than they lost" due to people dropping out of contact due to embarrassment and people crash-dieting right before the study period ended to save face!

What a complete mess we are in. We need to take a step back and adjust our collective mentality to approach the subject of healthy eating with a fresh perspective. There is no reason why any of us should suffer from excessive body fat, emotional stress, or disappointment on the subject of eating. I am advocating a variable, intuitive eating style that includes a tremendous variety of delicious foods and minimal (from one point of view anyway!) restrictions. Furthermore, I am not irresponsibly pitching the Primal Blueprint eating style as the end-all secret to good health and longevity; the best outcomes result from combining primal-style eating with the other Primal Blueprint behaviors. Ignoring them is a recipe for failure. For example, an extreme endurance athlete immersed in a stressful training program (burning carbs for hours on end every day) will probably crash and burn if he suddenly switches to eating Primal Blueprint style. For such an athlete, we must first address the issue of sensible training methods before turning our attention to dietary habits (details in the book *Primal Endurance*).

The Primal Blueprint works because it isn't a diet, it doesn't involve depriving or exhausting yourself, and because you make all the decisions about how to make it work best for you within the general guidelines laid out in this book. As with any diet or lifestyle modification, if you don't enjoy it and truly believe in what you're doing it can't be sustainable long term. The estimated two million sincere primal/paleo enthusiasts know that a Primal Blueprint-aligned lifestyle works. I believe the logic behind it is unassailable—and who could argue that we shouldn't be eating real, delicious food, exercising in a fun, intuitive manner, enjoying time in the sun, playing, getting enough sleep, using our brain creatively, and avoiding stupid mistakes? I trust that if you take the leap, the results will speak for themselves.

PRIMAL BLUEPRINT INTERNET RESOURCES

I've taken advantage of the infinite capacity of the Internet to augment this book with continually updated supporting material. The direct links are as follows:

Primal Blueprint Text References

marksdailyapple.com/the-book/references/primal-blueprint-text-references/

Primal Blueprint Suggested Reading

marksdailyapple.com/the-book/references/suggested-reading/

Primal Blueprint Shopping and Information Resources

marksdailyapple.com/the-book/references/primal-blueprint-resources/

Primal Blueprint Q&A: *Everything You Always Wanted to Ask… but Were Afraid to Know*

marksdailyapple.com/the-book/references/questions-and-answers/
   All About Grok
      Dispute About Recent Human Evolution

PRIMAL
BLUEPRINT
SUCCESS STORIES

Some of the most rewarding elements of the Primal Blueprint movement are the astonishing Success Story submissions we receive at MarksDailyApple.com each week. We publish a story every Friday, but the submissions have become so frequent we can only share a portion of them. Nevertheless, I read every single one and they touch me profoundly. It's mind blowing to realize how big the movement has become and how much momentum has been created from word of mouth on Internet blogs, forums, and local community meetup groups.

While I hope this book is everything you were looking for, I would love for you to take things further by joining the MarksDailyApple. com community. These success stories are a mere sampling of the hundreds you'll find online. Who knows? Maybe someday you'll be compelled to send us a story and photos to join the ranks of people who have transformed their lives living Primally.

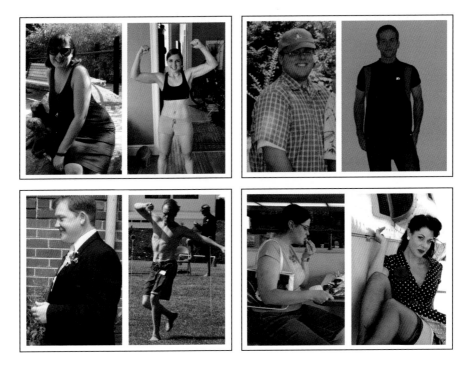

SUCCESS STORY:
MALIKA DUKE
Ft. Worth, TX

I was starting to think I'd have to settle for the 'fluffy mommy look' forever.

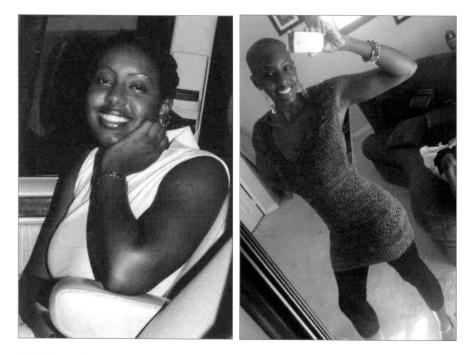

Malika submitted a sequence of stunning photos chronicling her Primal transformation over time. Describing her starting point in May of 2010, Malika says, "After having three kids, I was starting to believe that I'd have to settle for the 'fluffy mommy look' forever. I'd completed a double round of an intense 90-day home workout program that glamorized 'muscle confusion,' but I was not happy with the way my body looked afterward. Since I'd worked incredibly hard, I suspected that the problem lay in my diet."

"Interestingly, I was at the same age (32) where my father (eating a traditional Caribbean diet high in rice and beans) was first diagnosed with diabetes. The disease has rendered him legally blind, compromising his independence, self-worth, self-esteem, and enjoyment of life. Diabetes also took the life of my grandmother in 2008, and affects my sister, mother (high cholesterol and blood pressure), aunt, uncle, two cousins, and others in my family who refuse to seek change or entertain life after grains. My motivation to go primal was to have diabetes and related conditions stop with me in the family bloodline!" asserts Malika.

She continues, "We had some family arguments over such a sudden dietary change, particularly when the food bills got higher from eating uncured bacon, sausage, and farm-fresh eggs. After a short time, however, there wasn't much for my husband to argue about. I mean, come on—what red-blooded American male would argue for whole wheat pasta instead of spinach, tomato and onion in bacon fat with a big honking piece of rib-eye?!"

Body composition results for Malika and her family were immediate and dramatic. "I didn't have a scale to weigh that old fluffy mommy, but I dropped all the way down to my current 151 pounds (69 kilos), and I'm seeing muscles that I thought were lost forever! My husband seems to have recovered from his totally undiagnosed Irritable Bowel Syndrome, and he thanks me at least once a week for his newly uncovered eight-pack!

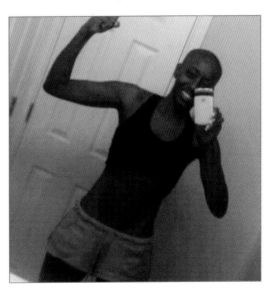

My ten- and eight-year-olds have leaned out from a pudgy 137 lbs (62 kg) and 110 lbs (50 kg), to 106 lbs (48 kg) and 84 lbs (38 kg), respectively. Things have gone so well that we've created a community to help women and families transition to a Primal Blueprint lifestyle!" Check out her website, featuring numerous helpful videos from Malika, FitRichWoman.com.

SUCCESS STORY:
NICK LASZLO
South San Francisco, CA

*I'm actually looking forward to turning 50,
and I've never felt or looked better!
What a sharp contrast from when I turned 40...*

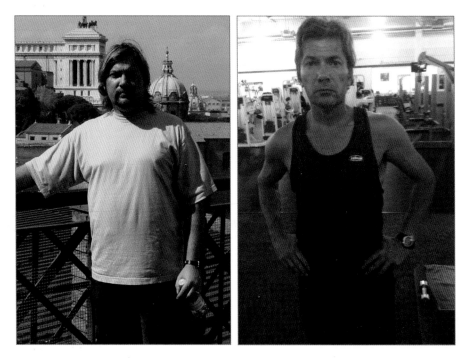

Nick, 49, is a recovered alcoholic, "former fattie," and former elite long distance runner. After reaching his peak as an athlete in his 20s, Nick sustained a series of injuries and burnout, and then "plunged into a 20-year exercise in self-pity," featuring substance abuse, pizza, fast food, high blood pressure, high cholesterol, and a long-term bout with Hepatitis C.

During his steady decline in health and fitness, Nick was cranking along in what he calls a "successful facade of a highly paid software engineer." Losing his job in March of 2010 inspired Nick to take action and turn his life around. He quit drinking and took a long look in the mirror, noticing how well 36 percent body fat obscured the elite athlete trapped inside. Nick laced up his running shoes again, thinking that running, his "trusted best friend from the past," would make everything right. Alas, it wasn't so easy to return to single digit body fat. He tried starvation diets, diet pills, and dangerous amounts of stimulants to no avail.

Good results started to happen as he dabbled in primal-style eating: He dropped 55 pounds (25 kilos), going from 36 percent to 6 percent body fat, and gaining eight pounds of muscle, and his blood work normalized. However, he still had bouts of binge eating and a sense that things weren't ideal. After discovering *The Primal Blueprint* at a bookstore one day in 2010 and implementing its principles, Nick enjoyed breakthroughs in energy, metabolism, general health, and competitive success as a masters (age-group) long distance runner.

While Nick puts in more miles training for master's competition than might typically be recommended by the Primal Blueprint, he is careful to moderate his pace, avoid chronic patterns, and also integrate primal-style strength and sprint workouts into his training regimen.

"Here I am today, looking forward to turning 50, and feeling tons better than when I was 40," commented Nick. "I currently earn my living as a personal trainer specializing in weight loss at a local health club. I give each new client a 'homework assignment' after our first appointment: Go out and buy Mark's book! *The Primal Blueprint* has changed my life and I know it will change theirs too."

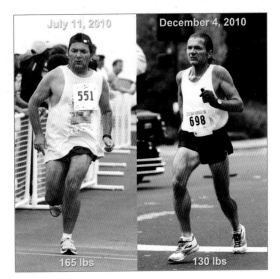

July 11, 2010   December 4, 2010

165 lbs   130 lbs

SUCCESS STORY:
MICHELLE MATANGI
New Plymouth, New Zealand

*I finally feel freed from my obsession
with food, and can do the odd 24-hour fast
with no problems.*

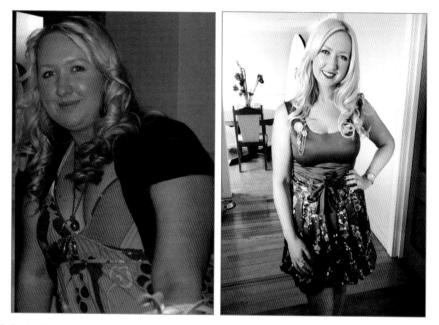

Michelle, aka "Dollface" the prolific primal blogger (primaljourney. blogspot.com), relates a compelling story of struggling for years to be healthy and fit. Her travails began a decade ago at age 21, with job stress, depression, weight gain, and of course the obligatory prescription meds from her physician. Michelle blames antidepressant medication for contributing to rapid weight gain, as she hit 87 kilograms (191 pounds) at 5'6". Upon adopting the Atkins Diet, she dropped many kilos in short order but didn't feel healthy. "Lot's of diet coke and artificially sweetened chocolate, and continued anxiety and depression," remembers Michelle.

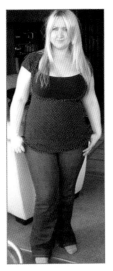

Michelle shifted gears, went back to grain-based eating, and endured several years of "constant hunger, and steady weight gain up to a morbidly obese 107 kilos (235 lbs). I was eating every 2-3 hours and constantly hungry!" Realizing she had done better on a low-carb program, Michelle intensified her Internet research and discovered MarksDailyApple.com. "I was glued to the site for days!" remembers Michelle. "I eliminated grain foods, and added plenty of veggies, protein, and fat. No diet coke this time, just soda water and herbal teas. Furthermore, as I got deeper into the Primal Blueprint, I realized it's all about lifestyle, not just dieting. I now weigh 69 kilos (152 lbs) and finally have my anxiety under control."

Michelle continues, "The primal way feels so natural—coming from a person who absolutely had to eat every two to three hours or I would get lightheaded and even dizzy! Now I can do the odd 24-hour fast with no problem. I finally feel freed from my obsession with food, and the handcuffs of my eating timetable. This is one of the best things about going primal."

Michelle takes to care to not let her stunning before/after transformation photos and her incredible passion for primal living get in the way of reality when communicating with others. Asked the secret to her succcess, she shoots straight: "Sometimes it feels impossible, stuck in a fat body, to imagine how you could ever be thinner. It can be a tough pill to swallow when you realize there is no magic pill, and you have to make some major changes if you want real results.

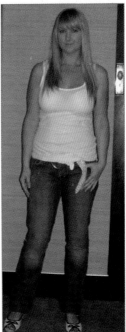

"Sure, I still face daily challenges in a world driven by conventional wisdom and refined foods everywhere. But when I make conscious choices and focus on the satisfaction of eating primal foods, it's easy to stay on track. That and I keep a pair of my old size 20 jeans around; they're a great reminder of where I've been and how far I've come!"

SUCCESS STORY:
DAVE PARSONS
Roosevelt, NJ

I EAT MARK'S APPLE EVERY DAY. IT MAKES IT OKAY TO BE WHO I AM… AND BE A MEMBER OF THE PRIMAL LIFE CLAN!

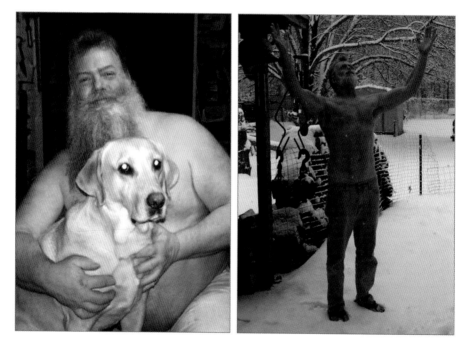

"Unconquerable Dave" as he is known at MarksDailyApple.com wows us with regular updates in his inimitable ALL CAPS writing style:

DEAR MARK, A PIC IS WORTH 1,000 WORDS… STARTED ~300 POUNDS… DOWN TO 200… NOW THERE AIN'T MUCH LEFT TO LOSE… I REMEMBER THIS SIZE WHEN I WAS 18 YEARS OLD. GROK ON AND THANK YOU FOR THE ILLUMINATION! LATER BROTHER. STAY IN THE LIGHT. GROK RULES!

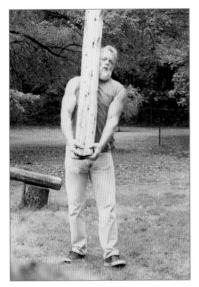

Dave, 54, first contacted me after losing 40 pounds (18 kilos) in six months. He related how his passion for cooking (SAD stuff) "just about slayed my entire family!" After four months of transitioning to primal-style eating, he got into the groove with a simple approach, "If I can't kill it, find it, or gather it, I don't eat it. Makes it real easy to eat well! My body tells me what it wants, and I listen. The wife and kids still around are impressed with my new attitude and look."

While most of Dave's early results came from primal eating with only mild exercise, he relates that as weight came off and energy increased, he was able to resume some significant strength training. "I like the primal approach way better than being a gym gorilla. I have my own outdoor primal gym of trees and rocks and stuff," Dave relates. Averse to the gym or not, Dave's progress reports include some impressive gym numbers, such as a 404-pound (183 kilo) deadlift and 18-inch biceps. It's hard to top Dave's images to capture the essence of living primally, but he makes a good attempt with words in closing a recent update:

"To steal words from Walt Whitman...
'I too am not a bit tamed, I too am untranslatable,
I sound my barbaric YAWP over the roofs of the world.'"

Everyone in the primal community hears your YAWP, Dave! May it echo to many more folks. Grok On, brother!

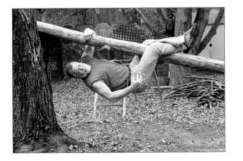
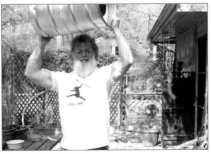

SUCCESS STORY:
DEANNA EBERLIN
Corning, NY

The biggest change in my life, beyond what I eat, how I exercise, or how I sleep, is the simple freedom that the Primal Blueprint has afforded me.

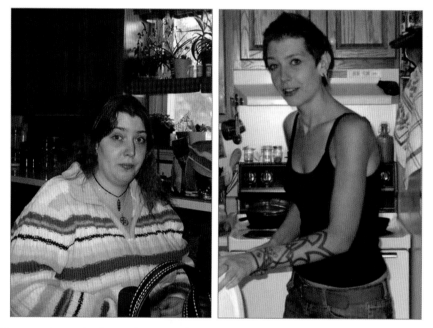

Deanna is one of our longest-duration success stories, still going strong over four years. Deanna relates that she started trending toward obesity in third grade, "the last time I felt normal." She reached 200 pounds (91 kilos) at age 18, feeling generally unhappy about life and her dead-end jobs. Fed up and tipping the scales at 250 pounds (114 kilos—"I stopped weighing myself after that"), Deanna kicked off a new direction by ditching grains and engaging in chronic cardio. On a diet of six treadmill miles and 1,800 calories a day, Deanna dropped to 140 pounds (64 kilos), at which point she reached a frustrating plateau.

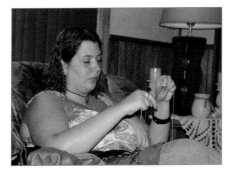

While Deanna's methods delivered substantial results on the scale, they were both short of her ultimate goal and seemed unsustainable over the long term. After some ruminating and Internet research, Deanna ultimately decided to "overcome my initial fat phobia" and begin transitioning to a primal lifestyle; not just diet, but optimal sleeping habits, more play, and ditching chronic cardio for a primal-aligned program. In only three months of going primal, Deanna lost that pesky final 15 pounds (7 kilos) to reach 125 pounds (57 kilos). "Half of my former bodyweight—how freaky is that?!" Beyond the body composition improvements, Deanna reports having more regulated daily energy levels,("I only eat two to three times per day instead of five to six"), high-energy mornings in the office (to the dismay of dragging coworkers!), and enjoyable evenings ("I don't pass out on the couch after dinner anymore").

We checked back with Deanna in early 2012, two years after her initial submission and four years into her Primal journey. "I've added five pounds of muscle, and have experienced some peripheral health benefits such as increased hair thickness and an improved complexion," Deanna related.

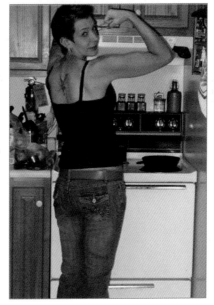

Currently Deanna is taking college courses in Health and Wellness. Her final thoughts extend out to readers with a few tips: "Focus on lifestyle change that is sustainable and forget the extreme stuff. Choose freedom: eat what you want, when you want; and if you don't feel like exercising one day, skip it. Finally, set ambitious goals. When I started I couldn't do a single pushup. Now I can do 20—real ones, not girlie! Believe in the power of the body to transform, and be patient with the process."

SUCCESS STORY:
WADE BAKER
Portland, OR

Within a month of eating primally, my lifelong
symptoms of asthma disappeared,
my gastric reflux abated, I dropped 15 pounds,
and ceased all prescription medication.

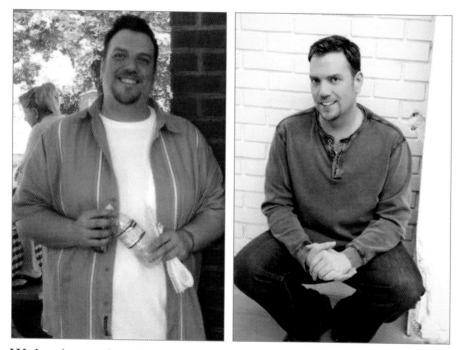

Wade relates a disturbing litany of health conditions prior to going primal. At 5'10" and 325 pounds, with a BMI of 47, Wade was taking three asthma medications, suffered from severe acid reflux (taking expensive prescription acid reducers), and strapped up to a CPAP machine each night to deal with his sleep apnea.

Having struggled his entire life with excess body fat, Wade embarked upon yet another weight-loss program in January of 2010, guided by a professional physical therapist, trainer, and nutritionist. "I committed myself feverishly to conventional wisdom: daily torturous battles with my body at the gym and a low-fat, high-fiber, high-carb diet. I experienced some modest initial results but had a sense that all those refined carbs were not healthy. I battled about this with my nutritionist/trainer, who swore that my instincts were wrong and that I would be doomed to failure if I broke from conventional wisdom," Wade relates.

After a couple months of unease, Wade recalls, "I followed my gut and set out full-steam ahead down my primal path. Within a month of ceasing my refined flour and sugar consumption and eating primally, I began to see immediate and dramatic results. My lifelong symptoms of severe asthma immediately disappeared, my painful gastric reflux abated, I dropped 15 pounds that first month, and I was able to cease all prescription medication."

Concurrent to his dietary changes, Wade backed off of his chronic cardio patterns, taking his exercise heart rate down to 70 percent of max and establishing a rhythm of cardio and strength workouts balanced by sufficient recovery.

In eleven months, Wade dropped 105 pounds, humming along at a steady rate of 8 to 12 pounds of body fat lost per month. "No asthma, no gastric reflux, no painful sleep-deprivation headaches, no weakness from chronic workouts, no lethargy from insulin crashes, and no more annoying CPAP machine to sleep!" reports Wade.

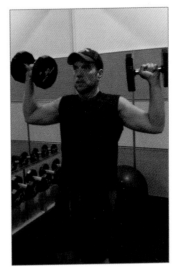

Wade has checked in several times since his initial report nearly two years ago. "My life has dramatically changed. I almost never go hungry, and have no cravings—even when I skip a meal, which I often do. I have lost a total of 137 pounds following the Primal Blueprint. I'm currently working with a personal trainer and getting into some heavy weights. My success has even convinced my trainer to start eating primally, and he now recommends it to his clients!"

SUCCESS STORY:
LARRY DIAMOND
Round Rock, TX

*Over 100 pounds lost, and things
just keep getting better and better.*

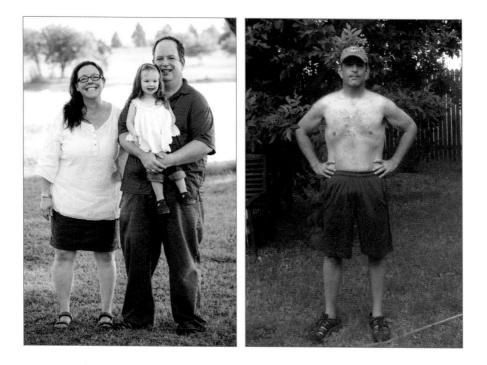

Most of his adult life, Larry, at 5' 9", was morbidly obese, weighing in at
250 to 300 pounds. "I'd like to say that becoming a parent [Larry and his
wife adopted a daughter in 2011] was was enough to lead to dramatic
changes to my daily eating and exercise habits. It wasn't."

But more changes than parenting were in store. His uncle, a father figure to him, developed dementia. He also had diabetes, as had Larry's grandmother who had eventually lost her life due to complications from the disease. In 2012, Larry and his wife became the sole caregivers for his uncle. Work, parenting, and his uncle's caregiving swallowed up all the couple's time. "I was gaining weight, profoundly saddened at my uncle's condition and just trying to stay afloat. Did I see my future in my uncle? Yes. Did I know what to do? No."

In May of 2013, he looked around at a crowded concert and realized he was one of the biggest people there. The fear of ending up like his uncle and becoming a burden to his wife and child shifted something inside him. His motivation kicked in.

But one thing bothered Larry. Why was he genuinely always hungry? So he googled it. His first Internet search led him to discussions about insulin, its key role in metabolism, fat storage versus burning, and blood sugar and hunger. His family history of diabetes and a bloodwork panel that indicated he was heading in the same direction were the impetus to stop buying bread and pasta, fast food, potato chips, and candy bars. But severe sleep apnea, back pain, and allergies still plagued him.

He read exhaustively about key players in modern nutrition theory: Ancel Keys and his Seven Country Study on diet and cardiovascular disease which led to the questionable public policies underlying our Standard American Diet, sports medicine doctor Professor Tim Noakes, Gary Taubes, Dr. David Perlmutter, Tom Naughton, and of course, Mark Sisson of the primal/paleo world and Mark's Daily Apple. "I started to have a coherent vision of what had gone so wrong the last 40 years for my family, for America, for global society."

Following the Primal Blueprint, Larry successfully dropped down to the high 170s (a weight not experienced since high school), and finally his ailments subsided. His taste buds, he claims, "are no longer dominated by sweetness, and the artificial and chemical." Larry's fitness routine also evolved, focusing on pushups, sit ups, burpees, planks, and squats. Inspired by the concept of incorporating play into fitness, Larry found that his daughter, at 30 pounds, was excellent for lifting. "Games in the backyard are play, bonding, and fitness combined. I hope to be climbing trees with my daughter when she is old enough."

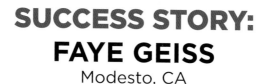

SUCCESS STORY:
FAYE GEISS
Modesto, CA

*At 87 years old, for the first time in my life
I feel beautiful both inside and out.*

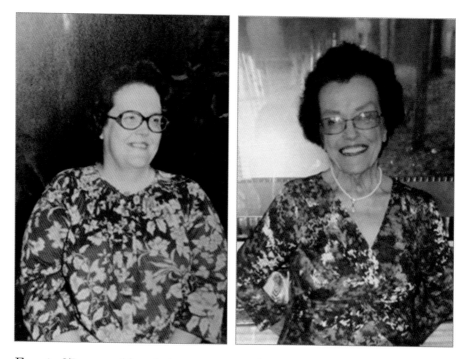

Faye is 87 years old and the youngest of 11 children who were raised on a cotton farm in California's Central Valley. "Everyone worked on the farm during the Depression," Faye said, "and ate what they grew." Self-conscious like many young teenagers, Faye once asked her teacher if she looked fat. "You are pleasingly plump," she was told.

At 17 she left home and moved to Santa Cruz to work at the Boardwalk, living on hot dogs and hamburgers. Four years later she met my husband of 64 years. They had four children: three daughters and a son. They ate a lot of beans, oats, and rice in order to make ends meet. "My husband and I worked in the restaurant business, he as a chef and myself as a waitress. Needless to say, we both worked long hours, and meals for us were whatever was quick for the family."

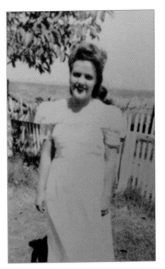

Eventually she became a stay-at-home mother. But boredom and loneliness crept in and food began to fill the void. "I never had a driver's license, and my husband worked 10 to 12 hours a day." After her children left home, empty nest syndrome spurred more emotional eating. Faye's attempts to diet and lose weight never seemed to work. In 1990, at the age of 63, Faye learned she was diabetic. Confused and scared, she did her best to follow the SAD eating recommendations for diabetics but still couldn't lose weight. Then came the onset of heart disease and a heart attack in 1999. She stepped up her efforts with fad diets, to no avail.

Faye's grandson, Aaron Fox, is the Chief Marketing Officer of Primal Blueprint. His parents had begun following this new lifestyle. "They gave me a copy of *The Primal Blueprint*, and as I began reading it something just clicked." Faye said. Once she began following the primal guidelines, her weight dropped from 220 to 130 pounds, without any sense of depri-

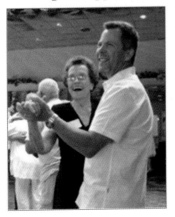

vation. "After a year of being primal, I moved to be closer to my daughter." Faye said. "My new doctor checked my blood work and took me off several medications, including insulin. I have been able to manage my diabetes by eating primally and exercising three times a week. At 87 years old, for the first time in my life I feel beautiful, both inside and out."

SUCCESS STORY:
ERIC ROSEBERG
Fox Lake, IL

I feel healthier, stronger, and more energetic.

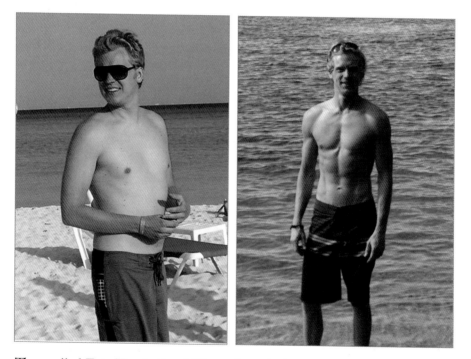

They called Eric "Lanky" and "Bones" as a kid. His poor diet didn't matter back then because he was so active, playing dodgeball, football, and basketball with the neighborhood kids. The weight didn't start piling on until after his first couple of years in college, thanks to what he calls "my horrible eating patterns.... I'm talking about daily fast food, tons of soda, any packaged food you can think of, and of course tons of beer." Nor did he remain physically active during those years, only half-heartedly attempting reps at the gym while socializing with friends.

But pictures from his honeymoon in 2010 motivated him to get into shape in time for vacation the following year. He started running the trails three to five days a week for a few miles or so and incorporated some fruits and vegetables into his diet, but still ate "a ton of processed, packaged foods and plenty of carbs to fuel my runs." Though he dropped a good 10 pounds, Eric lost momentum and started putting on weight again. A stint at the gym for chronic cardio workouts followed, but his diet still consisted of "the typical preservative-filled, packaged meals." Nevertheless, he dropped 15 pounds.

Yet random injuries plagued him, starting with runner's knee, so he bought expensive running shoes. Then a bulging disc in his lower back caused back pain and tingling down his leg. Exertion headaches caused by high blood pressure followed. "The doctor tried putting me on meds, but at 28 years old, I respectfully declined." He followed orders to reduce his sodium intake, only to realize that sodium is in everything, especially his favorite frozen meals. "I did the best I could and took some time off to reevaluate my lifestyle."

Not long after, he stumbled across Mark's Daily Apple and the paleo/primal lifestyle, and the pieces started falling into place. "I immediately signed up for Mark's newsletter and completely absorbed the 10 Primal Blueprint Laws." He cut out all processed foods, including fast food and packaged frozen meals. Grains, soda, and most sugars were tossed out the window. He added in more animal protein and eggs, fruits, vegetables, nuts, and healthy fats. Rather than compulsively counting calories, he now eats when hungry, and stops when he's full.

In addition, he quit the chronic cardio, focusing instead on weight training (squatting, deadlifting, pushing, pulling), light biking, and occasional sprints. "Needless to say, I feel great, and I haven't experienced any of the aforementioned injuries." After his blood pressure levels shifted into normal ranges, the same doctor who had wanted to prescribe him meds was floored by the improvement and told him to keep doing what he was doing.

Summary

1. Slow down cardio workouts to avoid falling into a chronic pattern. During most of your cardio workouts, exert discipline to keep your heart rate below your maximum aerobic heart rate, which is calculated using the simple formula 180 minus your age.
2. Take incremental steps to increase overall daily movement—work breaks, errands, evening strolls, etc. Even a five-minute walk or ascending a few flights of stairs builds habits that support a more active lifestyle.
3. Get out for extended outings once in a while and enjoy nature or urban adventures.
4. Integrate complementary flexibility/mobility work to counter all the time spent in fixed positions.

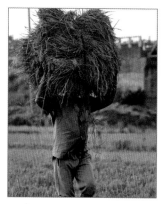

Law #4: Lift Heavy Things: Again, let's make things simple so there are no excuses or hurdles to making Law #4 a fun, comfortable, and consistent part of your lifestyle. The fitness/gym/bodybuilding scene is so laden with hype, complexity, intimidation, and "broscience" that even looking at a dumbbell or strapping into a spaceship-style strength-training contraption at the gym can be completely unappealing to all but the most fervent enthusiasts.

As a counterargument to the "broscience" that says you need "muscle confusion," workout days cross-referenced against specific body parts, or multimillion dollar, 30,000 square foot gyms and top-dollar personal trainers to develop an impressive physique, allow me to assert: *you can get extremely fit in just two intense workouts a week, lasting as little as 10 minutes and not more than 30 minutes.* No equipment is necessary (except perhaps a pull-up bar), as your own bodyweight for resistance is all that's required.

The Primal Essential Movements (PEMs) are four simple, safe, full-body functional exercises that can be done anywhere—backyard, park, or even a cramped motel room. These four exercises—pushups, pull-ups, squats, and planks—work the entire body in a functional manner to develop broad athletic competency. The PEMs are scalable to all levels of fitness through

SUCCESS STORY:
STEPHEN SANKARSINGH
Trinidad and Tobago

I rediscovered my health and love of real food.

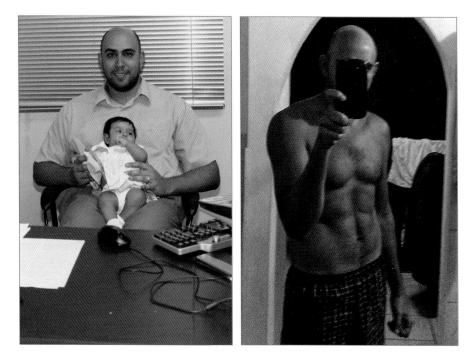

Growing up in Trinidad and Tobago, Stephen never quite took to sports like some of his classmates, opting for recreational basketball or body-boarding on the weekends. He was not a fat kid, but by the time he reached 6'2", his friends referred to him jokingly as T3 (for thin, tall, and terrible). His weekday diet consisted of three to four sandwiches with margarine and some type of meat (usually from a tin or a pack) a few times a day.

Sometimes he ate a home-cooked lunch, usually pasta or rice and some sort of chicken, on the weekends.

At 16, he cut back on physical activities to dedicate more time to studying, without making any real changes to his diet. By the time he was in college, the term "going for a sweat" meant playing video games, so most of his time was spent behind a computer. He married his college sweetheart after college, and four years later they brought a baby girl into the world. "People joked that of the two of us, I gained the most weight during our pregnancy."

Commuting to work in Trinidad and Tobago could take Stephen anywhere from one to two hours each way. Between family, work, and the commute, there wasn't much time left over. His weight increased from 185 pounds—what he thought would be his "set weight for life"—to 260.

Stephen worked in IT, though when asked what he did for a living, he responded, "I sit at a desk all day long waiting to be either diagnosed with diabetes or to experience my first myocardial infarction." His dad's experience as a type 1 diabetic had given Stephen a healthy fear of sweets, needles, and illness.

In mid-2012, he picked up martial arts and on the first day remembers laying on the ground after the 15-minute warmup waiting for oxygen to fill his burning lungs. He persevered, but after a year lost only 5 to 10 pounds. A friend advised Stephen that he could exercise all he liked, but he would never see any body changes until his diet changed.

One day, Stephen's mentor/adopted godfather noticed his pensive mood and asked what was up. Stephen noticed how much healthier and "baby smooth" the older man's feet looked. "My feet, on the other hand, were ashy and grey with cracks and webs, reminiscent of a well-mottled terrazzo floor." His mentor exclaimed, "You need a lifestyle change," directing him to Mark's Daily Apple.

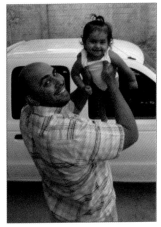

The first thing Stephen pulled up on Mark's Daily Apple was a picture of a delicious pork dish. "How could it possibly be health food? It was caramelized in its own heart-stopping saturated fat." But he began reading about grains, insulin, fats, carbs, protein, and cholesterol.

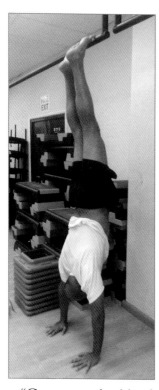

He waded through Mark's Definitive Guides. Eventually, things began making sense.

Stephen launched his primal lifestyle on September 1, 2013. The hardest part, he said, was figuring out what foods should replace bread and wheat. He even suffered through the "carb flu" (caused by the exotoxins produced when the "bad" gut bacteria die off from carb elimination).

But the weight started dropping at around two to three pounds per week. "It's not like I switched to primal overnight, this was a learning process," Stephen said about figuring out which foods to substitute for grains and sugars. He experimented with different egg dishes for breakfast. He loves lamb, but he wasn't yet sure about eating the fat. Instead he stored the fat in his freezer until he ran out of space. Then he learned how to render tallow to fry up vegetables.

"Gone was the blandness of vegetables, they were now lamb-fat infused. Now that I was primal, I could distinguish individual tastes. Garlic, peppercorns, ginger, rosemary, even salt makes food come alive. I wasn't even aware that I was missing it." Eating primally isn't always cheap he noted, but he'd rather eat more healthfully than brave going to a doctor

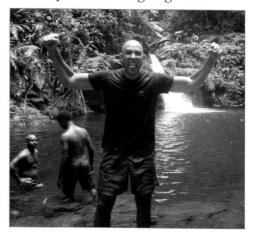

in Trinidad—though he happily reported that blood tests run a year after going primal proved "protective" or in the safe range.

"My mentor saw me in the market a couple months into this lifestyle change and pointed his gnarly finger at me, claiming that I owed him money for his advice, to which I said, in fact, he owed me money since none of my clothes fit anymore."

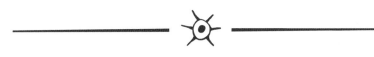

BE YOUR OWN SUCCESS STORY

The success stories and stunning photos here (and published every Friday at MarksDailyApple.com) are meant to inspire and motivate. However, if you are struggling to meet your diet and lifestyle goals, the good fortune of others can sometimes have the opposite effect. Here are some tips to get grounded, focused, and pursue success with lifestyle change on your own terms.

1. Adopt a positive attitude and a process-oriented mindset: Embark upon lifestyle change because it makes you feel good—enjoyable meals and workouts, more sleep, more energy. Instead of using the word "need" (I need more sleep, I need to ditch my ice cream habit, I need to exercise more), replace it with the word "deserve." Catch and reframe any negative thoughts into positive ones.

2. Get plenty of sleep: You can easily nullify devoted diet and exercise efforts if you aren't getting enough sleep. Fat reduction is primarily about hormone optimization. Insufficient sleep drives increased appetite and increased fat storage. More sleep can be better than more exercise.

3. Ditch sugars, grains, and bad oils: Adopt a zero tolerance policy for dietary poisons and stick to it for 21 days. Build some momentum, see how much better you feel, and soon you won't miss 'em—really!

4. Move more: Sure you'll want to perform your regular cardio sessions, lift heavy things, and sprint once in a while, but before worrying about all that, resolve to become more active throughout your day. Prolonged inactivity drives increased appetite and increased fat storage. Sound familiar?

5. Go with the flow: Read these stories carefully and you'll detect that the before/after success came as a natural byproduct of enjoyable lifestyle change. Conversely, when you obsess on your calorie count, scale numbers, or workout volumes, you'll be more likely to struggle, get discouraged, and fall off the track.

6. Take a "before" photo: Wherever you are, there's no time like the present to get started. Good luck!

TOO GOOD TO BE TRUE?

Hey, I thought the same thing upon receiving some of our more amazing photos (yep, they're real—we obtained signed affidavits from everyone). However, with even a basic understanding of gene expression, these photos and stories begin to make perfect sense—how someone like Deanna, enduring obesity since adolescence, can shed half of her bodyweight in a couple years, or how Nick can turn back the clock and rediscover athletic genes hidden for over two decades.

I know you love your morning granola and afternoon strawberry yogurt snack, but would you be open to tweaking some lifestyle staples for 21 days to see if things could get even better? Granted, it's easier said than done for creatures of habit like us, but I hope these stories will get you dreaming big!

Remember, your hand is on the dial 24/7. You can offend your genes with all manner of modern challenges: evening laptop sessions staring into a screen as bright to your eyes (and hormones) as the midday sun, or visits to a brightly-painted smoothie shop to obtain triple the amount of carbs Grok ate in a day in just 20 minutes of slurping and scarfing.

Or, you can try as best you can to deliver the experience your genes expect to make you healthy (eating meat, fish, fowl, eggs, nuts, and produce; lifting heavy things and doing some occasional all-out sprints; basking in the sun; hitting the sack soon after sunset), and reap the comprehensive benefits. The choice is yours!

INDEX

Kelly Korg suggested eating plan, 434
Ken Korg suggested eating plan, 430
Korg family, 79–80
tips, 487
breakthrough workouts, 440
Briffa, Dr. John, 97
Brown, Stuart, 54
budget, 488
family finances, 98
budgeting for better food, 214–216
buffering joint compounds, 268
bunny hopping, 510
butter, 243
Time magazine "Eat Butter" cover, 125, 291
butters (nuts, seeds), 220–223

C

caffeine, 98
coffee, 234–236
Ken Korg, 85–86
CAFO (concentrated animal feeding operation) animals, 206
calcium uptake, and cortisol, 240, 284
Calment, Jeanne, 246
calories
counting, 165
Kelly Korg suggested weight-loss plan, 433
Ken Korg suggested weight-loss plan, 428
cancer
hypomethylation, 35
sun exposure, 55–57
canola oil, 290–291
Carbohydrate Curve, 173–178, 425–426
maintenance zone, 175, 189
sweet spot, 175, 189, 416–420, 424–426, 448–450
variables to consider, 177–179
carbohydrates, 170, 172–179
blood glucose, 43–45
carb-neutral vegetables, 173
combined with fat intake, 182
high-carb eating pattern vs. primal eating pattern, 122
high-nutrient-value carbs, 107, 244–246
insulin response, 44, 105–107, 113–114, 170–171
insulin sensitivity/resistance, 114–117
lactose, 238–239
net carbs, 173
optimal intake amount. *See* Carbohydrate Curve

refeeding, 247
short-term effects of elevated glucose levels, 120–124
smoothies, 176
Standard American Diet, 106–107
sugar crashes, 44, 85, 153, 157
weight-loss macronutrient plan, 424–425
cardio
"180 minus age" formula, 335–337, 438
aerobic base building, 331–334
benefits of low-level aerobic activity, 330–331
chronic. *See* chronic cardio
conventional wisdom vs. Primal Blueprint, 5
primal approved exercise, 482
cardio machines, 356
casein, 238
Castelli, Dr. William, 127, 275
Celebrex, 83
cellular function, 104
Certified Organic, 206
cheese, 238
chemical-free label on meat, 207
chicken, 202–208
childhood obesity, 464–465
children
ADHD. *See* Attention Deficit Hyperactivity Disorder (ADHD)
life expectancy of modern children, 98–99
obesity, 98
recreation/leisure time, 88, 98
sleep, 96–97
television viewing, 99
walking to school, 97
chocolate. *See* dark chocolate
cholesterol, 124–127
animal foods, 198
atherosclerosis, 118–119, 124, 129–130, 132, 138
benefits, 128
conventional wisdom vs. Primal Blueprint, 3
Framingham Heart Study, 126–127
government guidelines, 125
heart disease, 133–138
interesterified fats, 294
Ken Korg, 81
lipoproteins, 127–135
Metabolic Syndrome, 141
statins, 81, 139–141
trans fats, 294

chronic cardio, 338–343, 488
compensation theory, 436
cortisol production, 339
chronic excessive insulin production, 43
cinnamon, 234
circadian rhythm, 373, 379
CLA (conjugated linoleic acid), 292
Clay, Brian, 320
coconut/coconut oil, 181, 223–225, 243, 480
cod liver oil, 396
coffee, 234–236, 484
cold water plunges, 95, 151, 381
commuting, 96
Ken Korg, 82–83
complementary flexibility/mobility practices, 343–346
condiments, 484
conventional wisdom, ix–xii, 14
diets/dieting, 513–515
vs. Primal Blueprint, 1–9
propaganda and flawed science regarding fat, 182–184
questioning, 92
cookbooks
Paleo Primer, 489
The Primal Blueprint Cookbook, 219, 224, 432
Primal Blueprint Quick & Easy Meals, 219, 224, 432, 489
Cooke, Denise, 178
CoQ10, 137
statins, 97, 139–140
Cordain, Dr. Loren, xx, 27, 39, 230, 238, 278, 296
cortisol, 48, 81, 121, 123, 286
chronic cardio, 339–341
sleep, 375, 452, 498
waking up, 76
Country of Origin Labeled (COOL), 207
CPK (creatine phosphokinase), 146
C-reactive protein, 142
Crisco, 291
criticism of primal/paleo, 39–40, 468–469
Cronometer.com, 173
CrossFit, 321, 344
cruciferous vegetables, 200
curcumin, 234
Cult Diets, xx
Curry, Stephen, 320–321
Cutler, Dr. Richard G., 65
cycling sprints, 512–513
form, 362
workout specifics, 361
CYP1A2 gene, 236